Provided as a service to medicine by Servier, makers of:

DIAMICRON® MR
gliclazide modified release

COVERSYLPLUS®
perindopril 4mg/indapamide 1.25mg

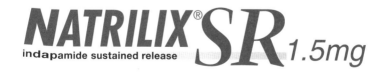

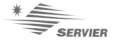

Servier Laboratories Pty Ltd.
8 Cato St, Hawthorn Victoria 3122 ABN 54 004 838 500

HOT TOPICS

Hypertension

Brent M. Egan, MD
Professor of Medicine and Pharmacology, Department of Medicine
Head, Hypertension Section, Division of General Medicine
Medical University of South Carolina
Charleston, South Carolina

Jan N. Basile, MD
Associate Professor of Medicine
Ralph C. Johnson Veterans Affairs Medical Center
Medical University of South Carolina
Charleston, South Carolina

Daniel T. Lackland, DrPH
Professor, Department of Biometry and Epidemiology
Director, Graduate Training and Education
Medical University of South Carolina
Charleston, South Carolina

HANLEY & BELFUS
An Affiliate of Elsevier

HANLEY & BELFUS, INC.
An Affiliate of Elsevier

The Curtis Center
Independence Square West
Philadelphia, Pennsylvania 19106

Note to the reader: Although the information in this book has been carefully reviewed for correctness of dosage and indications, neither the editors, nor the authors, nor the publisher can accept any legal responsibility for any errors or omissions that may be made. No warranty is expressed or implied with respect to the material contained herein. Before prescribing any drug, the reader must review the manufacturer's current product information (package inserts) for accepted indications, absolute dosage recommendations, and other information pertinent to the safe and effective use of the product described.

Library of Congress Control Number: 2003107485

HYPERTENSION: HOT TOPICS   ISBN 1-56053-578-4

Printed in the United States of America

Last digit is the print number: 9 8 7 6 5 4 3 2 1

Contents

Section I. General Evaluation of the Hypertensive Patient

1. Initial Evaluation of Blood Pressure   1
   John Kevin Hix, M.D., and Donald G. Vidt, M.D.

2. The Use of Home Blood Pressure Monitors in Practice   13
   Steven A. Yarrows, M.D.

3. Urine Microalbumin: For Diabetics Only?   23
   Sunita Sharma, M.D., and Eddie L. Greene, M.D.

Section II. Target Organ Evaluation in the Hypertensive Patient

4. Evaluation of Cardiac Structure and Function   37
   Alan Hinderliter, M.D.

5. Assessment of Renal Function in Hypertension   49
   Meryl Waldman, M.D., and Raymond R. Townsend, M.D.

6. Renal Artery Occlusive Disease in Hypertension   57
   James C. Stanley, M.D.

7. Carotid and Peripheral Vascular Disease   67
   Robert D. Brook, M.D., Henna Kalsi, M.D., and
   Alan B. Weder, M.D.

Section III. Screening and Diagnosis of Selected Secondary Causes of Hypertension

8. Sleep Apnea: The Not So Silent Epidemic   89
   Narayana S. Murali, M.D., Anna Svatikova, and
   Virend K. Somers, M.D., Ph.D.

9. Primary Aldosteronism   99
   Marion Wofford, M.D., MPH

Section IV. Management of Hypertension: Goals and Objectives

10. Treating to Goal Blood Pressure   105
    William J. Elliot, M.D., Ph.D.

11. High Normal Blood Pressure   119
    Stevo Julius, M.D., Sc.D.

12 Patient-related Barriers to Hypertension Control   129
    Miyong Kim, R.N., Ph.D., Martha Hill, R.N., Ph.D.,
    and Hwayum Lee, R.N., M.P.H.

13. Hypertension Control: Focus on Providers   137
    David Hyman, M.D., MPH

14. Culturally Congruent Medical Care   147
    B. Waine Kong, Ph.D., J.D., and Stephanie Kong, M.D.

Section V. Lifestyle Approaches: Translating Research into Practice!

15. Promoting Lifestyle Modification in the Office Setting   155
    Lawrence J. Appel, M.D., MPH, and
    Edgar R. Miller, M.D., Ph.D.

16. Dietary Cations and Hypertension   165
    Paul K. Muntner, Ph.D., MHS,
    Paul K. Whelton, M.D., M.Sc, and Jiang He, M.D., Ph.D.

17. Nutrition, Dietary Supplements, and Nutraceuticals
    in Hypertension   181
    Mark C. Houston, M.D., SCH

18 Comorbid Depression and Hypertension-related
    Chronic Medical Conditions   191
    Leonard E. Egede, M.D., M.S.

19. Management of Obesity   203
    Patrick Mahlen O'Neil, Ph.D., and Corby K. Martin, Ph.D.

20. Physical Activity for Patients with Hypertension   215
    Nancy S. Diehl, Ph.D., and Kelly R. Evenson, Ph.D.

21. Behavioral Approaches in Blood Pressure Reduction   223
    Thomas Pickering, M.D., D.Phil.

Section VI. Medical Therapy: Evidence-Based Approach to the Important Practical Issues

22. An Evidence-based Approach to Selecting Initial
    Antihypertensive Therapy   231
    Jan Basile, M.D.

23. Remedies for Single-Dose Therapy Failure   237
    Barry J. Materson, M.D., MBA

24. The Metabolic Syndrome   243
    William H. Bestermann, Jr., M.D.

25. Managing Hypertension in Diabetic Patients   249
    Peter D. Hart, M.D., and George L. Bakris, M.D.

26. Isolated Systolic Hypertension   263
    Stanley S. Franklin, M.D.

27. Management of Refractory Hypertension   277
    Lawrence R. Krakoff, M.D.

Section VII. Medical Therapy: Meeting Most Management Challenges

28. Hypertension and Congestive Heart Failure   285
    Alan H. Gradman, M.D., and A. Tareq Khawaja, M.D.

29. Managing Hypertension in Patients with Chronic
    Renal Insufficiency   297
    Crystal A. Gadegbeku, M.D.

30. Supine Hypertension with Orthostatic Hypotension   309
    Gary L. Schwartz, M.D.

31. Management of Renovascular Hypertension   325
    Michael J. Bloch, M.D., and Jan Basile, M.D.

32. Management of Transplant Hypertension   335
    C. Venkata S. Ram, M.D., and Pedro Vergne-Marini, M.D.

33. Management of Hypertensive Patients with
    Sexual Dysfunction   345
    Carlos M. Ferrario, M.D.

34. Novel Cardiovascular Risk Factors and Their Use in
    Clinical Practice   359
    Peter W. F. Wilson, M.D.

Section VIII. Update on Hypertension and CVD Prevention in Special Populations

35. Hypertension in Pregnancy 369
   Sandra J. Taler, M.D.

36. Preventing Cardiovascular Disease in Women 379
   Andrew P. Miller, M.D., Philippe Bouchard,
   and Suzanne Oparil, M.D.

37. Hypertension in African Americans 399
   Elijah Saunders, M.D., Wallace Johnson, M.D.,
   and Charlotte Jones-Burton, M.D.

38. Hypertension in Adolescents 411
   Bonita Falkner, M.D.

39. Hypertension in Surgical Patients 421
   Randa K. Noseir, M.D., and Thomas J. Ebert, M.D., Ph.D.

Section IX. Pharmacotherapeutic Considerations: Maximizing Opportunities and Minimizing Threats

40. Use of Nonsteroidal Anti-inflammatory Drugs in
   Hypertensive Patients 427
   Perry V. Halushka, Ph.D., M.D.

41. Amiloride-sensitive Hypertension 435
   David A. Calhoun, M.D.

42. Adverse Drug Reactions in Patients with Hypertension 443
   Domenic A. Sica, M.D.

INDEX 455

Contributors

Lawrence J. Appel, MD, MPH
Professor, Departments of Medicine, Epidemiology, and International Health, Johns Hopkins Medical Institutions, Baltimore; Johns Hopkins Hospital, Baltimore, Maryland

George L. Bakris, MD
Professor, Department of Preventive Medicine, Rush Medical College, Chicago; Director, Hypertension/Clinical Research Center, Rush-Presbyterian-St. Luke's Medical Center, Chicago, Illinois

Jan N. Basile, MD
Associate Professor of Medicine, Ralph C. Johnson Veterans Affairs Medical Center, Medical University of South Carolina, Charleston, South Carolina

William Henry Bestermann, Jr, MD
Low Country Medical Group, Beaufort; Adjunct Assistant Professor, Medical University of South Carolina, Charleston, South Carolina

Michael J. Bloch, MD
Assistant Professor, Department of Medicine, University of Nevada School of Medicine, Reno; Medical Director, St. Mary's Healthy Heart Risk Reduction Center, Reno, Nevada

Philippe Bouchard
Intern Scholar, Vascular Biology and Hypertension Program, University of Alabama, Birmingham, Alabama

Robert D. Brook, MD
Assistant Professor, Division of Cardiovascular Medicine–Hypertension, University of Michigan, Ann Arbor, Michigan

David A. Calhoun, MD
Associate Professor, Department of Medicine, Vascular Biology and Hypertension Program, University of Alabama, Birmingham, Alabama

Nancy S. Diehl, PhD
Assistant Professor, Departments of Rehabilitation Science and Psychiatry, Medical University of South Carolina, Charleston, South Carolina

Thomas J. Ebert, MD, PhD
Professor, Department of Anesthesiology, Adjunct Professor, Department of Physiology, Medical College of Wisconsin, Milwaukee; Staff Anesthesiologist, Veterans Affairs Medical Center, Milwaukee, Wisconsin

Brent M. Egan, MD
Professor of Medicine and Pharmacology, Department of Medicine, and Head, Hypertension Section, Medical University of South Carolina, Charleston, South Carolina

Leonard E. Egede, MD, MS
Assistant Professor, Department of Medicine, Division of Geriatrics, Medical University of South Carolina, Charleston, South Carolina

William J. Elliott, MD, PhD
Professor of Preventive Medicine, Internal Medicine, and Pharmacology, Department of Preventive Medicine, Rush Medical College, Chicago; Attending Physician, Rush-Presbyterian-St. Luke's Medical Center, Chicago, Illinois

Kelly R. Evenson, PhD
Research Assistant Professor, Department of Epidemiology, School of Public Health, University of North Carolina, Chapel Hill, North Carolina

Bonita Faulkner, MD
Professor of Medicine and Pediatrics, Department of Medicine, Division of Nephrology, Thomas Jefferson University, Philadelphia, Pennsylvania

Carlos M. Ferrario, MD
Professor and Director, Hypertension and Vascular Disease Center, Wake Forest University School of Medicine, Winston-Salem, North Carolina

Stanley S. Franklin, MD, FACP, FACC
Clinical Professor of Medicine, University of California, Irvine; Associate Medical Director, UCI Heart Disease Prevention Program, Irvine, California

Crystal A. Gadegbeku, MD
Assistant Professor, Department of Internal Medicine, Division of Nephrology, Medical University of South Carolina, Charleston, South Carolina

Alan H. Gradman, MD
Chief, Division of Cardiovascular Diseases, The Western Pennsylvania Hospital, Pittsburgh; Professor of Medicine, Temple University School of Medicine–Clinical Campus, Pittsburgh, Pennsylvania

Eddie L. Greene, MD
Associate Professor, Department of Internal Medicine, Division of Nephrology, Mayo Clinic and Mayo Medical School, Rochester, Minnesota

Perry V. Halushka, PhD, MD
Professor, Department of Pharmacology and Medicine, Dean, College of Graduate Studies, Medical University of South Carolina, Charleston, South Carolina

Peter D. Hart, MD
Director, Hypertension Clinic, and Senior Attending Physician, Cook County Hospital, Chicago; Assistant Professor, Department of Medicine, Rush Medical College, Chicago, Illinois

Jiang He, MD, PhD
Professor, Departments of Epidemiology and Medicine, Tulane University School of Public Health and Tropical Medicine, New Orleans, Louisiana

Martha Hill, RN, PhD
Dean and Professor, School of Nursing, Johns Hopkins University, Baltimore, Maryland

Alan Hinderliter, MD
Associate Professor of Medicine, Division of Cardiology, University of North Carolina, Chapel Hill, North Carolina

John Kevin Hix, MD
Fellow, Department of Nephrology and Hypertension, Cleveland Clinic Foundation, Cleveland, Ohio

Mark C. Houston, MD, SCH, FACP, FAHA
Associate Clinical Professor, Department of Medicine, Vanderbilt University School of Medicine, Nashville; Director, Hypertension Institute, and Chief, Division of Nutrition, Hypertension Institute, St. Thomas Hospital, Nashville, Tennessee

David J. Hyman, MD, MPH
Associate Professor, Departments of Internal Medicine and Family and Community Medicine, Baylor College of Medicine, Houston; Section Chief, Department of General Internal Medicine, Ben Taub General Hospital, Houston, Texas

Wallace Johnson, MD
Clinical Assistant Professor of Medicine, Section of Hypertension, University of Maryland School of Medicine, Baltimore, Maryland

Charlotte Jones-Burton, MD
Resident, Department of Medicine, University of Maryland School of Medicine, Baltimore, Maryland

Stevo Julius, MD, ScD
Professor, Departments of Medicine and Physiology, University of Michigan Medical Center, Ann Arbor, Michigan

Henna Kalsi, MD
Fellow and Lecturer, Division of Cardiovascular Medicine–Hypertension, University of Michigan, Ann Arbor, Michigan

A. Tareq Khawaja, MD
Cardiology Fellow, Department of Medicine, Division of Cardiovascular Diseases, Western Pennsylvania Hospital, Pittsburgh; Temple University School of Medicine–Clinical Campus, Pittsburgh, Pennsylvania

Miyong Kim, RN, PhD
Associate Professor, School of Nursing, Johns Hopkins University, Baltimore, Maryland

B. Waine Kong, PhD, JD
Chief Executive Officer, Association of Black Cardiologists, Inc., Atlanta, Georgia

Stephanie Kong, MD
President, MetroHealth Group of America, Atlanta, Georgia

Lawrence R. Krakoff, MD
Professor, Department of Medicine, Mount Sinai School of Medicine, New York, New York; Chief of Medicine, Englewood Hospital and Medical Center, Englewood, New Jersey

Daniel T. Lackland, DrPH
Professor, Department of Biometry and Epidemiology, and Director, Graduate Training and Education, Medical University of South Carolina, Charleston, South Carolina

Corby K. Martin, PhD
Instructor, Department of Health Psychology, Pennington Biomedical Research Center, Baton Rouge, Louisiana

Barry J. Materson, MD, MBA
Professor, Department of Medicine, University of Miami, Miami, Florida

Andrew P. Miller, MD
Fellow in Cardiology, Vascular Biology and Hypertension Program, University of Alabama, Birmingham, Alabama

Edgar R. Miller, III, MD, PhD
Assistant Professor, Departments of Medicine and Epidemiology, Johns Hopkins Medical Institutions, Baltimore; Staff, Johns Hopkins Hospital, Baltimore, Maryland

Paul K. Muntner, PhD, MHS
Assistant Professor, Departments of Epidemiology and Medicine, Tulane University School of Public Health and Tropical Medicine, New Orleans, Louisiana

Narayana S. Murali, MD
Instructor, Department of Medicine, Mayo Medical School; Resident, Department of Internal Medicine, Mayo Clinic and Mayo Foundation, Rochester, Minnesota

Randa K. Noseir, MD
Fellow, Department of Anesthesiology, Medical College of Wisconsin, Milwaukee, Wisconsin

Patrick Mahlen O'Neil, PhD
Professor, Department of Psychiatry and Behavioral Sciences, Director, Weight Management Center, Medical University of South Carolina, Charleston, South Carolina

Suzanne Oparil, MD
Director, Vascular Biology and Hypertension Program; Professor of Medicine, Departments of Physiology and Biophysics, University of Alabama, Birmingham, Alabama

Valory N. Pavlik, PhD
Associate Professor, Department of Family and Community Medicine, Baylor College of Medicine, Houston, Texas

Thomas Pickering, MD, DPhil
Professor of Medicine and Director, Integrative and Behavioral Cardiovascular Health Program, Zena & Michael A. Wiener Cardiovascular Institute, Mount Sinai School of Medicine, New York, New York

C. Venkata S. Ram, MD, MACP, FACC
Director, Texas Blood Pressure Institute, Dallas; Director, Medical Education and Clinical Research, Dallas Nephrology Associates, Dallas; Clinical Professor of Internal Medicine, University of Texas Southwestern Medical School, Dallas, Texas

Elijah Saunders, MD, FACC, FACP
Professor, Department of Medicine, University of Maryland School of Medicine, Baltimore; Head, Section of Hypertension, Division of Cardiology, University of Maryland Hospital, Baltimore, Maryland

Gary Lee Schwartz, MD
Associate Professor, Department of Internal Medicine, Mayo Medical School, Rochester; Chair, Division of Hypertension, Mayo Clinic, Rochester, Minnesota

Sunita Sharma, MD
Resident, Department of Internal Medicine, Mayo Clinic, Rochester, Minnesota

Domenic A. Sica, MD
Professor of Medicine and Pharmacology, Department of Internal Medicine, Division of Nephrology; Chair, Section of Clinical Pharmacology and Hypertension, Virginia Commonwealth University / Medical College of Virginia Hospitals and Physicians, Richmond, Virginia

Virend K. Somers, MD, PhD
Professor of Medicine and Consultant, Divisions of Cardiovascular Disease and Hypertension, Mayo Clinic and Mayo Foundation, Rochester, Minnesota

James C. Stanley, MD
Professor and Head, Section of Vascular Surgery, Department of Surgery, University of Michigan Medical School, Ann Arbor, Michigan

Anna Svatikova
Graduate Student, Department of Molecular Science, Mayo Clinic and Mayo Foundation, Rochester, Minnesota

Sandra J. Taler, MD
Assistant Professor of Medicine, Department of Internal Medicine, and Consultant, Divisions of Hypertension and Nephrology, Mayo Clinic, Rochester

Raymond R. Townsend, MD
Professor of Medicine, University of Pennsylvania School of Medicine, Philadelphia; Director, Hypertension Program, University of Pennsylvania Health System, Philadelphia, Pennsylvania

Pedro Vergne-Marini, MD, FACP, FACC
Director, Transplant Program, Methodist Hospital, Dallas; Clinical Professor of Medicine, University of Texas Southwestern Medical School, Dallas, Texas

Donald G. Vidt, MD
Consultant, Department of Nephrology and Hypertension, Cleveland Clinic Foundation, Cleveland, Ohio

Meryl Alaine Waldman, MD
Fellow, Renal Electrolyte & Hypertension Division, University of Pennsylvania, Philadelphia, Pennsylvania

Alan B. Weder, MD
Professor, Division of Cardiovascular Medicine–Hypertension, University of Michigan, Ann Arbor, Michigan

Paul K. Whelton, MD, MSc
Professor, Department of Epidemiology, Senior Vice President for Health Sciences, Department of Medicine, Tulane University School of Public Health and Tropical Medicine, New Orleans, Louisiana

Peter W.F. Wilson, MD
Professor, Department of Medicine, Boston University School of Medicine, Boston, Massachusetts

Marion Ridgway Wofford, MD, MPH
Associate Professor of Medicine and Director, Division of Hypertension, University of Mississippi Medical Center, Jackson, Mississippi

Steven A. Yarows, MD, FACP
Associate Professor, Department of Internal Medicine, Division of Hypertension, University of Michigan, Ann Arbor, Michigan

Foreword

In this book, a superb collection of authors noted both for their clinical and teaching skills take the reader on a tour of the most challenging areas of hypertension management. They successfully synthesize a daunting body of knowledge and translate it into practical reading for a broad audience. This "translation" of research is a difficult task in any area. In hypertension, it is particularly challenging. A vast body of research has illuminated our understanding and led to better management options for patients. Indeed, hypertension-related morbidity and mortality rates have dramatically improved over the last 25 years. Yet after more than a century of intensive research, the mystery of the cause of hypertension still eludes complete solution. The science is extensive and complex. The research results are broad and deep. Thus the need for this "translation."

The chapters herein allow practical consideration of complex science and therefore are of benefit and usefulness to a broad range of readers. The busy clinician, who has no hope of keeping abreast of the "latest" in the myriad of journals devoted to work in hypertension, will gain insight in the application of recent research to better manage patients. The authors, who generally walk in both the world of research and of clinical practice, distill the literature into understandable language. Clinicians from all the disciplines involved in hypertension management will benefit, including primary care physicians, specialty and subspecialty physicians, nurses, nurse practitioners, pharmacists, and nutritionists. Students of these disciplines will benefit from this approach, as well.

Hypertension Hot Topics should also benefit scientists interested in gaining a greater appreciation for the translation of basic research and clinical trials into patient care. The researcher will gain a broader understanding of principles in hypertension outside the focus area of his or her own research interests, which can lead to greater insights and better research.

I encourage readers to take this opportunity to broaden their understanding of hypertension. This book illuminates a broad range of clinically relevant topics in hypertension and will help improve the blood pressure management and overall health of our patients.

Daniel W. Jones, MD
VICE CHANCELLOR FOR HEALTH AFFAIRS
DEAN, SCHOOL OF MEDICINE
UNIVERSITY OF MISSISSIPPI MEDICAL CENTER
JACKSON, MISSISSIPPI

Preface

Hypertension is a major public health problem and the most common ICD-9 code addressed by the primary care clinician serving adult patients in the outpatient setting. It is also frequently encountered in the outpatient and inpatient settings of both medical and surgical services. Due to the burgeoning epidemic of obesity and sedentary lifestyles, hypertension and the metabolic syndrome no longer predominantly affect middle-aged and older adults, but also young adults and teenagers. Blood pressures requiring medical attention are estimated to affect ~60,000,000 individuals in the U.S. alone. Recent estimates place hypertension control rates at 31%, though clinical trials suggest that control rates of 60–70% are attainable. The medical literature contains a treasure of evidence-based information that can be used to improve control of blood pressure and associated disorders of carbohydrate and lipid metabolism.

However, the literal weight of the medical literature is growing exponentially. Practitioners are faced with the monumental challenges of understanding and implementing the information, providing healthcare services for an evermore diverse and aging population, and deriving an income and meeting overhead expenses against a tide of increasingly complex regulation and decreasing reimbursement. Despite these formidable challenges, clinicians recognize the benefits of translating research into practice efficiently and effectively, and demonstrate their commitment to remaining current. They know that success in applying evidence-based medicine can have dramatic health benefits and cost savings. Nevertheless, there is often a gap of a decade or more between the science and the practice of medicine, and implementation is frequently suboptimal. Examples abound and include appropriate use of aspirin in patients at risk for CHD, use of ACE inhibitors, and more recently ARBs, in patients with heart failure and/or nephropathy, beta-blockers and "statins" post MI, and beta-blockers in systolic heart failure.

This book is intended to serve as a rapid reference guide for the practicing clinician in a variety of medical settings, from pediatric to geriatric as well as medical and surgical, who has a desire to implement contemporary, evidence-based approaches in the evaluation and treatment of patients with hypertension and the metabolic syndrome. *The chapters are written so that answers to a variety of common and clinically important questions encountered in the daily management of hypertensive patients can be quickly identified and the practical implications for management readily applied.*

The "Hot Topics" selected for this book include issues that are just now moving from the research to the clinical arena; recent discoveries that are impacting the diagnostic and therapeutic approach to management of long-recognized clinical entities; and hypertension-related questions that are commonly encountered but infrequently addressed. The authors are an eclectic group of clinicians-educators-scientists. Each author is not only an established expert but also a gifted teacher and communicator. We retained each author's individual style, personality, and passion.

In an effort to enhance the utility of this book as a daily and ready reference, the book is organized in nine sections, each of which addresses a thematically important Hot Topic. The book begins with a section on general evaluation, followed by sections on evaluation of key target organs and selected secondary causes of hypertension that are relatively common but often overlooked (sleep apnea, primary aldo) and rarely considered (neurovascular compression). The rationale for the goals of therapy, the challenge of high-normal blood pressures (more recently termed "pre-hypertension"), and the critical interface between the patient and provider is then discussed. The therapeutic alliance is absolutely fundamental to therapeutic success, and this rarely illuminated topic is moved from behind the scenes to center stage, with insight on the provider's role in patient adherence, including cultural competence.

Moving forward, the range of useful lifestyle changes available for reducing blood pressure and improving cardiovascular health is addressed succinctly and yet in-depth. An exploration of pharmacotherapeutic approaches to hypertension covers selection of initial antihypertensive therapy, what to do when the first prescription doesn't control blood pressure, and management of the metabolic syndrome, diabetic hypertension, and isolated systolic hypertension. Management of treatment-refractory and -resistant hypertension and referral guidelines are also covered. The range of commonly encountered patients with complicated hypertension, including patients with heart failure, renal insufficiency and renal vascular disease, orthostatic hypotension (with supine hypertension), transplant hypertension, sexual dysfunction, and diabetes, is described.

The next group of chapters addresses hypertension and CVD prevention in special populations, including pregnant women, African Americans, adolescents, and surgical patients. *Hypertension Hot Topics* concludes with an exploration of special pharmacological considerations.

It is our sincere hope that this book will provide you with timely information that will enhance your care of patients with hypertension and related risk factors.

Brent M. Egan, MD
Jan Basile, MD
Daniel Lackland, DrPH
EDITORS

ACKNOWLEDGMENTS

The editors are indebted to Ms. Jacqueline M. Mahon, whose diligent perseverance was critical in keeping everyone on task and whose editorial and publishing expertise are clearly evident and greatly appreciated in the final product. We are deeply indebted to the chapter authors who accepted the invitation to write based on their sincere commitment to patient care and professional education. We are particularly appreciative of Ms. Kim Edwards, Administrative Assistant, for her unwavering support in managing more details than were imagined at the start of this project. Finally, we are forever grateful to our patients, who provide many valuable lessons.

HOT TOPICS

chapter
1

Initial Evaluation of
Blood Pressure

John Kevin Hix, M.D. and Donald G. Vidt, M.D.

Blood pressure (BP) is a continuous physiologic trait, which, at elevated levels, is strongly associated with cardiovascular and renal disease. The high prevalence of elevated BP in the general population makes the identification and treatment of affected patients a top priority for clinicians. Key concepts in identifying patients who suffer from hypertension include the accurate determination of the BP using proper office-based sphygmomanometery and the identification of that subset of patients in whom ambulatory or home BP measurements may be useful. The majority of diagnosed hypertensive patients have no identifiable or reversible underlying cause for the disease at this time; however, a careful history, physical, and laboratory evaluation assists physicians in risk stratification of the hypertensive population and helps them identify patients with potentially treatable underlying diseases.

BP in humans is a quantifiable physiologic trait, which, in population studies, has a normal distribution with slight skew.[1] High BP contributes to coronary artery disease, stroke, and renal disease. The deleterious effects of BP elevations are seen even within the "normal" range and seem to be continuous with increasing pressures. There is no sharp distinction between normal and pathologic BP. However, as a practical matter, a consensus agreement as to what BPs are tolerable and what BPs represent hypertension (and require intervention) has been outlined in The Sixth Report of the Joint National Committee on Prevention, Detection, Evaluation, and Treatment of High Blood Pressure (JNC VI) (Table 1).[2] The treatment of hypertensive patients remains a primary goal in the effort to reduce morbidity and mortality from cardiovascular disease, stroke, and kidney disease. Identification of patients with hypertension requires health care providers to be familiar with the ap-

TABLE 1. JNC VI Classification of Hypertension		
Category	Systolic BP (mm Hg)	Diastolic BP (mm Hg)
Optimal	< 120 and	< 80
Normal	< 130 and	< 85
High-normal	130–139 or	85–89
Hypertension, stage 1	140–159 or	90–99
Hypertension, stage 2	160–179 or	100–109
Hypertension, stage 3	≥ 180 or	≥ 110

plication, use, and limitations of the technologies available for noninvasive measurements of BP.

The initial evaluation of hypertensive patients most often occurs in the outpatient setting and is often done by a primary care provider. (Table 2). The initial evaluation is a multifocal approach designed both to evaluate the hypertension itself and to identify any underlying—and potentially treatable—causes for the hypertension. As is appropriate for any initial patient visit, the recommended practice is a thorough history, physical examination, and basic laboratory workup.

Identification of Elevated Blood Pressure

The initial evaluation and identification of hypertensive patients starts with measurement of the BP. Typically, this occurs in the office setting, although the patient may have already had high BP identified outside of the clinician's office by other means.

The successful management of any hypertensive patient requires that the measurement of the BP be accurate, reproducible, and highly

TABLE 2. Goals of the Initial Evaluation of Hypertensive Patients
1. **Establish the diagnosis:** The presence and severity of the patient's hypertension must be established at the initial visit. This is best done by recording the BP using the proper equipment and technique, as outlined in this chapter.
2. **Stage the disease:** Using the criteria outlined in Table 1, the level of hypertension is staged. This guides immediate management.
3. **Rule out secondary hypertension:** This includes an initial history, physical examination, and laboratory workup focused on identifying any underlying disorders that may be the cause of (or may be contributing to) the hypertension.
4. **Identify target-organ changes:** This extends the initial history, physical examination, and laboratory workup to identify any ongoing end-organ damage from the hypertension as well as to establish baselines for end-organ function.

correlated with the patient's actual average BP.[3] Efforts to address the limitations of office measurements have resulted in two techniques that measure BP in more "natural" settings. These techniques are home BP monitoring (HBPM) and ambulatory BP monitoring (ABPM).

Home Blood Pressure Measurement

The prevalence of hypertension and the need for continuing assessment of the efficacy of interventions have led to the development of techniques for measuring BP at home. One consistent finding in studies that compare HBPM readings with those obtained in the clinical setting is that HBP readings are generally lower than their clinical counterparts. In fact, studies have documented high specificity of HBP monitoring in detecting "white coat hypertension."[11]

Ambulatory Blood Pressure Monitoring

ABPM is another method of obtaining information about BP in a patient outside the clinical setting. Typically, this is done by having the patient fitted with a device that independently measures and records the individual's BP at specified intervals (or a number of times) during a certain period. The most common selection is a 24-hour time period. During this time, the patient is able (and encouraged) to complete his or her usual daily activities. The BP readings are recorded and later analyzed.

The devices used in ABPM share some similarities with those used for HBPM. The data that ABPM yields are dependent on the device and the software used to analyze the data. The Association for the Advancement of Medical Instrumentation (AAMI) is the institution entrusted with the validation of instruments to be used for ABPM.

The establishment of "normal" and "hypertensive" values for BP readings obtained by means of ABPM remains a consensus definition at this time because we lack true randomized, large-scale studies to definitively identify these values. However, it is known that BPs obtained by means of ABPM generally are lower than those obtained in the clinical setting. Commonly used ABPM "normal" values for BP are ≤ 135/85 mm Hg (daytime) and ≤ 120/70 mm Hg (nighttime).[12]

The ability of ABPM to display readings taken throughout the day allows its use in unique circumstances in which isolated readings in the clinical setting may be regarded as suboptimal (Table 3).

BP values on ABPM in hypertensive patients seem to correlate better with end-organ damage effects than do measurements obtained in the clinical setting. Reviews of multiple cross-sectional and longitudinal studies comparing correlations of end-organ damage with ABPM or office-based measurements revealed that ABPM has nearly always been shown to have a more significant relationship with end-organ damage

TABLE 3. Special Situations for Ambulatory Blood Pressure Monitoring

Setting	Role for ABPM
"White coat hypertension"	Identifies patients who seem to exhibit hypertension only within the clinical setting and who remain normotensive outside the clinical office. This reinforces the diagnosis of hypertension in patients inclined to believe they have "white coat hypertension" yet who remain hypertensive outside the clinical setting.
High-normal BP	More accurate diagnosis and appropriate management of patients whose BP remains in question despite multiple clinical readings
Nocturnal hyphrtension	BP declines in most people during the night; the presence of elevated nocturnal BP may have important clinical relevance
Monitoring drug effects	ABPM provides important data regarding efficacy and duration of the response to therapy and BP values in relation to symptoms
Resistant hypertension	ABPM provides data for assessing efficacy and duration of therapy and complicating factors such as "white coat hypertension"

regardless of the organ evaluated.[13,14] In one randomized study,[15] ABPM was associated with equal inhibition of left ventricular enlargement despite less intense medical therapy compared with clinical measurement of BP. Although definitive data are still being gathered, it seems that just as BP is a continuous and variable physiologic parameter, the ability of ABPM to secure multiple data points during routine patient activity allows for crucial refinement in the estimation of the level of threat high BP represents to target organs. ABPM also allows for tighter control over the amount of pharmacologic intervention used to reduce the threat of end-organ damage.

Medical History

The medical history should not differ significantly from that obtained for any patient interview. However, several areas should be covered when assessing a hypertensive patient for the first time (Table 4). Additionally, some specific clues in the history might suggest an underlying cause to the hypertension (Table 5). The goals of the history include:

1. The identification of symptoms or conditions that may cause or

contribute to hypertension. Specific examples are summarized below in Table 4.

2. The identification of conditions that help to risk stratify the patient and guide therapy. These include diabetes, heart failure, coronary artery disease or risk factors for coronary disease, vascular disease, neurologic disease (including strokes), and pregnancy.

3. The identification of other factors that may influence diagnosis or treatment, including current medications (prescription and other), lifestyle factors, and prior therapy.

TABLE 4. The Medical History	
Historical Cue	**Significance**
Presentation of hypertension	Evaluate the time course and presentation of the hypertension. Obtain the last normal BP. List symptoms that may point to a possible underlying cause.
Age	Hypertension in young individuals raises concern for a secondary cause. Isolated systolic hypertension has significant prognostic importance and treatment concerns, and is seldom secondary.
Race	Young white patients are more likely than ethnic minorities to have an underlying secondary cause for their hypertension.
Gender	Pregnancy can impact diagnostic testing and treatment.
Medical history	Particular attention should be paid to history of cardiac disease, renal disease, and stroke or neurologic disorder.
Surgical history	Pay attention to abdominal and vascular surgeries.
Family history	Important hereditary conditions include kidney disease such as PKD (polycystic kidney disease), MSK (medullary sponge kidney), and family history of the MEN (multiple endocrine neoplasia) syndrome.
Social history	Ethanol use can increase BP. Cocaine use is a potent effector of hypertension. Smoking increases the risk of hypertension.
Medications	A detailed list of prescription and nonprescription medications with attention to those medications that can raise BP is important.
Review of systems, general	Changes in weight, nutrition, alcohol, nicotine, and caffeine intake; presence of symptoms suggestive of heart disease, stroke or neurologic disease, diabetes, vascular disease, or edema or skin changes.

TABLE 5. Historical Clues

Historical Cue	Significance
History of renal disease	Hypertension secondary to renal insufficiency
	Renal artery stenosis
Paradoxical hypertension after beta-blocker use	Pheochromocytoma
Headaches, palpitations, sweating, dizziness, pallor, or flushing with episodic or sustained hypertension	Pheochromocytoma
	Thyroid disorder
	Drug abuse (e.g., cocaine)
	Carcinoid syndrome
Lethargy, constipation, slow and sustained reflexes on examination	Hypothyroidism
Low or low normal potassium on routine laboratory examination	Hyperaldosteronism
Edema, full facies, stria	Cushing's disease
	Nephrotic syndrome
	Renal failure
Pulse or BP differences between limbs	Coarctation of the aorta
Bounding pulse	High output heart disease, hyperthyroidism
Anemia	Chronic renal failure
	Autoimmune disorders associated with thyroid disease, kidney disease
Difficulty undergoing surgery or anesthesia	Pheochromocytoma
Dizziness or paroxysmal hypertension associated with torso movements, exertion, or coitus	Pheochromocytoma
Family history of MEN	Pheochromocytoma
Autoimmune disease or family history of it	Chronic renal failure
	Autoimmune disorders associated with thyroid disease, kidney disease

Physical Examination

Each patient requires a complete physical examination, starting with a BP obtained in the proper manner and in at least both arms (preferably both arms and one leg in the initial evaluation). Areas of particular concern include the following:

1. Neurologic assessment is done to exclude any sequelae of previous stroke and, particularly in patients with markedly elevated BP, to exclude ongoing end-organ damage.

2. Funduscopic examination evaluates for end-organ damage. The grading of fundus is difficult to do effectively in the primary care setting,

but the exclusion of exudates, hemorrhage and papilledema is crucial and should be undertaken in the initial visit. Then a formal consultation with a specialist can be sought, particularly for patients with uncertain findings and in all diabetic patients.

3. The cardiovascular examination seeks to document cardiac murmurs, S3 or S4 gallop, arrhythmias, and pulmonary rales. Additional evidence can be obtained from estimation of the size and force of the point of maximal impulse (PMI), the size of the heart, and the adequacy of the peripheral circulation. Careful assessment of the pulse and presence of bruits in the major vascular beds is essential for the evaluation of renal artery stenosis and coarctation.

4. An abdominal examination features special attention to the identification of bruits, exclusion of enlarged or polycystic kidneys, and estimation of the abdominal aorta size and pulse characteristics.

5. An extremity examination includes attention to the presence of edema, assessment of pulses, and signs of embolic or peripheral vascular disease.

Laboratory Investigation

The initial laboratory evaluation of hypertensive patients is an extension of the previously discussed approach, in which attempts are made to identify target end-organ damage and obtain clues as to the origin of secondary hypertension (Table 6). In fact, most patients with hypertension have primary (essential) hypertension, so an exhaustive workup to identify a secondary cause is unrewarding. However, if clues obtained during the routine history and physical examination or by way of the routine workup raise suspicion for secondary hypertension, further guided workup to identify the underlying disorder is needed. Table 7 presents the basic workup appropriate for all patients with newly diagnosed hypertension, and Table 8 provides an optional workup for those suspected of having an underlying cause to their hypertension.

TABLE 6. Clinical Clues to Selected Secondary Causes of Hypertension[2,17]

Secondary Cause	History	Physical Examination	Laboratory Evaluation
Pheochromocytoma	Paroxysmal hypertension, dizziness, palpitations, headache, nausea, vomiting, "sense of doom," worse with abdominal manipulations, postcoital or with abdominal torsion, episodes of hyper- or hypotension related to anesthesia or surgery; can have paroxysmal hypertension with beta-blockade; family or personal history suggestive of MEN syndrome	Flushing or pallor, tachycardia, bounding pulses; may be normo- or hypertensive on presentation; usually hypertensive during paroxysms; abdominal palpation may incite paroxysm	Elevated urine and plasma catecholamine level
Renal artery stenosis	Usually hypertension is severe, resistant to drug treatment, and often presents relatively acutely in previously normotensive individuals; age usually < 35 or > 55 years; may have history of renal insufficiency, particularly after ACE (angiotensin-converting enzyme inhibitor) or ARB (angiotensin receptor blocker) administration; often a history of vascular disease	Adominal bruit or bruits across other vascular beds suggestive of vascular disease	Duplex ultrasound or angiogram of the renal vessels; laboratory data may confirm the presence of renal insufficiency, often with bland urine sediment
Hypothyroidism	Dry skin, hair loss, weight gain, constipation, cold intolerance, cognitive slowing, menstrual irregularity; may be asymptomatic in elderly individuals	Round, full face; slow speech; hoarseness; muscle weakness; delayed relaxation on reflex testing; cold skin; coarse, brittle hair; normal or faint cardiac impulse; cardiac enlargement; bradycardia; edema	Low thyroid hormone levels, high thyroid-stimulating hormone (TSH) level
Hyperthyroidism	Lability, irritability, palpitations, muscle weakness, weight loss, diarrhea, heat intolerance, menstrual irregularity	Tremor, fine hair, onycholysis, eyelid lag, proptosis, tachycardia, atrial fibrillation, wide pulse pressure	Elevated thyroid hormone levels, suppressed TSH level

	Symptoms	Signs	Laboratory findings
Cushing's disease	Weakness, weight gain, amenorhea	Moon facies, acne, supraclavicular fat pad, purple stria on abdomen or thighs, edema	Increased plasma cortisol, increased urinary 17 keto- and hydroxysteroids
Coarctation of the aorta	Usually none; epistaxis, intermittent claudication, dizziness, or headaches may occur; occasionally seen in patients with Turner's syndrome	Diminished pulse or BP in the vessels distal to coarctation (femoral, sometimes L brachial); bruits over ribs	Electrocardiogram shows left ventricular hyperplasia (LVH); chest radiograph may show notching of lower rib borders; angiography is diagnostic
Hyperparathyroidism	Muscle weakness, nausea, anorexia, constipation, weight loss, polyuria, polydipsia, deafness, parasthesias, bone pain; suggested by triad of peptic ulcer, urinary calculi, and pancreatitis	Band karatitis, hypotonia, weakness	Hypercalcemia, hypophosphatemia, hypercalciuria, elevated alkaline phosphate level
Hyperaldosteronism	Often none; weakness, paralysis, or paresthesias may be present	Weakness; Chvostek or trousseau's sign (rare)	Hypokalemia or low normal potassium level
Renal parenchymal disease	Varies, from none to overt uremic; may have history of renal disease, diabetes, urinary tract infections, abdominal surgeries, prostate disease or family history of polycystic kidney or other renal disease; many drugs can cause or worsen renal disease	Varied; weakness, anorexia, weight changes, edema, palpable enlarged kidneys	Urinalysis may reveal blood, protein, or leukocytes; sediment examination may reveal casts, oval fat bodies, or dysmorphic cells; however, completely bland sediment does not exclude diagnosis; proteinuria should be quantified with 24-hour urine; basic chemistry panel reveals elevated blood urea nitrogen (BUN) or creatinine in many patients, although calculation of creatinine clearance may be needed in elderly patients or those with low muscle mass to identify those with normal serum creatinine by laboratory examination but reduced glomerular filtration rate; renal with ultrasound, renal biopsy, and urine electrolytes may assist

TABLE 7. Primary Laboratory Work-up for All Patients

Procedure	Purpose
Urinalysis and sediment review	Identifies possible renal disease or end organ dysfunction
Basic chemistry, including potassium, fasting glucose, BUN, and creatinine	Evaluate for renal disease; low or low normal potassium may be seen in hyperaldosteronism; fasting glucose can assess for presence of diabetes
Complete blood count	Evaluate for polycythemia, which can cause secondary hypertension
Fasting lipid panel	Risk stratification for patients with dyslipidemia
Electrocardiogram	Risk stratification in patients with coronary artery disease; evaluate for LVH

TABLE 8. Optional Laboratory Work-up: Select Patients

Procedure	Purpose
TSH, T4 level	Screen for those with presentation suggestive of underlying thyroid disorder
Plasma catecholamines, 24-hour urinary catecholamines	Biochemical screen for pheochromocytoma, considered diagnostic if plasma > 2000 pg/mL and suspicious if > 500 pg/mL
Plasma cortisol or urinary keto- and hydroxysteroids	Screen for those with presentation suggestive of Cushing's disease
Microalbuminuria or 24-hour urine protein	Evaluation of patients with diabetes or proteinuria by urinalysis; patients suspected of having nephrotic syndrome
Duplex ultrasound of renal vessels	Evaluate patients suspected of having renal artery stenosis
Echocardiogram	Further risk stratification and evaluation of patients with presentation suggestive of heart failure or cardiomegaly
Parathyroid hormone	Patients with known metabolic bone disease, hypercalcemia, or presentation suggestive of hyperparathyroid disease

References

1. Carretero OA, Oparil S: Essential hypertension: part 1: definition and etiology. Circulation 2000; 101: 329–335.
2. JNC VI The Sixth Report of the Joint National Committee on Prevention, Detection, Evaluation, and Treatment of High Blood Pressure Arch Intern Med 1997, 157: 2413–2446.
3. Prisant LM, Alpert BS, Robbins CB, et al: American National Standard for nonautomated sphygmomanometers: summary report. Am J Hypertens 1995, 8:210–213.
4. Perloff D, Grim C, Flack J, et al: Human blood pressure determination by sphygmomanometry. Circulation 1993, 88:2460–2467.

5. Weber MA: Hypertension Medicine. Humana Press, 2001.
6. Gillespie A, Curzio J: Blood pressure measurement: assessing staff knowledge. Nurs Stand 1998, 12:35–37.
7. O'Brien E, Beevers G, Lip GYH: Blood pressure measurement: Part IV- Automated sphygmomanometry: self blood pressure measurement. Br Med J 2001, 322:1167–1170.
8. Staessen JA, O'Brien ET, Lutgarde T, Fagard, RH: Modern approaches to blood pressure measurement. Occ Envir Med 2000, 57:510–520.
9. O'Brien ET, Petrie J, Littler W, et al: The British Hypertension Society protocol for the evaluation of automated and semi-automated blood pressure measuring devices with special reference to ambulatory systems. J Hypertens 1990, 8:607–619.
10. White WB, Berson AS, Robbins C, et al: National standard for measurement of resting and ambulatory blood pressures with automated sphygmomanometers. Hypertension 1993, 21:504–509.
11. McAlister FA, Straus SE: Measurement of blood pressure: an evidence based review. Br Med J 2001, 322:908–911.
12. O'Brien E, Beevers G, Lip GYH: Blood pressure measurement: part III—automated sphygmomanometry: ambulatory pressure measurement. Br Med J 2001, 322:1110–1114.
13. Verdecchia P: Prognostic value of ambulatory blood pressure: current evidence and clinical implications. Hypertension 2000, 35:844–851.
14. Mancia G, Parati G: Ambulatory blood pressure monitoring and organ damage. Hypertension 2000, 36:894–900.
15. Staessen JA, Byttebier G, Buntinx F, et al: Antihypertensive treatment based on conventional or ambulatory blood pressure measurement: a randomized controlled trial. JAMA 1997, 278:1065–1072.
16. Yarows SA, Julius S, Pickering TG: Home blood pressure monitoring. Arch Intern Med 2000, 160:1251–1257.
17. DeGowin, RL, DeGowin & DeGowin's Diagnostic Examination, 6th ed. New York: McGraw-Hill, 1994.

The Use of Home Blood Pressure Monitors in Practice

chapter 2

Steven A. Yarows, M.D., FACP

Home blood pressure monitors (HBPMs) have been endorsed by patients, yet their utility remains an enigma to many physicians. Most HBPMs are purchased by patients without physician advice, which may reflect their providers' limited understanding of this method of measurement. Physicians are taught in medical school the basic technique of auscultatory blood pressure (BP) measurement without mention of the oscillatory technique. Despite physician leadership, most BP measurements in hospitals are performed by automated devices based on the oscillometric technique.

Types of Monitors

HBPMs may use either the auscultatory or oscillometric technique. The **auscultatory method** generally requires that someone, often the patient, has calibrated equipment as well as adequate dexterity, vision, hearing, and training to obtain reliable readings. The aneroid "dial" gauge is a fragile combination of metal and plastic that is subject to damage from dropping and metal fatigue (Fig. 1). This author's experience indicates that the aneroid gauges that are used at home are less accurate than the fixed office aneroid gauges, most likely a result of increased damage from dropping of these portable devices.[1] Elderly patients often have declining vision, hearing, and hand coordination, further affecting the accuracy of BP measurement. Approximately 20 to 45 minutes of instruction are needed to properly teach auscultatory measurement, which is usually not possible in a busy primary care practice.[2–4]

The **oscillometric technique,** which is used by most automated devices, has largely replaced the auscultatory method for home BP monitoring. The oscillometric technique uses electronic sensors and circuit boards to measure the peak oscillations of the artery during deflation of the cuff, which reflects the mean arterial pressure (Fig. 2). The systolic BP and diastolic BP are calculated from the measured mean arterial pressure. Each company

Figure 1. **A,** An aneroid monometer. **B,** Magnification shows the delicate mechanism.

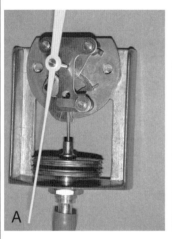
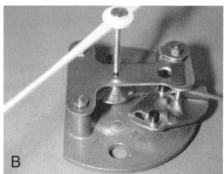

has its own secretive proprietary algorithm that calculates systolic and diastolic BP. Companies also develop new models with new algorithms. Thus, even within the same company, different algorithms may be used. The variation between monitors is similar to the variation between different health care providers, and most patients use only a single oscillometric machine.[5] The variation between nurses, for the same patient, is 6 mm Hg for systolic BP and 10 mm Hg for diastolic BP with the auscultatory technique.[6,7] Additionally, this technique eliminates the rounding up or down (zero terminal preference) that is common with the auscultatory technique. Patients using an oscillometric machine do not need to learn auscultation, which is the most difficult part of BP measurement.[8]

Figure 2. Oscillometric readings from deflating the BP cuff.

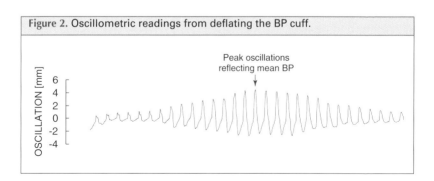

Electronic sphygmomanometers are either fully automatic (containing an electronic pump) or semi-automatic (which requires the patient to manually inflate the cuff). Both devices electronically calculate the systolic and diastolic BP. The fully automatic devices are approximately $50 more than the manually inflated devices but are easier to use, especially for patients with arthritis in their hands. The electronic devices are required to withstand 10,000 inflation/deflation cycles by current standards, which should allow the units to be used for at least 5 years (although not tested), which would make this cost difference relatively minor.[9] The electronic devices contain circuit boards with a built-in pressure sensor (Fig. 3). Long-term usage of an electronic measuring device could result in a malfunction with this circuit board, resulting in a lack of a reading or error report, but inaccurate measurements would not occur. Inaccurate readings over time could result from a pressure sensor malfunction, change in the individual's arm size, or heart rhythm.

Electronic monitors may measure the BP from the upper arm, wrist, or finger. The upper arm cuffs are most commonly used because of the similarity to auscultatory monitors, in addition to numerous published calibration studies. Both the wrist and finger measurements fluctuate depending on the position of the monitor relative to the heart. The correction of the measured BP based on arm position is to subtract 2 mm Hg for every inch (2.54 cm) that the BP cuff is below the horizontal plane of the heart and the addition of 2 mm Hg for measurements above heart level.[10] Finger manometers are not recommended by any professional organizations because of a lack of calibration data and increased variation from peripheral vasoconstriction and potential atherosclerotic disease.[11,12]

Figure 3. Front display (**A**) and rear component (**B**) of a Sunbeam 7654 electronic monitor.

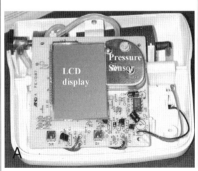
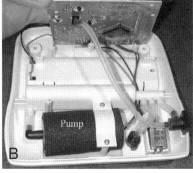

Accuracy

Before accuracy standards were developed, HBPMs were usually found to be inaccurate. The industry is regulated by the Federal Drug Agency (FDA) in the United States, which uses the Association for the Advancement of Medical Instrumentation (AAMI) standards for sphygmomanometers.[9] Other countries use the standards of the British Hypertensive Society Working Party on Blood Pressure Measurement (BHSWP).[13,14] Combination and simplification of these two guidelines have been proposed. However, new devices usually report accuracy according to both current guidelines.[15-17]

Some of the major manufacturers have published reports on instrument accuracy in peer-reviewed journals, which has allowed physicians to recommend accurate machines to patients (Table 1). Smaller manufacturers do not publish their data. Many electronic models from various companies are sold with different names and model numbers than the published models, which makes it difficult for physicians to recognize approved machines. The author recommends that patients purchase only approved models.

The author has tested patients' previously purchased HBPMs over 2.5 years and found an accuracy of 0.3 mm Hg ($\pm$2.3 mm Hg) for the 91 electronic HBPMs with an overall 92% accuracy, as defined within $\pm$3 mm Hg.

Normal Home Readings

Home BP measurements are performed during different circumstances than office and ambulatory BP readings. Several published reports have shown that the average HBPM is 9/6 mm Hg lower than the

TABLE 1. Published and Approved Oscillometric Models via AAMI and BHS Standards	
Model	**Reference**
Home Upper Arm	
Omron HEM 705CP	O'Brien[45]
Omron HEM 735C	O'Brien[45]
Omron HEM 713C	O'Brien[45]
Omron HEM 737 Intellisense	O'Brien[45]
A&D UA-767	Rogoza et.al.[49]
Office Upper Arm	
Omron HEM-907 (AAMI only)	White and Anwar[50]
BPM-100	Wright et.al.[51]
Omron Healthcare, Vernon Hills, IL; A & D Engineering, Milpitas, CA	

office BP measurements and minimally different (2 mm Hg higher for systolic BP and 1 mm Hg lower for diastolic BP) when compared with daytime ambulatory monitoring.[18] As a result, the HBPM "normal" averages need to be adjusted accordingly. Based on reports from two large databases, a Task Force concluded that home BP readings below 135/85 mm Hg reflect normal readings and are equivalent to office BP readings of below 140/90 mm Hg.[12] If an individual patient has a lower office BP goal, the HBPM goal should be adjusted by subtracting 9/6 mm Hg compared with the office goal.

When to Use and When to Avoid Home Blood Pressure Monitors

HBPMs are most useful for monitoring and adjusting therapy for a known hypertensive patient. The numerous measurements that can be attained offer advantages over the limited and relatively expensive office readings. Ambulatory BP monitoring could also be used, but is impractical because of its expense, especially for serial monitoring over time.[19] HBPM better predicts end-organ damage than office BP measurement does, although the data are not as extensive as office BP measurements.[20,21] HBPM also better predicts mortality.[22,23]

The oscillometric technique used both in the office and at home is becoming more common in multicenter clinical trials because of the lack of observer training and inter-observer variation in BP measurement.[24–27] A recent trial (The Treatment of Hypertension According to Home or Office Blood Pressure [THOP]) should soon clarify the benefits of antihypertensive treatment guided by self-measured BP versus treatment based on conventional BP measurement.[28]

HBPM helps patients cope and understand the fluctuations of BP and the treatment of hypertension.[29,30] Patients who use HBPM may have better control of their hypertension and improved compliance, although studies are limited and have mixed results based on older, non-oscillometric monitors.[31–38] Although data are very limited, HBPM can also be cost effective.[39]

HBPM should be avoided in patients with marked irregular heart rates, such as atrial fibrillation, because of a lack of data regarding accuracy of measurements with this condition.[40]

How to use Home Blood Pressure Monitors in Clinical Practice

A patient handout that describes the purchase and proper usage of HBPMs was developed for improved patient education and to save provider time.[41] The handout indicates common errors in the measurement of BP. Patients are instructed regarding proper cuff size, rest period before measurement, and avoidance of talking and crossing legs during the measurement. Health care providers should underscore the importance of proper cuff size and instruct patients to use only upper arm HBPM.

Included with the handout is a chart to graph the readings with the expected normal range highlighted. It is easier to appreciate trends and averages of the measurements in graph form than randomly placed numbers on the back of a shopping list or on a scroll of napkins (Fig. 4). Patients who are starting a new medication or having adjustments in medication dosing regimen are instructed to measure their BP twice a day in the morning and before dinner for 2 to 4 weeks, depending on the medication.[5] Stable hypertensives are told to monitor BP on the first day of the month and more frequently if the readings are elevated. The charts are faxed or mailed to the physician's office, and necessary therapy adjustments are performed with the cycle repeated until adequate hypertension control is achieved.

Newer HBPM with memory and optional computer links allow graphical display and statistical analysis of the data and may limit patient reporting bias, although they are much more costly.[43] Automatic trans-

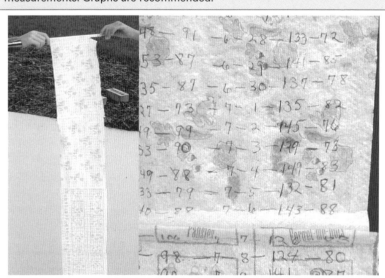

Figure 4. An ill-advised method (using paper towels) for recording home BP measurements. Graphs are recommended.

mission of BP data over telephone lines may eventually become the standard method of hypertension monitoring.[44]

Key Points

∽ HBPMs have become popular because of direct consumer marketing and despite lack of physician endorsement.

∽ The oscillometric models have replaced the more cumbersome auscultatory models over the past decade.

∽ Studies by several manufacturers and in the author's office indicate that many of these devices are accurate and relatively inexpensive.

∽ HBPM may not be accurate in patients with irregular heart rates, and more research is needed to determine their accuracy.

∽ Patient handouts offer an easy approach to teach proper usage of the automated HBPM and also to indicate expected usage and proper reporting techniques to the health care provider.

References

1. Yarows SA, Qian K: Accuracy of aneroid sphygmomanometers in clinical usage: University of Michigan experience. Blood Pressure Monitoring 2001, 6:101–106.

2. Armstrong R, Barrack D, Gordon R: Patients achieve accurate home blood pressure measurement following instruction. Aust J Adv Nurs 1995, 12:15–21.

3. Mejia A, Julius S: Practical utility of blood pressure readings obtained by self-determination. J Hypertens 1989, 7(suppl 3):53–57.

4. Yarows SA: Home blood pressure monitoring in primary care. Blood Pressure Monitoring 1998, 3(suppl 1):11–17.

5. Yarows SA, Staessen JA: How to use home blood pressure monitors in clinical practice [editorial]. Am J Hypertens 2002, 15(part 1):93–96.

6. Kay LE: Accuracy of blood pressure measurement in the family practice center. J Am Board Fam Pract 1998, 11:2528.

7. Rocha JC, Rocha AT, Magossi AMG, et al: Evaluation of the technique for taking blood pressure by health care workers in an University Hospital [abstract] Am J Hypertens 1988, 11(part 2):66.

8. Armstrong R, Barrack D, Gordon R: Patients achieve accurate home blood pressure measurement following instruction. Aust J Adv Nurs 1995, 12:15–21.

9. Electronic or automated sphygmomanometers. Developed by Association for the Advancement of Medical Instrumentation. Approved October 16, 1992. American National Standards Institute, Inc., 330 Washington Boulevard, Suite 400, Arlington, Virginia.

10. Ramsey M: Blood pressure monitoring: automated oscillometric devices. J Clin Monitoring 1991, 7:56–67.

11. Raamat R, Jagomagi K, Talts J: Different responses of Finapres and the oscillometric finger blood pressure monitor during intensive vasomotion. J Med Engineer Technol 2000, 24:95–101.

12. White WB, Asmar R, Imai Y, et al: Task force VI: Self-monitoring of the blood pressure. Blood Pressure Monitoring 1999, 4:343–351.
13. O'Brien E, Petrie J, Littler W, et al: The British Hypertension Society protocol for the evaluation of automated and semi-automated blood pressure measuring devices with special reference to ambulatory systems. J Hyperten 1990, 8:607–619.
14. O'Brien E, Petrie J, Littler W, et al: Short report: An outline of the revised British Hypertension Society protocol for the evaluation of blood pressure measuring devices. J Hypertens 1993, 11:677–679.
15. O'Brien E: Modification of blood-pressure measuring devices and the protocol of the British Hypertensive Society. Blood Pressure Monitoring 1999, 4:53–54.
16. O'Brien E: Proposals for simplifying the validation protocols of the British Hypertension Society and the Association for the Advancement of Medical Instrumentation. Blood Pressure Monitoring 2000, 5:43–45.
17. O'Brien E, De Gaudemaris R, Bobrie G, et al: Devices and validation. Blood Pressure Monitoring, 2000, 5:93–100.
18. Yarows SA, Julius S, Pickering T: Home blood pressure monitoring. Arch Intern Med 2000, 160:1251–1257.
19. Yarows SA: Ambulatory Blood Pressure Monitoring JAMA 1998, 279:196.
20. Ibrahim MM, Tarazi RC, Dustan HP, Gifford RW Jr: Electrocardiogram in evaluation of resistance to antihypertensive therapy. Arch Intern Med 1977, 137:1125–1129.
21. Kleinert HD, Harshfield GA, Pickering TG, et al: What is the value of home blood pressure measurement in patients with mild hypertension? Hypertension 1984, 6:574–578.
22. Sakuma M, Imai Y, Tgsuji I, et al: Predictive value of home blood pressure measurement in relation to stroke morbidity: a population based study in Ohasama, Japan. Hypertens Res 1997, 20:167–174.
23. Tsuji I, Imai Y, Nagai K, et al: Proposal of reference values for home blood pressure measurement: prognostic criteria based on a prospective observation of the general population in Ohasama, Japan. Am J Hypertens 1997, 10(4 pt1):409–418.
24. Hannson L, Zanchetti A, Carruthers SG, et al: Effects of intensive blood pressure lowering and low dose aspirin in patients with hypertension: principal results of the Hypertension Optimal Treatment (HOT) randomized trial. Lancet 1998, 351:1755–1762.
25. Trial of Preventing Hypertension using Candesartan Cilexetil in patients with high normal blood pressure (TROPHY), unpublished, current study Astra-Zenecca.
26. Denolle T, Waeber B, Kjeldsen S, et al: Self-measurement of blood pressure in clinical trials and therapeutic applications. Blood Pressure Monitoring 2000, 5:145–149.
27. Kjeldsen SE, Hedner T, Jamerson K, et al: Hypertension Optimal Study: home blood pressure in treated hypertensive subjects. Hypertension 1998, 31:1014–1020.
28. Blood Pressure Monitoring 1998; 3(suppl. 1):S29–S35
29. Krecke HJ, Fleischmann C, Bokmann M: Distribution and acceptance of self measurement of blood pressure in the Hamburg area: Verbreitung und Akzeptanz der Blutdruckselbstmessung im Grossraum Hamburg. Schweiz Rundsch Med Prax. 1989, 78:1336–1342.
30. Krecke HJ, Lutkes P, Maiwald M, Schultze-Rupp A: Self-measurement of blood pressure in hypertensive subjects in Germany: results of a questionnaire in Spring/early Summer 1993. Blutdruckselbstmessung bei Hypertonikern in Deutschland. Ergebnisse einer Umfrage im Fruhling/Fruhsommer 1993. Schweiz Rundsch Med Prax. 1994, 83:895–900.
31. Johnson AL, Taylor DW, Sackett DL, et al: Self-recording of blood pressure in the management of hypertension. Can Med Assoc J 1978, 119:1034–1039.

32. Midanik LT, Resnick B, Hurley LB, et al: Home blood pressure monitoring for mild hypertensives. Public Health Reports 1991, 106:85–89.
33. Stahl SM, Kelley CR, Neill PJ, et al: Effects of home blood pressure measurement on long-term control. Am J Public Health 1984, 74:704–709.
34. Carnahan JE, Nugent CA: The effects of self-monitoring by patients on the control of hypertension. Am J Med Sci 1975, 269:69–73.
35. Midanik LT, Resnick B, Hurley LB, et al: Home blood pressure monitoring in hypertesnion. Public Health Rep 1991, 106:85–89.
36. Edmonds D, Foerster E, Groth H, et al: Does self-measurement of blood pressure improve patient compliance in hypertension? J Hypertens 1985, 3(suppl)31–34.
37. Haynes RB, Sackett DL, Gibson ES, et al: Improvement of medication compliance in uncontrolled hypertension. Lancet 1976, 1:1265–1268.
38. Nessman DG, Carnahan JE, Nugent CA: Increasing compliance: patient-operated hypertension groups. Arch Intern Med 1980, 140:1427–1430.
39. Soghikan K, Casper SM, Fireman BH, et al: Home blood pressure monitoring: effect on use of medical services and medical care costs. Medical Care 1992, 30:855–865.
40. Yarows SA: Response to letter to the editor: blood pressure monitoring in atrial fibrillation using electronic devices. Arch Intern Med 2001, 161:294.
41. http://www.med.umich.edu/intmed/hypertension/homebp.htm
42. Reference deleted.
43. Myers MG: Reporting bias in self-measurement of blood pressure. Blood Pressure Monitoring 2001, 6:181–183.
44. Rogers MAM, Small D, et al: Home monitoring service improves mean arterial pressure in patients with essential hypertension. Ann Intern Med 2001, 134:1024–1032.
45. O'Brien E: State of the market in 2001 for blood pressure measuring devices. Blood Pressure Monitoring 2001, 6:171–176.
46. Rogoza AN, Pavlova TS, Sergeeva MV: Validation of A&D UA-767 device for the self-measurement of blood pressure. Blood Pressure Monitoring 2000, 5:227–231.
47. White WB, Anwar YA: Evaluation of the overall efficacy of the Omron office digital blood pressure HEM-907 monitor in adults, Blood Pressure Monitoring 2001, 6:107–110.
48. Wright JM, Mattu GS, Perry TL, et al: Validation of a new algorithm for the BPM-100 electronic oscillometric office blood pressure monitor. Blood Pressure Monitoring 2001, 6:161–165.

Urine Microalbumin: For Diabetics Only?

Sunita Sharma, M.D., and
Eddie L. Greene, M.D.

chapter

3

General Aspects

Microalbuminuria is a major cardiovascular risk factor and indicates increased susceptibility to both cardiovascular and renal disease.[1-3] Estimates suggest that microalbuminuria is present in 7% to 8% of the general U.S. population and in 10% to 25% of patients with essential hypertension.[1,3] Microalbuminuria in hypertensive patients is directly linked to the development and progression of chronic renal disease, left ventricular hypertrophy, endothelial dysfunction and peripheral vascular disease, serum lipid abnormalities, and hyperinsulinemia.[1-3]

Microalbuminuria plays an important role in the development and progression of diabetic and nondiabetic renal disease. Given the increasing age, obesity, and ethnic diversity of the U.S. population, clinicians are likely to treat increasing numbers of patients who have one or more cardiovascular risk factors, including microalbuminuria. This chapter provides a frame of reference for clinicians to better understand the pathogenesis and clinical implications of microalbuminuria during the diagnostic work-up. Understanding the implications will allow implementation of therapeutic plans that are tailored to improve the patient's cardiovascular risk profile.

Definition of Microalbuminuria

Microalbuminuria indicates a urinary albumin excretion (UAE) of 30 to 300 mg/24 hours or 20 to 200 µg/min, which exceeds the 95% confidence interval determined for the normal population.[4] A minimum of three timed urine collections within the ranges noted constitutes a definitive diagnosis of microalbuminuria. The urine samples should be sterile and obtained within a period of 6 to 12 weeks. Repeated measurements reduce false-positive and -negative results. The sustained presence of urinary albumin excretion at these levels predicts an increased likelihood for the development of overt and progressive renal failure.[4] The detection of microalbuminuria in a spot urine sample is discussed later in this chapter.

23

Prevalence

Data from the third National Health and Nutrition Examination Survey (NHANES-III) suggest that 11% of men and 12% of women in the general U.S. population have microalbuminuria.[3] The data indicate a significant increase in microalbuminuria in elderly patients, particularly those older than age 60 years. NHANES-III data suggest that approximately 30% of patients with diabetes and approximately 16% of patients with essential hypertension have chronic microalbuminuria.[3] When data from the NHANES-III cohort are compared with previous surveys, the prevalence and incidence of microalbuminuria continue to rise. The increased numbers of patients with microalbuminuria may be a forerunner of an increasing burden of future cardiovascular disease.

Key Points

☞ Microalbuminuria occurs commonly and is being increasingly recognized clinically.
☞ The presence of microalbuminuria reflects increased risk for cardiovascular morbidity and mortality.
☞ The prevalence of microalbuminuria is substantially increased in both the diabetic and hypertensive patient populations.

Effects of Age, Gender, and Ethnicity on Microalbuminuria

Surprisingly, a high prevalence of microalbuminuria has been found in children age 6 to 19 years, for unclear reasons. The lowest prevalence of microalbuminura exists among those age 20 to 39 years, with a dramatic increase in prevalence after age 40 years.[3] Clinically significant microalbuminuria may affect approximately 6% of people of European origin and approximately 5% to 6% of U.S Hispanics. As many as 20% of African Americans may have high urinary albumin excretion rates.[5]

Postulated mechanisms to explain the increased prevalence of microalbuminuria in African Americans include defects in endothelial nitric oxide synthesis and its bioavailabilty and increases in intraglomerular capillary pressure, both of which can lead to chronic declines in renal reserve over time, possibly as a result of chronic glomerular remodeling.[6] Ethnic minorities may be more likely to have microalbuminuria at the time diabetes or hypertension is diagnosed.[7-9] Whether this reflects underutilization of or poor access to health care, or additional pathophysiologic mechanisms, remains undetermined. Nevertheless, the clinical significance of microalbuminuria in significant numbers of minority patients with hypertension is underscored by the accompanying disparities in target organ disease, clinical outcomes, and overall patient survival.

Studies suggest that links may exist between the presence of the metabolic syndrome and microalbuminuria in African Americans.[10] The presence of microalbuminuria represents another common concomitant risk factor and places these patients at very high risk for earlier and possibly more severe cardiovascular disease.[10]

Key Points

- ⊙ The prevalence of microalbuminuria varies as a function of age, with the highest rates found in patients older than age 40 years.
- ⊙ The prevalence of microalbuminuria is elevated in ethnic minority populations and particularly in African Americans.
- ⊙ The metabolic syndrome is common in African Americans and is frequently accompanied by microalbuminuria, which further magnifies cardiovascular risk.

Mechanisms Involved in the Normal Renal Handling of Albumin

Albumin and other proteins filtered by the kidney are degraded during their passage through the nephron into multiple small peptide fragments before they are excreted in the urine. These fragments may not be easily detected by current methods used to measure urinary albumin excretion,[11] leading to underestimation of urinary albumin excretion. Healthy individuals purportedly excrete approximately 25 mg of albumin and up to 1300 mg of protein fragments per day.[12] Passage of proteins into the glomerular filtrate depends on several factors, including the electric charge, molecular size, molecular weight of the protein, and the size and distribution of pores within the glomerular basement membrane.[11] Filtered proteins are taken up and degraded within intracellular lysosomes in glomerular epithelial and tubular cells.[12] Two proteins highly expressed in the proximal tubule are cubulin and megalin. Both are involved in the reuptake and lysosomal targeting of filtered albumin for eventual degradation. Functional or structural defects in these proteins lead to greater quantities of albumin reaching distal segments of the nephron, where they may instigate local tubulointerstitial injury.[13]

Key Points

◌➣ Albumin and other large proteins filtered by the glomerulus are usually degraded into multiple peptide fragments.
◌➣ Defective mechanisms involving reuptake and degradation of filtered proteins play a major role in urinary protein losses.
◌➣ The passage of proteins into the glomerular filtrate may depend on several interacting factors, including (but not necessarily limited to) electric charge, molecular size, and weight of the protein
◌➣ Glomerular pore size in the glomerular basement membrane may also serve as a barrier to major loss of protein in the urine.

Measurement of Renal Albumin Excretion and Microalbuminuria in the Clinical Setting

Measurement of urinary albumin excretion can be obtained by various methods including radioimmunoassay, immunoturbidometry, nephelometry, and enzyme-linked immunosorbent assay (ELISA). Although specific guidelines to quantify microalbuminuria are still being developed, office dipstick testing, using devices such as the Micral-Test urine dipstick, may be sensitive and specific. The Micral-Test urine dipstick uses an immunoassay on the test strip. After immersion of the strip in the patient's urine for 5 seconds, the resulting color change after 5 minutes is used to quantify the amount of urinary albumin by comparison to known standards. Urinary albumin levels greater than 20 mg/L are deemed a positive result. Use of the Micral-Test dipstick in busy primary care offices is an excellent way to quickly and efficiently screen at-risk patients and may reduce cost.[14,15] A useful approach and algorithm is suggested in Figure 1.[16,38]

Albumin excretion rates may vary as much as 40% to 100% during an average day.[4] Normal albumin excretion may be 25% greater during the day than at night. Variability in urinary albumin excretion is decreased when first morning voided urine is used for measurement.[4,15]

Dehydration, physical exercise, major alterations in dietary protein intake, and acute febrile illnesses can influence albumin excretion. If a specimen shows positive results for microalbuminuria, it is critical to ensure that none of the aforementioned conditions or other problems are present that will invalidate the test. The test should be repeated following the resolution of an intervening illness. A positive result for microalbuminuria on two separate occasions within a 3 to 6-month period in the absence of other concurrent illness that causes transient proteinuria is highly suggestive for chronic microalbuminuria. Further work-up

Figure 1. Initial approach to the evaluation of microalbuminuria and proteinuria.

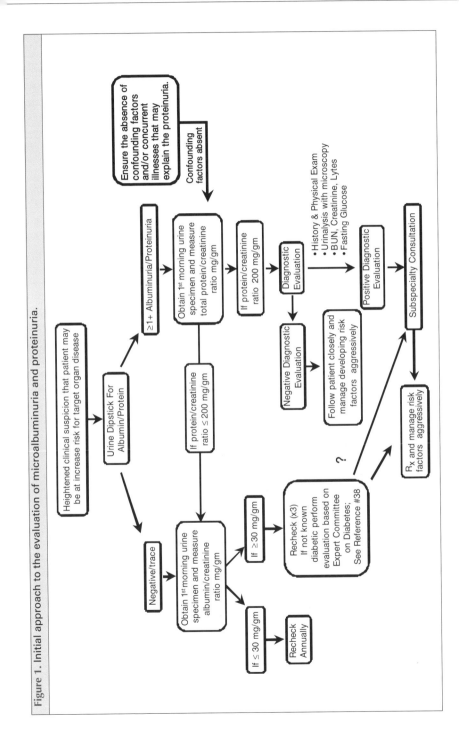

and therapy should be pursued at this point. Because of the potential for significant variability in a single random measurement of urinary albumin excretion, the 24-hour urine collection remains the gold standard for gauging urinary albumin excretion.[4,15] However, patient adherence with the 24-hour urine collection is often suboptimal and has led to the evaluation of simpler alternatives. The albumin/creatinine ratio (ACR) from the first void morning urine sample may offer a reliable alternative to the 24-hour urine sample.[16,17] The sensitivity and specificity of the calculated ACR to detect clinically relevant microalbuminuria is reported to be 98% and 89%, respectively.[18] An ACR greater than 3.0 mg/mmol is abnormal.[4] Recent recommendations have been made to change the diagnosis of microalbuminuria using the ACR to values greater than 4.4 mg/mmol in women and greater than 2.5 mg/mmol in men.[18,19] However, gender-specific standards have not been universally accepted and require additional studies.

Key Points

- ∞ Microalbuminuria is defined as a UAE within the range of 30 to 300 mg/24 hours or 20 to 200 μg/min.
- ∞ Urinary albumin excretion can be variable, and potential confounding factors include dehydration, exercise, dietary protein intake, and febrile illnesses.
- ∞ The gold standard for measuring urinary albumin excretion is 24-hour urine collection.
- ∞ The ACR calculated from the first morning void can provide a reliable and convenient alternative for measuring UAE when collecting a 24-hour urine is not feasible.
- ∞ Standards are still being established for the use of the urine dipstick for determination of microalbuminuria.

Clinical Aspects

Pathogenesis

Because hypertensive patients with microalbuminuria are at increased risk of developing target organ disease, an appreciation of the pathophysiologic mechanisms underlying microalbuminuria assists clinicians in providing precise preventive, diagnostic, and therapeutic measures to lower urinary albumin excretion.

Hypotheses to explain microalbuminuria in essential hypertension implicate both hemodynamic and nonhemodynamic factors, which may interact. Glomerular capillary hemodynamic alterations accompany elevations in the intraglomerular hydrostatic pressure. Well recognized are elevations in systolic blood pressure (BP) that are transmitted to the glomerulus when preglomerular arteriole myogenic tone is compromised. Normally, glomerular hydrostatic pressure is tightly regulated by the intrinsic myogenic tone of the afferent and efferent arterioles. Autoregulation by the afferent arteriole also limits the transmission of elevated systemic BP to the glomerulus. In this way, maintenance of the normally low intraglomerular hydrostatic pressure is accomplished with little day-to-day variation.

In the presence of hypertension and other intrinsic renal diseases, efferent and afferent arteriolar vascular tone can be influenced by many factors, including circulating and intrarenal peptides such as angiotensin II and endothelin, alterations of sympathetic nerve output, alterations in redox status, defective nitric oxide synthesis, and low bioavailability of nitric oxide.[20,21] The altered glomerular hemodynamic function caused by hypertension can ultimately lead to chronic glomerular injury. Mesangial cell secretion of cytokines such as transforming growth factor (TGF) β1 may amplify renal injury. A study of urinary TGFβ1 in African Americans strongly suggested a role for this cytokine in the pathogenesis of hypertensive renal disease.[22] In addition, excessive renal TGFβ1 may reduce intracellular lysosomal activity, thereby interfering with the normal pathways involved in filtered albumin degradation.[23]

Also of note is the association of persistent systemic hypertension and increases in glomerular hydrostatic pressure with progressive tubulointerstitial disease. These findings imply that the presence of increased urinary albumin excretion in patients with essential hypertension may be both a marker of underlying renal injury and an important measure of cardiovascular risk and prognosis.[11]

Key Points

- ☞ Systemic and intraglomerular hemodynamic changes contribute to the pathophysiology and effects of microalbuminuria in essential hypertension.
- ☞ Compromised intrinsic myogenic tone and alterations in autoregulatory mechanisms of the afferent arteriole occur in some forms of essential hypertension and contribute to increases in glomerular hydrostatic pressure.
- ☞ Hypertension may be associated with elevations in renal TGFβ1. Pathophysiologic alterations caused by TGFβ1 may alter renal albumin excretion.

Key Points (*Continued*)

↪ Chronic elevations in intraglomerular hydrostatic pressure may permanently alter the architecture of the glomerulus and tubulointerstitium, thereby contributing to both microalbuminuria and progressive renal disease.

Microalbuminuria in Essential Hypertension

Reports estimate that the prevalence of microalbuminuria in patients with essential hypertension ranges from 6% to 40%. In addition, microalbuminuria is strongly associated with the presence of early end-organ damage in nondiabetic hypertensive patients, including left ventricular hypertrophy and increased carotid artery wall thickness. Major cardiovascular events associated with microalbuminuria in hypertensive patients include the development of left ventricular hypertrophy, coronary artery disease (74%), peripheral vascular disease (44%), and fatal and nonfatal coronary events.[25]

The increased cardiovascular risk in hypertensive patients with microalbuminuria is multifactorial. Higher BP levels occur in hypertensive patients with microalbuminuria. Moreover, the nocturnal dip in BP is either blunted or absent in hypertensives with microalbuminuria and may increase the likelihood of earlier end-organ damage.[26]

Key Points

↪ Microalbuminuria is associated with increased cardiovascular risk in patients with essential hypertension.
↪ Microalbuminuria may be associated with increased BP, left ventricular hypertrophy, and carotid artery thickness.
↪ An attenuation or loss of the nocturnal dipping response in BP levels can be associated with microalbuminuria and contribute to end-organ damage and injury.

Relationship Between Microalbuminuria and Serum Lipids

Lipid abnormalities in hypertensive patients are associated with microalbuminuria. *In vitro* and *in vivo* animal and human studies indicate that hyperlipidemia can directly and indirectly contribute to the pathophysiology of microvascular and macrovascular renal injury.[27] Glomerular injury caused by oxidized lipids and elevated fatty acids can lead to microalbuminuria and possibly potentiate excessive protein losses. Elevations in urinary albumin excretion are associated with elevations in serum triglycerides, elevated low-density lipoprotein cholesterol, and low high-density lipoprotein cholesterol levels.[27] Although the specific pathogenesis of hyperlipidemia in individuals with microalbuminuria and proteinuria is currently not well understood, increased lipid intake as well as increased compensatory hepatic lipoprotein and lipid synthesis in response to increased urinary protein losses may figure prominently.[28]

Key Points

- ⤷ Hyperlipidemia occurs commonly in patients with microalbuminuria
- ⤷ Increased lipid intake or increased hepatic lipid synthesis may play prominent roles.

Insulin-resistance Syndrome and Microalbuminuria

Obesity is increasingly recognized as a major contributor to the epidemic of cardiovascular disease and possibly to the recent increases in renal disease.[29,30] Elevations in urinary albumin excretion are associated with increases in body mass index (BMI) and waist-to-hip ratios in some populations.[31] The metabolic, or insulin-resistance, syndrome is characterized by hyperinsulinemia, insulin resistance, central obesity, hyperlipidemia, and increased urinary albumin excretion.[29] Evidence demonstrates a direct link between the insulin-resistance syndrome and microalbuminuria in hypertensive patients. In nondiabetic hypertensive patients with microalbuminura, whole-body glucose utilization is decreased and may lead to increased concentrations of serum insulin.[5] Nonesterified fatty acids are also elevated in patients with the insulin resistance syndrome and may contribute to vascular dysfunction via synergism with angiotensin II through the induction of oxidative stress in the vasculature. Studies also suggest that features associated with insulin resistance increase the activity of the renin-angiotensin system and the risk of developing end-organ damage.[29]

Key Points

- ⤷ Increased urinary albumin excretion is associated with increases in both BMI and waist-to-hip ratios.
- ⤷ The metabolic risk factor cluster is characterized by insulin resistance, central obesity, hyperinsulinemia, and hyperlipidemia and is associated with microalbuminuria.

Key Points (*Continued*)

☞ The metabolic risk factor cluster and microalbuminuria contribute to target organ damage.

Effect of Smoking

Evidence indicates a link between smoking and the development of proteinuria and progressive renal disease in both diabetic and nondiabetic cohorts, including patients with essential hypertension.[32] The reduction in glomerular filtration rate (GFR) may be as much as 3.2 mL/min for every 10 pack/years smoked in active smokers.[32] Astute clinicians emphasize smoking cessation, particularly for those at high risk of developing renal and cardiovascular disease.

Key Points

☞ Smoking is linked to the development of renal disease in both diabetic and nondiabetic populations.

☞ GFR may be reduced by as much as 3.2 mL/min for every 10 pack/years of cigarette use in smokers.

☞ Efforts targeted at smoking cessation in all patients and particularly those with increased cardiovascular risk are essential to lower risk and prevent premature cardiovascular disease.

Treatment

Both lowering of the urinary albumin excretion rate and optimal BP control should be the cornerstones of the therapeutic approach in hypertensive patients with microalbuminuria and proteinuria, particularly in those at greatest risk for the progression of renal disease.[33] Several studies suggest that blocking the renin-angiotensin-aldosterone system (RAAS) using angiotensin-converting enzyme (ACE) inhibition, angiotensin receptor (AT_1) antagonists, or both attenuate urinary protein excretion beyond that attributable to lowering systemic BP alone. The results from several clinical trials, including AASK,[24] MDRD,[34] HOPE,[35] Micro-HOPE,[36] HOT,[37] all support this notion. Reasonable goals for target BP for those without diabetes who have microalbuminuria is 135/80 mm Hg and lower in individuals with diabetes and frank proteinuria to 125/75 mm Hg.[33] If BP is effectively lowered to the target goal, most effective antihypertensive regimens will also lower urinary protein excretion. Dihydropyridine calcium channel blockers may be an exception. Residual microalbuminuria during antihypertensive therapy may be predictive of the subsequent rate of loss of renal function.

Specific blockade of RAAS may have independent cardiovascular and renal protective effects in addition to the effects attributable to the lowering of systemic BP alone.[33] Substantial reduction in proteinuria is likely to contribute greatly to these additional effects. Evidence suggests that RAAS blockade reduces proteinuria in part by a reduced GFR, a decrease in the filtration fraction, and a reduction of glomerular basement membrane permselectivity. All of these changes decrease urinary albumin excretion to an extent greater than that attributable to the reduction in BP alone. Salt restriction and diuretic therapy may also be useful adjuncts in some patients, particularly in African Americans.

Key Points

- ⊛ ACE inhibition and angiotensin receptor blockade represent key therapeutic targets to treat and prevent microalbuminuria.
- ⊛ Transient small reductions in the GFR and the filtration fraction contribute to the decline in microalbuminuria.
- ⊛ Multidrug combinations, including diuretics accompanied by salt restriction, may often be necessary for optimal BP control.

Conclusions

Microalbuminuria is a risk marker for target organ injury and a major risk factor for both cardiovascular and renal disease in diabetic and nondiabetic patients with essential hypertension. It is crucial for clinicians to determine the UAE rate in hypertensive patients and to implement appropriate therapy when urinary albumin excretion is elevated. An ACR calculated from urine albumin levels obtained during a first morning void is a simple clinical measurement easily performed in the ambulatory or outpatient setting; it provides a good approximation of the patients's urinary albumin excretion. Reducing both systemic and intraglomerular pressures are important components of therapy for patients who have microalbuminuria. RAAS blockade (ACE inhibition, angiotensin II receptor antagonism or both) is an important component of the therapeutic regimen.

References

1. Mimran A, Ribstein J, DuCalier G: Microalbuminuria in essential hypertension. Curr Opin Nephrol Hypertens 1999, 8:359–363.
2. Lydakis C, Lip GYH: Microalbuminuria and cardiovascular risk. Quart J Med 1998, 91:381–391.
3. Jones CA, Francis ME, Eberhardt MA, et al: Microalbuminuria in the US population: Third National Health and Nutrition Examination Survey. Am J Kidney Dis 2002, 39:445–459.
4. Bianchi S, Bigazzi R, Campese VM: Microalbuminuria in essential hypertension: significance, pathophysiology, and therapeutic implications. Am J Kidney Dis 1999, 34:973–995.
5. Kohler KA, McClellan WM, Ziemer DC, et al: Risk factors for microalbuminuria in black Americans with newly diagnosed type 2 diabetes. Am J Kidney Dis 2000, 36:903–913.
6. Earle KA, Mehrotra S, Dalton RN, et al: Defective nitric oxide production and functional renal reserve in patients with type 2 diabetes who have microalbuminuria of African and Asian compared with White origin. J Am Soc Nephrol 2001, 12:2125–2130.
7. Kiang X, Srinivasan SR, Radhakiishnamurthy B, et al: Microalbuminuria in young adults related to blood pressure in a biracial (black-white) population. The Bogalusa Heart Study. Am J Hypertens 1994, 7:794–800.
8. Summerson JH, Bell RA, Konen JC: Racial differences in the prevalence of microalbuminuria in hypertension. Am J Kidney Dis 1995, 26:577–579.
9. Chelliah R, Sagnella GA, Markandu N, MacGregor GA: Urinary protein and essential hypertension in black and white people. Hypertension 2002, 39:1064–1070.
10. Srinivasan SR, Myers L, Berenson GS: Risk variables of insulin resistance syndrome in African-American and Caucasian young adults with microalbuminuria: the Bogalusa heart study. Am J Hypertes 2000, 13:1274–1279.
11. Russo LM, Bakris GL, Comper WD: Renal handling of albumin: a critical review of basic concepts and perspective. Am J Kidney Dis 2002, 39:899–919.
12. Grieve KA, Balazs NDH, Comper WD: Protein fragments have been considerably underestimated by various protein assays. Clin Chem 2001, 47:1717–1719.
13. Christensen EI, Birn H: Megalin and cubulin: synergistic endocytic receptors in the proximal tubule. Am J Physiol 2001, 280(suppl F):562–573.
14. Davidson MB, Smiley JF: Relationship between dipstick positive proteinuria and albumin:creatinine ratios. J Diabet Complications 1999, 13:52–55.
15. Gerber LM, Johnston K, Alderman MH: Assessment of a new dipstick test in screening for microalbuminuria in patients with hypertension. Am J Hypertens 1998, 11:1321–1327.
16. Approach to Diabetic Nephropathy: A Position Paper of the American Diabetes Association on Clinical Practice Recommendations for 2003. Diabetes Care. 2003, 26(suppl 1):94–98.
17. Bennett PH, Haffner S, Kasiske BL, et al: Screening and management of microalburninuria in patients with diabetes mellitus: recommendations to the scientific advisory board of the National Kidney Foundation from an ad hoc committee of the council on diabetes of the National Kidney Foundation. Am J Kidney Dis 1995, 25:107–112.
18. Connell SJ, Hollis S, Ties Zen KL, et al: Gender and clinical usefulness of the albumin-creatinine ratio. Diabetic Med 1994, 11:32–36.
19. Mattix HJ, Hsu CY, Shaykevich S, Curhan G: Use of albumin/creatinine ratio to de-

tect microalbuminuria: implications of sex and race. J Am Soc Nephrol 2002, 13:1034–1039.

20. Neal L, Greene EL: Pathophysiology of chronic progressive renal disease in the African American patient with hypertension. Am J Med Sci 2002, 323:72–77.

21. Williams IL, Wheatcroft SB, Kearney MT: Obesity, atherosclerosis, and the vascular endothelium: mechanisms of reduced nitric oxide bioavailability in obese humans. Internat J Obesity 2002, 26:754–764.

22. Suthanthiran M, Li B, Song JO, et al: Transforming growth factor-beta 1 hyperexpression in African-American hypertensives: a novel mediator of hypertension and/or target organ damage. Proc Natl Acad Sci USA 2000, 97:3479–3484.

23. Russo LM, Osicka TM, Bonnet F, et al: Albuminuria in hypertension is linked to altered lysosomal activity and TGF-beta1 expression. Hypertension 2002, 39:281–286.

24. Agodoa LY, et al: Effect of ramipril vs amlodipine on renal outcomes in hypertensive nephrosclerosis: a randomized controlled trial. JAMA 2001, 285:2719–2728.

25. Pedrinelli R, Dell'Omo G, Di Bello V, et al: Microalbuminuria, an integrated marker of cardiovascular risk in essential hypertension. J Hum Hypertens 2002, 16:79–89.

26. Bianchi S, Bigazzi R, Baldari G, et al: Diurnal variations of blood pressure and microalbuminuria in essential hypertension. Am J Hypertens 1994, 7:23–29.

27. Sahadevan M, Kasiske BL: Hyperlipidemia in kidney disease: causes and consequences. Curr Opin Nephrol Hypertens 2002, 11:323–329.

28. Shearer GC, Stevenson FT, Atkinson DN, et al: Hypoalbuminemia and proteinuria contribute separately to reduced lipoprotein catabolism in the nephrotic syndrome. Kidney Int 2001, 59:179–189.

29. Egan, BM, Greene EL, Goodfriend TL: Insulin resistance and cardiovascular disease. Am J Hypertens 2001, 14:(suppl)116–125.

30. Kambham N, Markowitz GS, Valeri AM, et al: Obesity-related glomerulopathy: an emerging epidemic. Kidney Int 2001, 59:1498–1509.

31. Metcalf P, Baker J, Scragg R, et al: Microalbuminuria in a middle-aged workforce. Diabetes Care 1993, 16:1485–1493.

32. Briganti EM, Branley P, Chadban SJ, et al: Smoking is associated with renal impairment and proteinuria in the normal population: the AusDiab kidney study. Am J Kidney Dis 2002, 40:704–712.

33. Sowers, JR, Epstein M, Frohlich ED. Diabetes, hypertension, and cardiovascular disease: an update. Hypertension 2001, 37:1053–1059.

34. Klahr S: Primary and secondary results of the modification of diet in renal disease study. Miner Electrolyte Metab 1996, 22:138–142.

35. Yusuf S, Sleight P, Pogue J, et al: Effects of an angiotensin-converting-enzyme inhibitor, ramipril, on cardiovascular events in high-risk patients: the Heart Outcomes Prevention Evaluation Study Investigators. N Engl J Med 2000, 342:145–153.

36. The Heart Outcomes Prevention Evaluation Study Investigators: Effects of ramipril on cardiovascular and microvascular outcomes in peoples with diabetes mellitus: results of the HOPE study and MICRO-HOPE substudy. Lancet 2000, 355:253–259.

37. Ruilope LM, Salvetti A, Jamerson K, et al: Renal function and intensive lowering of blood pressure in hypertensive participants of the hypertension optimal treatment (HOT) study. J Am Soc Nephrol 2001, 12:218–225.

38. Keane WF, Eknoyan G: Proteinuria, Albuminuria, Risk, Assessment, Detection, Elimination (PARADE): A Position Paper of The National Kidney Foundation. Am J Kid Dis 1999, 33:1004–1010.

SECTION II
Target Organ Evaluation in the
Hypertensive Patient

chapter
4

Evaluation of Cardiac Structure and Function

Alan Hinderliter, M.D.

The primary goal in the treatment of patients with hypertension is to reduce cardiovascular morbidity and mortality. The approach to therapy in an individual patient should be guided by the absolute risk of death or disability from a cardiovascular event, which is determined largely by the presence of target organ damage from high blood pressure (BP). Thus, an important element of the evaluation of hypertensive patients is an assessment of clinical or preclinical hypertensive heart disease.

Left ventricular hypertrophy (LVH) is the principal cardiac manifestation of hypertension. Increased left ventricular (LV) mass can be identified in nearly 30% of unselected hypertensive adults and in the majority of those with long-standing, severe hypertension. As illustrated in Figure 1, the most important clinical consequence of LVH is congestive heart failure (CHF). More than 90% of patients with heart failure have antecedent hypertension, and data from the Framingham Heart Study suggest that high BP accounts for almost half of the population burden of this disorder. Heart failure develops as a consequence of the myocyte hypertrophy and ventricular fibrosis that characterize hypertensive LVH and may be caused by either abnormal diastolic properties or impaired contractile function of the LV.

The electrocardiogram (ECG) and echocardiogram have been invaluable tools in elucidating the epidemiology, pathophysiology, and natural history of hypertensive heart disease, and they can be used clinically to detect LVH, assess LV diastolic function, and quantify LV systolic function. This chapter discusses the spectrum of hypertensive heart disease and reviews the value of ECGs and echocardiography in determining prognosis and guiding management.

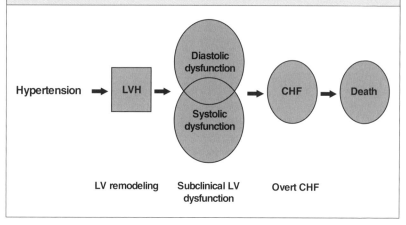

Figure 1. Progression of hypertension to LVH, LV systolic or diastolic dysfunction, congestive heart failure, and death. (Adapted from Vasan RS, Levy D: The role of hypertension in the pathogenesis of heart failure. A critical mechanistic overview. Arch Intern Med 156:1789–1796, 1996.)

Left Ventricular Hypertrophy

Hypertensive LVH develops primarily in response to increased ventricular afterload caused by elevated peripheral vascular resistance and arterial stiffness. Hemodynamic overload stimulates an increase in the synthesis of contractile elements and an increase in myocyte size. These cellular changes are accompanied by fibroblast proliferation and deposition of extracellular collagen, which contribute to ventricular stiffness and myocardial ischemia. Evidence suggests that this interstitial fibrosis is stimulated by angiotensin II and aldosterone, independent of pressure overload.

LVH is more prevalent in men than women and more common in African Americans than in whites with similar levels of BP. Increasing age, obesity, high dietary sodium intake, and diabetes are also associated with cardiac hypertrophy.

Evaluation

Features of LVH on the ECG include increased magnitude and duration of the QRS complex; leftward shift of the QRS axis; repolarization changes; and P-wave morphologies suggesting left atrial enlargement. Published criteria for LVH rely on some combinations of these features (Table 1). ECGs are inexpensive, widely available, and reproducible. However, although most studies have demonstrated a high degree of specificity for ECG LVH, the sensitivity of this technique is limited.

TABLE 1.	Electrocardiographic Criteria of LVH

Voltage Criteria

$S_{V1} + R_{V5}$ or $R_{V6} > 35$ mm
$R_I + S_{III} > 25$ mm
RaVL > 11 mm

Romhilt Estes Point Score

5 points = left ventricular hypertrophy
4 points = probable left ventricular hypertrophy

1. Amplitude   3 points
    Any of the following:
    (a) Largest R or S wave in the limb leads ≥ 20 mm
    (b) S_{V1} or S_{V2} wave in V_1 or $V_2 \geq 30$ mm
    (c) R_{V5} or R_{V6} wave in V_5 or $V_6 \geq 30$ mm
2. ST-T segment "strain" pattern
    Without digitalis   3 points
    With digitalis   1 point
3. Left atrial enlargement   3 points
    (terminal negativity of $P_{V1} \geq 1$ mm in depth and
    ≥ 0.04 sec in duration)
4. Left axis deviation $-30°$ or more   2 points
5. QRS duration ≥ 0.09 sec   1 point
6. Intrinsicoid deflection in V5 and V6 ≥ 0.05 sec   1 point

Cornell Criteria

For men:
    RaVL + $S_{V3} > 35$ mm
    or
    RaVL + $S_{V3} > 22$ mm and
        a) $T_{V1} \geq 0$ mm (for age < 40 years)
        b) $T_{V1} \geq 2$ mm (for age ≥ 40 years)
For women:
    RaVL + $S_{V3} > 25$ mm
    or
    RaVL + $S_{V3} > 12$ mm and
        a) $T_{V1} \geq$ mm (for age < 40 years)
        b) $T_{V1} \geq 2$ mm (for age ≥ 40 years)

Echocardiographic manifestations of LVH include increased LV wall thickness and calculated LV mass. M-mode echocardiography has been anatomically validated for the measurement of LV mass and has been used extensively in studies of hypertensive heart disease. Reliable measurements can also be obtained using two-dimensional echocardiography. Several factors, however, limit the usefulness of routine echocardiographic measurements of LV mass in designing therapy or assessing the effects of treatment in individual patients. First, no uniform method for correcting LV mass for body size is available. Many studies have indexed LV mass to height or body surface area; more recently, height^2, height$^{2.7}$, and lean body mass have been advanced as superior indices. Second, even with careful attention to technical detail, significant variability exists in individual measurements of LV mass.

Prevalence and Prognosis

Whether determined by ECG or echocardiography, LVH is a powerful predictor of cardiovascular morbidity and mortality, both in the general population and in patients with hypertension. In the Framingham Heart Study, for example, ECG evidence of LVH was present in 6% of adults and, after adjusting for potential confounders, was associated with a two-fold greater risk of cardiovascular morbidity or mortality.[1] In a subsequent study from Framingham, echocardiographic criteria for LVH were fulfilled in 16% of men and 21% of women, and the adjusted relative risks for all-cause mortality were 1.5 to 2.0.[2] The prognostic implications of LVH are even more striking in patients with hypertension. Studies in large cohorts of hypertensive patients have demonstrated ECG evidence of LVH in 9% to 44% of participants and have found a two- to fourfold greater risk of cardiovascular morbidity and all-cause mortality associated with LVH. Studies using echocardiographic measures of LV mass have demonstrated a similarly increased risk of cardiovascular events in hypertensive patients with LVH.[3]

Although LVH (i.e., an increase in left ventricular mass) is recognized as an important risk factor for cardiovascular morbidity and mortality, the pattern of hypertrophy may also be of prognostic significance. As illustrated in Figure 2, four geometric patterns of hypertensive heart disease can be defined based on the indexed LV mass and the ratio of wall thickness to LV internal dimension (i.e., relative wall thickness). Concentric hypertrophy is characterized by an increase in LV mass caused by increased relative wall thickness. Eccentric hypertrophy is defined as an increased LV mass caused partly by chamber dilatation, with a normal relative wall thickness. Increased relative wall thickness with a normal LV mass is termed concentric remodeling. Some studies suggest that cardiovascular events occur most frequently in those with concentric hypertrophy, and patients with eccentric hypertrophy or concentric remodeling have an intermediate risk of cardiovascular morbidity. Thus, incremental prognostic information may be gained by assessing LV geometry as well as mass.[4,5]

Diastolic Dysfunction

Alterations in LV filling are an early manifestation of hypertensive heart disease. Asymptomatic diastolic dysfunction is commonplace in

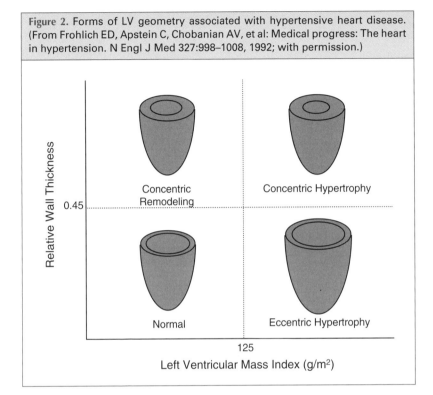

Figure 2. Forms of LV geometry associated with hypertensive heart disease. (From Frohlich ED, Apstein C, Chobanian AV, et al: Medical progress: The heart in hypertension. N Engl J Med 327:998–1008, 1992; with permission.)

individuals with mildly elevated BP and may even precede the development of LVH. The term "diastolic dysfunction" describes an abnormal mechanical property of the heart, which may or may not be associated with symptoms. Some patients with hypertension develop diastolic heart failure, a syndrome characterized by pulmonary congestion and decreased tissue perfusion associated with an isolated or predominant abnormality in diastolic function. Studies suggest that one third to one half of patients treated for CHF have diastolic dysfunction and a normal or nearly normal ejection fraction (EF).

LV filling may be impaired because of abnormalities in active myocardial relaxation or in passive ventricular stiffness. Relaxation is an active, energy-requiring process that occurs at the onset of diastole and reflects the time course and extent of cross-bridge dissociation after systolic contraction. It is governed in part by the activity of the sarcoplasmic reticulum calcium ATP-ase enzyme (SERCA), which removes calcium from the cytosol. SERCA is downregulated in pressure-overload hypertrophy, leading to impaired relaxation. LV compliance is a passive property that influences LV filling later in diastole. Increased LV wall thickness and interstitial collagen deposition are key determinants of compliance and contribute to myocardial stiffness in hypertension.

Evaluation

Doppler echocardiography is the most widely used noninvasive means of assessing LV diastolic function. Pulsed-wave Doppler measures of diastolic transmitral flow and of pulmonary vein flow characterize left atrial and LV filling. The Doppler flow profiles associated with progressive abnormalities are shown in Figure 3.

Normal diastolic function is characterized by ventricular filling predominantly in early diastole, resulting in a higher peak E wave (early filling) than A wave (late filling) in the transmitral flow profile. With impaired relaxation, relatively more ventricular filling is contributed by atrial contraction, resulting in a lower E to A ratio, and the deceleration time of the E wave is prolonged. When decreased LV compliance results in elevated diastolic LV pressure and left atrial pressure, the E wave again becomes dominant, with rapid deceleration in a "pseudonormal" pattern. Finally, in a "restrictive" pattern, almost all filling occurs early in diastole with a very short deceleration time.

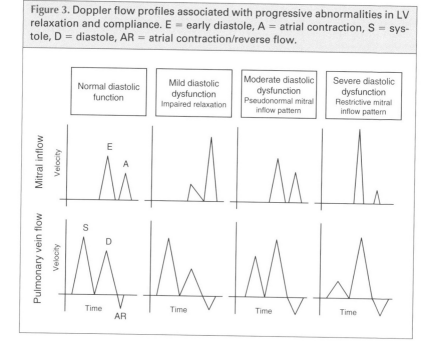

Figure 3. Doppler flow profiles associated with progressive abnormalities in LV relaxation and compliance. E = early diastole, A = atrial contraction, S = systole, D = diastole, AR = atrial contraction/reverse flow.

Pulmonary vein flow consists of two waves, one occurring in systole (S) and one occurring in diastole (D). Increased left atrial pressure impairs atrial filling during ventricular systole, and the pulmonary vein flow occurs predominantly in diastole. Thus, diastolic-dominant pulmonary vein flow helps distinguish pseudonormal or restrictive filling patterns from normal transmitral flow profiles.

Although valuable indices of LV diastolic function, Doppler variables can be influenced by many factors other than LV relaxation and compliance. Age, heart rate, loading conditions, LV systolic function, atrial function, and mitral regurgitation all affect transmitral and pulmonary vein flow velocities. Doppler parameters cannot fully characterize the complex phenomenon of LV diastolic function, and measures of transmitral and pulmonary vein flow should be evaluated in the context of the clinical setting and in conjunction with an assessment of LV structure and systolic function.

Several new Doppler techniques may enhance our ability to noninvasively evaluate LV diastolic function. Color M-mode Doppler echocardiography permits quantification of early diastolic flow propagation into the LV, a measure that is diminished in the presence of impaired relaxation or compliance. Doppler tissue imaging characterizes motion of the mitral annulus. In patients with abnormal LV filling properties, the relationships between early and late diastolic velocities are altered. Both of these methods are relatively independent of preload and, when used in combination with transmitral flow patterns, may prove useful in defining the stage of diastolic dysfunction.

Prevalence and Prognosis

Several studies in the general population and in hypertensive patients suggest that abnormalities in Doppler indices of LV filling identify patients at increased cardiovascular risk. In the Strong Heart Study, a population-based cohort survey in 13 American Indian communities, pulsed-wave Doppler interrogation of mitral inflow was used to categorize subjects with normal diastolic function, impaired relaxation (E/A < 0.6), or a restrictive filling pattern (E/A > 1.5). Mitral E/A > 1.5 was observed in 3% of subjects and was associated with a twofold increased all-cause mortality and threefold increased cardiac mortality. E/A < 0.6 was noted in 16% of subjects and predicted a twofold increase in all-cause and cardiac mortality, although this association was not significant after adjusting for covariates.[6] Redfield et al.[7] studied more than 2000 randomly selected residents of Olmsted County, Minnesota, by pulsed-wave Doppler of mitral inflow and pulmonary vein flow and by Doppler tissue imaging of the mitral annulus. The prevalence of CHF was 2%, and of these 44% had an EF > 50%. Overall, 28% of the population had Doppler evidence of diastolic dysfunction; this was moderate or severe in about 7%. After controlling for age, gender, and EF, the risk of all-cause mortality was eight times greater in subjects with mild diastolic dysfunction and 10 times greater in those with moderate or severe abnormalities in LV filling.[7] The risk conferred by impaired LV relaxation in patients with hypertension was investigated in the PIUMA study. After controlling for age, heart rate, BP, LV mass, and other confounders, subjects with E/A less than the median had a relative risk for cardiovascular events of nearly 1.6.[8]

Systolic Dysfunction

If excessive levels of BP persist for a prolonged period, myocyte loss and fibrosis contribute to ventricular remodeling and contractile dysfunction. Compensatory mechanisms, including remodeling of the peripheral vasculature and activation of the sympathetic nervous system and renin-angiotensin system, accelerate the deterioration in myocardial contractility. The ultimate result is a decompensated cardiomyopathy and heart failure caused by systolic dysfunction.

Diagnosis

Left ventricular systolic performance can be evaluated using a host of M-mode, two-dimensional, and Doppler echocardiographic measures. Global LV function is most often quantified as EF, or the percent of LV diastolic volume that is ejected in systole. Although EF is an imperfect measure of ventricular contractility because of its dependence on loading conditions, it remains popular among clinicians because of its familiarity, conceptual simplicity, and relative ease of measurement.

Measurement of EF requires quantification of LV volumes in end diastole and end systole. Ventricular volumes can be estimated from M-mode dimensions by approximating the LV as a prolate ellipse. This method assumes that the M-mode dimension accurately represents a minor dimension of the LV, that the two short axes of the LV are equal, and that the LV contracts uniformly. Because these assumptions are often erroneous, measurement of EF by M-mode echocardiography is inaccurate in many patients. Two-dimensional echocardiography permits more accurate quantification of volumes in ventricles that are irregularly shaped or exhibit regional abnormalities in contractile function. Several well-validated methods use measurements of long- or short axis dimensions or the short axis area, and values are calculated assuming a geometric model. A more attractive technique is based on **Simpson's rule.** With this method, the LV is divided into slices of known thickness, and the volume of the chamber is calculated as the sum of the volumes of the slices (Fig. 4). A modification of Simpson's rule uses the apical two-chamber and four-chamber views of the LV. The endocardial borders of the two views are digitally traced, and a computer uses Simpson's rule to calculate volumes.[9]

Two-dimensional measurements of EF are reproducible and correlate closely with measurements using other established methods. The principal limitation of this method is the need to identify the endocardial border. Even in experienced laboratories, suboptimal endocardial definition may preclude quantification of EF in over > 20% of subjects.

Prevalence and Prognosis

The prevalence and prognosis of impaired LV systolic function in the general population are not well established. Several recent surveys using echocardiography (ECG) suggest that 3% to 6% of adults in industrialized societies have a depressed LV ejection fraction (LVEF). In the Echocardiographic Heart of England Screening study, performed in a representative population > 45 years of age, LV systolic dysfunction (i.e., EF < 40%) was diagnosed in 1.8% of participants. Borderline LV dysfunction (i.e., EF 40% to 50%) was observed in an additional 3.5%. Nearly 50% of those with LV dysfunction had a history of hypertension,

Figure 4. Determination of LV volume by Simpson's rule. (From Rogers EW, Feigenbaum H, Weyman AE: Echocardiography for quantitation of cardiac chambers. In Yu PN, Goodwin JF (eds): Progress in Cardiology, vol. 8. Philadelphia, Lea and Febiger, 1979; with permission.)

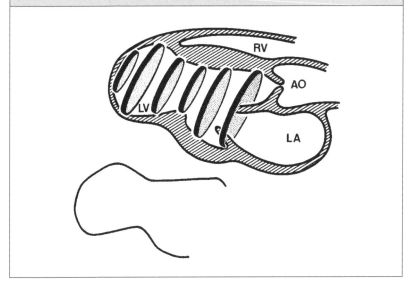

and nearly 50% had no symptoms.[10] Similarly, the prevalence of systolic dysfunction (i.e., EF < 50%) was 6% in the Olmsted County study, with moderate or severe dysfunction in 2%. Only 45% of those with moderate or severe systolic dysfunction and 20% of those with mild dysfunction had symptoms of heart failure.[7]

Depressed LV systolic function is associated with a poor prognosis whether or not symptoms are present. In the Studies of Left Ventricular Dysfunction (SOLVD) trials, asymptomatic participants with EF < 35% (mean = 28%) and an average age of 59 years had an annual mortality rate of nearly 5%.[11] Annual all-cause mortality was approximately 10% in patients with New York Heart Association (NYHA) class II or III symptoms.[12] In the Olmsted County study, each 5% decrement in LVEF was associated with a 20% greater risk of all-cause mortality.[7]

Data from the Framingham Heart Study underscore the prognostic significance of heart failure in patients with hypertension. High BP preceded the development of symptoms in > 90% of patients. In individuals between the ages of 65 and 74 years with the onset of heart failure between 1990 and 1999, 1-year mortality was 28% in men and 24% in women.[13] The diagnostic criteria for heart failure in the Framingham study were based on history, physical examination, and chest radiograph and did not include a measurement of LV systolic function. Whether patients with heart failure caused by systolic dysfunction have a worse prognosis than those with heart failure and a normal EF is unclear. Studies in younger cohorts suggest a higher mortality in patients with reduced EF, but more recent data in elderly patients suggest a grim prognosis in individuals with heart failure regardless of systolic function.

Evaluation of Individual Hypertensive Patients

Expert panels recommend an ECG as a part of the routine evaluation of patients with high BP. In large part due because of its expense, however, the use of echocardiography in this setting is controversial. Echocardiography is significantly more sensitive than ECGs in detecting LVH. However, studies from experienced centers suggest a test–retest variability of 35 to 65 g in measurement of LV mass, and this inherent variability limits the utility of echocardiography in the evaluation of individual patients.

Potential uses of echocardiographic measurements of LV mass include monitoring the effects of treatment and assessing the need for therapy in patients with borderline or stage 1 hypertension and no other cardiovascular risk factors. Because the variability in LV mass measurements exceeds the expected decrease in mass with treatment, there is little role for echocardiography in assessment of LVH regression in individual patients. Phillips and et al.[14] have proposed an algorithm for initiation of therapy in patients with borderline or stage 1 hypertension based on a derived probability of LVH for any measured value of LV mass. Intensive treatment is recommended if LV mass index > 110 g/m^2, a value that suggests a $> 20\%$ probability of LVH.[14] This approach may be appropriate for selected patients at centers with experience and expertise in quantification of LV mass, but its widespread application would come at considerable expense. Whether risk stratification with echocardiography leads to improved patient outcomes has not yet been tested.

In patients with hypertension and the syndrome of heart failure, echocardiography is indicated to assess LV mass and geometry, LV filling characteristics, and LV systolic function. The presence of any abnormality in LV structure or function attributable to high BP suggests the need for intensive antihypertensive therapy. The choice of BP lowering drugs will be influenced by the LV EF. The optimal treatment of heart failure with normal LV systolic function is not well established. Patients with a depressed EF benefit from therapy with angiotensin-converting enzyme inhibitors, beta-blockers, aldosterone antagonists, and diuretics.

Summary

An essential component of the evaluation of hypertensive patients is an assessment of clinical or preclinical hypertensive heart disease. Although less sensitive for detecting LVH than sophisticated imaging techniques, the ECG is an inexpensive tool that can identify patients at high risk of cardiovascular events and should be a part of the initial evaluation of all patients with high BP. Echocardiography provides an assessment of LV mass and geometry, LV filling characteristics, and LV systolic function. Because of expense and the inherent variability in LV mass measurements, the routine use of echocardiography in asymptomatic hypertensive patients is controversial. In hypertensive patients with symptoms of heart failure, however, assessment of diastolic and systolic function is instrumental in designing the optimal treatment regimen. Future advances in diagnostic techniques will undoubtedly enhance our ability to characterize LV structure and function and assess the risk of cardiovascular events in individual patients.

References

1. Kannel WB, Abbott RD: A prognostic comparison of asymptomatic left ventricular hypertrophy and unrecognized myocardial infarction: The Framingham Study. Am Heart J 111:391–397, 1986.

2. Levy D, Garrison RJ, Savage DD, et al: Prognostic implications of echocardiographically determined left ventricular mass in the Framingham Heart Study. N Engl J Med 322:1561–1566, 1990.
3. Vakili BA, Okin PM, Devereux RB: Prognostic implications of left ventricular hypertrophy. Am Heart J 141:334–341, 2001.
4. Koren MJ, Devereux RB, Casale PN, et al: Relation of left ventricular mass and geometry to morbidity and mortality in uncomplicated essential hypertension. Ann Intern Med 114:345–352, 1991.
5. Verdecchia P, Schillaci G, Borgioni C, et al: Prognostic value of left ventricular mass and geometry in systemic hypertension with left ventricular hypertrophy. Am J Cardiol 78:197–202, 1996.
6. Bella JN, Palmieri V, Roman MJ, et al: Mitral ratio of peak early to late diastolic filling velocity as a predictor of mortality in middle-aged and elderly adults. The Strong Heart Study. Circulation 105:1928–1933, 2002.
7. Redfield MM, Jacobsen SJ, Burnett JC, et al: Burden of systolic and diastolic ventricular dysfunction in the community. JAMA 289:194–202, 2003.
8. Schillaci G, Pasqualini L, Verdecchia P, et al: Prognostic significance of left ventricular diastolic dysfunction in essential hypertension. J Am Coll Cardiol 39:2005–2011, 2002.
9. Schiller NB, Shah PM, Crawford M, et al: Recommendations for quantitation of the left ventricle by two-dimensional echocardiography. J Am Soc Echocardiogr 2:358–367, 1989.
10. Davies MK, Hobbs FDR, Davis RC, et al: Prevalence of left-ventricular systolic dysfunction and heart failure in the Echocardiographic Heart of England Screening study: A population based study. Lancet 358:439–444, 2001.
11. The SOLVD investigators: Effect of enalapril on mortality and the development of heart failure in asymptomatic patients with reduced left ventricular ejection fractions. N Engl J Med 327:685–691, 1992.
12. The SOLVD investigators: Effect of enalapril on survival in patients with reduced left ventricular ejection fractions and congestive heart failure. N Engl J Med 325:293–302, 1991.
13. Levy D, Kenchaiah S, Larson MG, et al: Long-term trends in the incidence of and survival with heart failure. N Engl J Med 347:1397–1402, 2002.
14. Phillips RA, Diamond JA: Left ventricular hypertrophy, congestive heart failure, and coronary flow reserve abnormalities in hypertension. In Oparil S, Weber MA (eds): Hypertension: a Companion to Brenner and Rector's The Kidney. Philadelphia, W.B. Saunders, 2000, pp 244–276.

Assessment of Renal Function in Hypertension

chapter

5

Meryl Waldman, M.D., and
Raymond R. Townsend, M.D.

Impaired renal function occurs more commonly in hypertensive patients than in normotensive individuals. Chronic kidney disease (CKD) can both contribute to and result from elevated blood pressure (BP). Milder degrees of CKD are often subtle and overlooked until more severe disease ensues. Earlier detection of CKD can facilitate the implementation of appropriately aggressive therapy to prevent or at least slow progression to end-stage renal disease. This chapter provides important and practical advice on detecting CKD at early stages from data commonly obtained in the evaluation of hypertensive patients.

Renal Function in Hypertensive Patients

The development of CKD (i.e., loss of renal function) is more common in hypertensive than normotensive individuals.[1] When evaluating a hypertensive patient, whether early in the course of hypertension or after years of therapy, assessment of renal function is important for three reasons. First, hypertension may result from or contribute to CKD.[2] Second, some medications such as thiazide diuretics are less effective antihypertensives at usual doses when CKD is present, so a change in therapy can improve BP control.[3] Third, CKD is a risk factor for progressive loss of kidney function and is an independent risk factor for cardiovascular (CV) disease.[4] Of note, detection of early or mild CKD is crucial because it can lead to more appropriately aggressive treatment to arrest or slow progression to more severe CKD and reduce CV disease.[2] Serum creatinine level, the most commonly used measure for assessing renal function, is often incorrectly interpreted in patients with mild CKD.

Using a case-based format, this chapter reviews how to estimate kidney function from simple demographic, anthropometric, and laboratory

This work was supported by NIH Grant K24-DK-02684

tests and how to interpret electrolytes and basic urinary findings (other than microalbuminuria, which is covered in Chapter 3) that can impact therapeutic goals and selection of medications.

Case Study

A 58-year-old African-American woman has just moved to your community and is establishing health care. She is 5'3" and weighs 140 pounds. She has had hypertension for 15 years and takes a combination diuretic/angiotensin-converting enzyme (ACE) inhibitor tablet daily. Her seated BP averages 136/84 mm Hg, and her examination results are otherwise normal. She has a serum creatinine level of 1.3 mg/dL, potassium level of 3.5 mEq/L, serum bicarbonate level of 30 mEq/L, and uric acid level of 6.1 mg/dL. She has 1+ proteinuria. What do these findings tell you?

Renal Function

The main function of the kidneys is to clear waste products, which occurs primarily by glomerular filtration. Renal clearance of inulin or iothalamate remains the gold standard for measuring glomerular filtration rate (GFR), but these tests are expensive and cumbersome to perform. Serum creatinine level is a clinically useful surrogate for GFR, but several factors must be appreciated to correctly interpret the values.

Creatinine is produced in proportion to muscle mass and is cleared from the blood in proportion to kidney function. People with large muscle mass produce more creatinine than individuals with smaller muscle mass. As kidney function declines, higher serum creatinine levels occur to balance daily creatinine production and excretion. For example, a patient has a serum creatinine level of 1.0 mg/dL and a GFR of 100 mL/min. Her creatinine excretion is 1.0 mg/min or 1440 mg/d. If her GFR declines to 25 mL/min, then serum creatinine will increase to 4.0 mg/dL to maintain creatinine excretion.

Several formulae have been developed in an attempt to use simple laboratory, demographic, and anthropometric data to estimate kidney function. These estimates, although imperfect, are useful. Formulae for estimating GFR are outlined in Table 1 and are available online. Returning to the 58-year-old African American woman in your office, her estimated GFR is 47 mL/min using the Cockroft-Gault, 54 mL/min by the Modification of Diet in Renal Disease Study (MDRD), and 55 mL/min using the AASK equations. The MDRD and AASK formulae provide a more accurate kidney function estimate than the Cockroft when compared with a gold standard such as iothalamate clearance.[7,8] Her estimated kidney function, despite the unimpressive serum creatinine level of 1.3 mg/dL, shows her to be in the moderate CKD range (Table 2).[9]

To more precisely estimate GFR using either the MDRD or AASK equations, an adjustment for body size is required (see Table 2); otherwise,

TABLE 1.	Formulae for Estimating Kidney Function			
	Reference	Formula	Advantages	Limitations
GFR	Cockcroft and Gault[2]	$\dfrac{[140\text{-Age}] \times Kg[\times .85(F)]}{72 \times Cr}$	Simple; common	No ethnic correction
GFR: MDRD	Levey et al.[8]	$1.86 \times Cr^{-1.154} \times Age^{-0.203}$ $[\times 0.742\,(F)][\times 1.212(AA)]$	Validated in CKD	Not validated in normal individuals or diabetics
GFR: AASK	Lewis et al.[7]	$329 \times Cr^{-1.096} \times Age^{-0.294}$ $[\times 0.736(F)]$	Validated in CKD	Only valid in AA patients
BSA (Mostellar formula)		$(m^2) = ([Ht\,(cm) \times Wt\,(kg)]/3600)^{\frac{1}{2}}$		

Age = age in years; Kg = weight in kilograms; Cr = serum creatinine. Multiplicands within brackets are only used if the condition applies to that patient (e.g., see "(F)"—multiply by this term only if female; see "(AA)"—multiply by this term only if African-American). Validated in CKD = formula derived from iothalamate GFR measurements. AA = African-American, F = female.

these formulae assume a body surface area (BSA) of 1.73 m^2. BSA calculators are both published[10] and available online.[5,6] Based on her height and weight (see footnote to Table 1), her BSA is 1.68 m^2. After calculating her GFR and determining her BSA, we multiply her GFR value by her BSA (1.68 m^2) and divide by the standard 1.73 m^2, which yields a GFR of 52 mL/min/1.73 m^2 by MDRD and 53 mL/min/1.73m^2 by AASK. These values remain in the moderate CKD range (see Table 2).

Armed with this information, we would now place greater emphasis on BP control in preserving this patient's renal function and would monitor her serum creatinine and urinary findings more closely. We typically maximize ACE inhibitor dosage in hypertensive patients to lower systolic BP to less than 130 mm Hg and reduce proteinuria.[2]

Electrolyte Findings

A targeted review of key electrolyte and urinary findings is outlined in Table 3. This patient's potassium level is at the lower end of normal. Although the ACE inhibitor should lessen the potassium loss from the di-

TABLE 2.	Classification of Kidney Function[9]	
Stage	Description	GFR Range, mL/min/1.73 m^2
1	Normal	≥ 90
2	Mild CKD	60–89
3	Moderate CKD	30–59
4	Severe CKD	15–29
5	Kidney failure	< 15 or dialysis

TABLE 3. Common Renal Laboratory Findings in Hypertensive Patients

Test	Range*	Interpretation and Considerations
Creatinine	—	Indicates level of kidney function (see Table 2 for classification); strongly recommend converting serum level into a GFR value to estimate kidney function (see Tables 1 and 2)
Potassium	Low	May indicate aldosterone excess, diuretic therapy, intercurrent illness such as gastrointestinal (GI) virus; occasionally signals hereditary disorder such as Bartter's, Gitelman's, or Liddle's syndrome
	High	Usually associated with some degree of kidney function impairment; can be from drug therapy such as ACE inhibitors, angiotensin receptor blockers, beta blockers, potassium-sparing diuretics, NSAIDs, and potassium supplements
Bicarbonate	Low	Indicates the presence of metabolic acidosis, which may be secondary to respiratory disease (hyperventilation); the presence of kidney tubule disorders such as renal tubular acidosis or lower GI losses (diarrhea); or may occur with the loss of buffering daily dietary acid intake from CKD.
	High	Indicates presence of metabolic alkalosis, which may be secondary to primary or secondary forms of aldosterone excess; whereas the former are primary adrenal disorders, the latter are usually from either diuretic therapy or (occasionally) severe renal artery stenosis or other high renin activity state
Uric acid	Low	Usually indicates a hereditary enzyme enzyme disorder of reduced xanthine oxidase activity
	High	Usually indicates enhanced proximal tubule reabsorption activity resulting from volume depletion, often from diuretic therapy (loop diuretics or thiazide diuretics) May also reflect increased renal vascular resistance: some cases, increased uric acid levels are the result of neoplastic disorders with high cell turnover
Urinalysis: blood	Positive	Occasionally false-positive values after muscle damage (myoglobinuria); when red blood cells are present in the sediment it indicates bleeding from either the glomeruli, tubules, ureters, bladder, or urethra; when proteinuria is present, if the patient does not have a urinary tract infection, red blood cells are usually a sign of parenchymal renal disease
Protein	$\geq +1$	Proteinuria may indicate presence of parenchymal renal vascular disease (nephrosclerosis); heavy proteinuria ($\geq 3+$) usually indicates a glomerular disease, most commonly diabetes but a variety of other glomerular disease may be present; a simple spot urine sample sent for protein-to-creatinine ratio is very helpful to gauge the amount of proteinuria; when this ratio is greater than 500 mg protein per gram creatinine, guidelines suggest treating BP to a goal value of $\leq$ 125/75 mm Hg

*Range = numeric values of "normal" vary from laboratory to laboratory; please consult your local laboratory for the range of normal for each test covered in this table.

uretic, a high sodium diet reduces this benefit and may also blunt the capacity of ACE inhibition to reduce proteinuria.

Two other considerations are warranted regarding this patient's potassium level. Some patients with modest aldosterone excess may present without overt hypokalemia but may have a tendency to low potassium when taking a diuretic. Also, the benefits of diuretic therapy in stroke prevention decline when hypokalemia is present.[11]

This patient's serum bicarbonate concentration of 30 mEq/L is at the upper end of normal and borders on mild metabolic alkalosis. This likely represents a modest contraction alkalosis from the thiazide diuretic. Diuretics often stimulate aldosterone production that augments renal tubular sodium reabsorption and hydrogen ion secretion, resulting in metabolic alkalosis. Plasma renin activity is useful in distinguishing between hypokalemia resulting from primary aldosterone excess or a secondary aldosterone excess attributable to diuretic therapy. Renin activity is normal to elevated with diuretics and suppressed in primary aldosterone excess. In fact, a simple measure of plasma renin activity indexed against a serum aldosterone concentration can clarify whether a primary or secondary aldosterone excess may be present.[12]

The patient's uric acid level is also slightly elevated. Her mild hyperuricemia may reflect one of three processes: (1) modest volume depletion from diuretic therapy can increase proximal renal tubular reabsorption of uric acid; (2) higher renal vascular resistance can also enhance renal tubular uric acid reabsorption, which underlies hypertension in some minority populations, including African Americans[13]; or (3) the elevated uric acid level could be the result of her CKD.

Urinalysis Findings

Three items are of interest in evaluating the urinalysis of a patient with hypertension. Glycosuria detected by dipstick usually indicates the presence of undiagnosed or inadequately treated diabetes mellitus. The detection of blood in the urine by dipstick (hematuria), particularly with the presence of red blood cells shown in the microscopic examination, may reflect inflammation of the glomeruli (glomerulonephritis). However, kidney stones, urinary tract infections, urothelial tumors, trauma, and use of some drugs may also cause hematuria. Proteinuria, as in this case, is usually a marker of underlying kidney disease. The 1+ can be translated to a daily urinary protein loss of roughly 300 to 500 mg/day. In the patient presented, this degree of proteinuria typically reflects nephrosclerosis.[14] Proteinuria is an important prognostic sign because it predicts further renal function loss,[15] and is an established harbinger of cardiovascular disease.[16] A better estimate of this patient's proteinuria would be obtained by sending a spot urine for a protein-to-creatinine ratio. This is particularly important in diabetics, because BP treatment goals in these patients incorporate recommendations to reduce urine protein excretion and slow the rate of progression in diabetic nephropathy.[17-19] In the absence of diabetes, the role of proteinuria in this range is less well defined as a treatment endpoint per se; readers are referred to a recent and excellent overview of nondiabetic proteinuria for further treatment considerations.[20]

Key Points

☞ Renal dysfunction is relatively common in hypertensive patients and can be assessed from routine laboratory, demographic, and anthropometric data.

☞ Early detection of renal dysfunction is useful in guiding treatment and establishing more stringent therapeutic goals to slow or arrest the loss of renal function as well as the excess cardiovascular morbidity and mortality.

☞ Drug therapy for hypertension can affect serum electrolytes and acid-base balance, and understanding this information can facilitate appropriate changes in treatment.

References

1. Klag MJ, Whelton PK, Randall BL, et al: Blood pressure and end-stage renal disease in men. Clin Nephrol 1996, 334:13–18.
2. The sixth report of the Joint National Committee on prevention, detection, evaluation, and treatment of high blood pressure. Arch Intern Med 1997, 157:2413–2446.
3. Brater DC: Use of diuretics in cirrhosis and nephrotic syndrome. Semin Nephrol 1999, 19:575–580.
4. Sarnak MJ, Levey AS. Cardiovascular disease and chronic renal disease: a new paradigm. Am J Kidney Dis 2000, 35(suppl 1):117–131.
5. http://www.halls.md/body-surface-area/bsa.htm
6. http://www.nephron.com/mdrd/default.html
7. Lewis J, Agadoa L, Cheek D, et al: Comparison of cross-sectional renal function measurements in African Americans with hypertensive nephrosclerosis and of primary formulas to estimate glomerular filtration rate. The African-American Study of Kidney Disease and Hypertension (AASK). Am J Kidney Dis 2001, 38(2): 744–753.
8. Levey ASGT, Kusek JW, Beck GJ: A simplified equation to predict glomerular filtration rate from serum creatinine [abstract]. J Am Soc Nephrol 2002, 11:155.
9. Anonymous: KDOQI Clinical practice guidelines for chronic kidney disease: evaluation, classification, and stratification. Am J Kidney Dis 2002, 39 (suppl 2):1–266.
10. Mosteller RD: Simplified calculation of body surface area [letter]. N Engl J Med 1987, 317:1098.
11. Franse LV, Pahor M, Di B, et al: Hypokalemia associated with diuretic use and car-

diovascular events in the Systolic Hypertension in the Elderly Program. Hypertension 2000, 35:1025–1030.

12. Gallay BJ, Ahmad S, Xu L, et al: Screening for primary aldosteronism without discontinuing hypertensive medications: plasma aldosterone-renin ratio. Am J Kidney Dis 2001, 37:699–705.

13. Messerli FH, Frohlich ED, Dreslinski GR, et al: Serum uric acid in essential hypertension: an indicator of renal vascular involvement. Ann Intern Med 1980, 93:817–821.

14. Murphy C: Hypertensive emergencies. [review] Emerg Med Clin North Am 1995, 13:973–1007.

15. Remuzzi G, Bertani T: Pathophysiology of progressive nephropathies. Clin Nephrol 1998, 339:1448–1456.

16. Kannel WB, Stampfer MJ, Castelli WP, Verter J: The prognostic significance of proteinuria: the Framingham study. Am Heart J 1984, 108:1347–1352.

17. Lewis EJ, Hunsicker LG, Bain RP, Rohde RD: The effect of angiotensin-converting-enzyme inhibition on diabetic nephropathy. Collaborative Study Group. Clin Nephrol 1993, 329:1456–1462.

18. Brenner BM, Cooper ME, De Zeeuw D, et al: Effects of losartan on renal and cardiovascular outcomes in patients with type 2 diabetes and nephropathy. N Engl J Med 2001, 345:861–869.

19. Lewis EJ, Hunsicker LG, Clarke WR, et al: Renoprotective effect of the angiotensin-receptor antagonist irbesartan in patients with nephropathy due to type 2 diabetes. N Engl J Med 2001, 345:851–860.

20. Jafar TH, Stark PC, Schmid CH, et al: Proteinuria as a modifiable risk factor for the progression of non-diabetic renal disease. Kidney Internat 2001, 60:1131–1140.

21. Cockcroft DW, Gault MH: Prediction of creatinine clearance from serum creatinine. Nephrolog 1976, 16:31–41.

Renal Artery Occlusive Disease in Hypertension

chapter

6

James C. Stanley, M.D.

Renovascular hypertension (RVH) secondary to renal artery occlusive disease is the most common form of surgically correctable hypertension.[21,22] A stenosis causing an 80% reduction in renal artery cross-sectional area, a so-called critical stenosis, induces a pressure and flow gradient sufficient to cause increased renin release from the kidney.[25] Renin is a proteolytic enzyme that acts on angiotensinogen to form angiotensin I, which, when acted upon by angiotensin-converting enzyme (ACE), forms angiotensin II. Angiotensin II causes elevations in systemic blood pressure (BP) by its direct vasoconstrictive effect on blood vessels and indirectly by increasing aldosterone production, with its resultant increase in sodium and water retention that expands the circulating vascular volume.[25] The most common occlusive diseases that affect the renal arteries are arteriosclerosis and arterial fibrodysplasia.

Pathology

Arteriosclerosis affecting the renal artery accounts for 95% of reported cases of RVH (Fig. 1). Nearly 30% of patients who exhibit arteriosclerosis of the coronary, cerebral, mesenteric, or extremity circulation have evidence of renal artery arteriosclerosis. This is particularly the case in black patients, who are more likely than others to exhibit severe extrarenal arteriosclerotic vascular disease.[17] *Arterial fibrodysplasia* is the second most common type of renal artery occlusive disease, accounting for about 5% of reported cases of RVH (Fig. 2).[23,26] These two lesions and their subtypes have distinctive features (Table 1).

Clinical Features

The frequency of RVH approaches 2% when diastolic BP is > 100 mmHg. With more severe diastolic BP elevations, ≤ 5% of patients have RVH. It is important to become suspicious of a renovascular cause of BP

57

Figure 1. Severe arteriosclerotic aortic spill-over disease affecting the renal artery orifice and abdominal aorta.

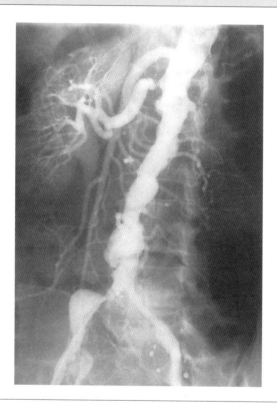

elevations when the patient's age, gender, and disease progression do not suggest the existence of essential hypertension. A decision algorithm based on the presenting severity of hypertension and presence or absence of clinical and laboratory evidence of RVH is of value in planning effective care of these patients (Fig. 3).

Major clinical findings that suggest a diagnosis of RVH include systolic and diastolic upper abdominal bruits; initial diastolic BP > 115 mmHg; a sudden worsening of mild to moderate essential hypertension; rapid onset of high BP after age 50 years; and development of hypertension during young adulthood, especially in women. Hypertension resistant to drug therapy is also more likely to be associated with this form of secondary hypertension. Deterioration in renal function while the patient is receiving multiple antihypertensive drugs, especially ACE inhibitors, may be the first evidence of renal artery stenotic disease. This usually occurs

Figure 2. Medial fibroplasia. Serial stenoses alternating with mural aneurysms, producing a string-of-beads appearance in the midportion and distal main renal artery.

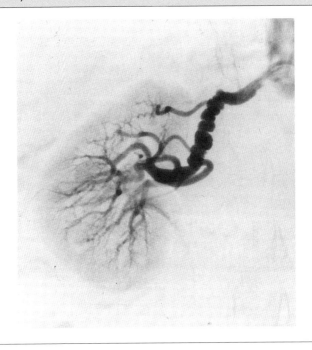

when the entire renal mass is at risk, as in the case of bilateral disease or unilateral disease in the solitary kidney. Lastly, recurrent heart failure with flash pulmonary edema and impaired renal function in a hypertensive patient suggests underlying renovascular occlusive disease.

Diagnosis

Most diagnostic and prognostic tests for RVH assess either the anatomic stenosis or derangements of renal function attributed to the stenosis. No tests are perfect, and the accuracy of any, at best, approaches 90%.

Conventional arteriography remains the standard by which other diagnostic imaging studies are compared. Clearly, collateral vessels circumventing a renal artery stenosis are evidence of the lesion's hemodynamic and functional importance. Intraarterial digital substraction arteriography allows use of smaller quantities of iodinated contrast agents and thus lessens the potential of contrast-induced nephrotoxicity.

Lesion Type	**Gender**	**Mean Age (years)**	**Anatomic Localization**	**Morphology**
Arteriosclerosis				
Renal	Male:female ratio of 2:1	55	Proximal renal artery, uncommon bilateral	Excentric or concentric focal stenoses with posterior extension into distal artery
Aortorenal			Ostial and adjacent aorta, 75% bilateral	
Arterial fibrodysplasia				
Intimal fibroplasias	No gender prediction	Children, young adults	Midrenal artery, uncommonly bilateral	Focal or tubular stenoses
Medial fibrodysplasia	Female	35	Mid and distal renal artery, 60% bilateral, segmental involvement in 25%	Serial stenoses with intervening mural aneurysms, string-of-beads appearance
Perimedial dysplasia	Female	45	Mid and distal renal artery, 25% bilateral, segmental involvement uncommon	Serial stenoses without mural aneurysms

TABLE 1. Classification of Renal Artery Occlusive Disease

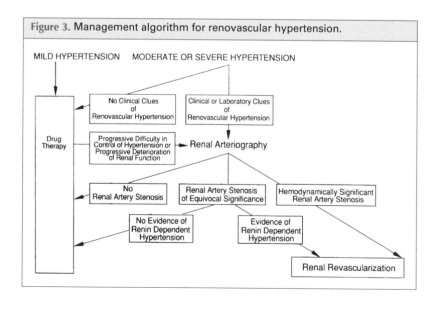

Figure 3. Management algorithm for renovascular hypertension.

Magnetic resonance angiography, especially with breathhold techniques and gadolinium enhancement, provides high-resolution images of diseased renal arteries in many patients with reported sensitivity and specificity for significant stenosis in the range of 90% to 95%.[11,19] Its noninvasiveness makes it an attractive test, but phase drop not attributed to stenotic disease is common, causing these studies to often overestimate the severity of renal artery narrowings.

Deep abdominal renal artery ultrasonography may identify approximately 90% of hemodynamically significant renal artery narrowings, defined by peak systolic velocities in the range of 180 to 200 cm/sec, or when the ratio of the renal artery velocity to that in the aorta approaches 3.5.[9,13] Unfortunately, ultrasonography does not discriminate among renal artery stenoses ranging from 60% to critical 80% narrowings. Another shortcoming of ultrasonography is that occluded accessory or segmental renal arteries may not be recognized, thus contributing to false-negative assessments.

Hypertensive urography is not a good diagnostic test for RVH because of its limited sensitivity in the range of 50% to 75%.[30,31] Bilateral or segmental disease often interferes with the recognition of gross differences in contrast excretion between the two kidneys. In a large series of patients with proven RVH, urograms showed normal findings in 52% of adults with arterial fibrodysplastic disease and 28% of adults with atherosclerotic lesions.[26] Nevertheless, when urographic abnormalities are present, they may suggest the presence of renal artery stenotic disease.

Isotopic renography allows both renal imaging and analysis of the washout curve of a number of radioactive tracers. The specificity and sensitivity of these studies are both about 75%. Administration of ACE inhibition improves both the sensitivity and specificity to approximately 90% to 95% by blunting the compensatory effects of angiotensin II and rapidly reducing glomerular filtration in the presence of reduce renal plasma flow in the affected kidney (or kidneys).[15] Despite its reported utility, false-negative isotopic study results in the presence of proven RVH have continued to limit widespread use of these tests.

Renin activity of peripheral and renal venous blood is a recognized means of detecting functionally important renal artery disease.[24] Peripheral blood renin assays have a reported sensitivity in the range of 50% to 80% for detecting RVH.[31] Indexing the renin assay to sodium balance or measuring plasma renin activity before and measuring its increase 1 hour after oral captopril appears to increase the sensitivity for detecting renal artery stenosis. Measurement of renal vein renin activity and relationship to systemic (vena cava) concentrations also enhances sensitivity and carries predictive information regarding the likelihood of a BP response to revascularization. However, renal vein renin sampling is undertaken only in unusual circumstances in contemporary practice.[21,22]

Management of Renal Arterial Disease

For Information on *medical therapy,* refer to Chapter 31 for additional details.

Percutaneous Transluminal Angioplasty

The minimally invasive nature of renal artery percutaneous transluminalangioplasty (PTA) offers certain advantages over operative intervention. To justify PTA, the physiologic and hemodynamic significance of the renal artery stenosis should be documented before initiating endovascular therapy. The patient should have adequate renal cortical reserves to recover renal function postintervention. PTA of a clinically insignificant renal artery stenosis as an added procedure accompanying catheterizations for nonrenal disease, a so-called "drive-by" angioplasty, has no legitimate place in contemporary practice.

Arterial Fibrodysplasia

Patients with renal artery fibrodysplasia benefit the most and incur the fewest complications after renal PTA.[3,20] Successful PTA in these patients carries a primary patency rate of 87% after more than 3 years of follow-up.[29] Patients with medial fibrodysplasia without segmental arterial involvement are the most likely to be successfully treated. Perimedial dysplasia and intimal fibroplasia are often resistant to dilatation. In general, PTA for fibrodysplastic RVH results in a cure in 50%, improvement in 40%, and failure in 10% of patients.

Arteriosclerosis

The presence of aortic spillover arteriosclerosis versus isolated renal artery arteriosclerosis has an important impact on PTA's long-term clinical results. PTA alone, without adjunctive stent placement results in an initial technical success rate of 70% to 80% in patients with arteriosclerotic disease limited to the renal artery. Ostial spillover lesions treated by PTA alone have even lower initial technical success rates of only 30% to 50%. Stenting is near mandatory with PTA in these patients, and it results in a reported 2-year secondary patency rate of 92% (see Chapter 31 for more additional information on renal artery stenting).[10] Others have documented 5-year primary and secondary patency rates of 84% and 92%, respectively.[2] PTA for arteriosclerotic RVH results in a cure in 20%, improvement in 60%, and failure in 20% of patients. These outcomes are not as salutary as after surgical therapy, but the mortality and morbidity rates after PTA are lower than after open operation. PTA with stenting for progressive ischemic nephropathy is not generally accepted to be effective at reversing renal failure in these patients. In part, this may reflect contrast nephrotoxicity or embolization associated with PTA, or it may simply represent poor selection of patients whose renal failure is not related to impaired blood flow.

Arterial Reconstructive Surgery

Operative treatment of patients with renovascular occlusive disease has become standardized.[1,4,7,16,22,27] *Aortorenal bypass* in adults with fibrodysplastic or arteriosclerotic occlusive disease is most often performed using reversed autologous saphenous vein. Dacron or Teflon grafts may also be used in reconstructing these vessels. *Endarterectomy* is often the preferred means of treating patients with proximal renal artery arteriosclerotic disease.[5,7,14,28] The two techniques most often used are (1) transaortic renal endarterectomy through an axial aortotomy or the transected infrarenal aorta and (2) direct renal artery endarterectomy.

Surgical treatment of patients with RVH affords excellent outcomes. Differences among most individual experiences reflect variations in the prevalence of the different renovascular disease categories. In general, renal revascularization for fibrodysplastic RVH results in a cure in 55%, improvement in 35%, and failure in 10% of patients. Operative mortality for fibrodysplastic patients is close to 0%. Surgical therapy for arteriosclerotic revascularization hypertension results in cure in 35%, improvement in 50%, and failure in 15% of patients. Operative mortality for arteriosclerotic patients is < 1% when unassociated with renal failure or concomitant aortic surgery but approaches 3% in the latter.

Renal preservation and maintenance of renal function are important in assessing surgical outcomes.[6,8,12,18] Nephrectomy does not offer the same benefit as revascularization. Improved renal function after revascularization is most likely to occur among select patients who exhibit arteriosclerotic disease with a relatively sudden onset of renal function impairment and no evidence of coexisting renal parenchymal disease.

References

1. Anderson CA, Hansen KJ, Benjamin ME, et al: Renal artery fibromuscular dysplasia: results of current surgical therapy. J Vasc Surg 22:207–216, 1995.
2. Blum U, Krumme B, Flugel P, et al: Treatment of ostial renal artery stenoses with vascular endoprostheses after unsuccessful balloon angioplasty. N Engl J Med 336:459–465, 1997.
3. Bonelli FS, Mckusick MA, Textor SC, et al: Renal artery angioplasty: Technical results and clinical outcome in 320 patients. Mayo Clin Proc 70:1041–1052, 1995.
4. Cambria RP, Brewster DC, L'Italien G, et al: Simultaneous aortic and renal artery re-

construction: evolution of an eighteen-year experience. J Vasc Surg 21:916–925, 1994.

5. Dougherty MJ, Hallett JW Jr, Naessens J, et al: Renal endarterectomy vs. bypass for combined aortic and renal reconstruction: Is there a difference in clinical outcome? Ann Vasc Surg 9:87–92, 1995.

6. Hallett JW Jr, Textor SC, Kos PB, et al: Advanced renovascular hypertension and renal insufficiency: Trends in medical comorbidity and surgical approach from 1970–1993. J Vasc Surg 21:750–760, 1995.

7. Hansen KJ, Starr SM, Sands RE, et al: Contemporary surgical management of renovascular disease. J Vasc Surg 16:319–331, 1992.

8. Hansen KJ, Thomason RB, Craven TE, et al: Surgical management of dialysis-dependent ischemic nephropathy. J Vasc Surg 21:197–211, 1995.

9. Hansen KM, Tribble RW, Reavis SW, et al: Renal duplex sonography: Evaluation of clinical utility. J Vasc Surg 12:227–230, 1990.

10. Henry M, Amor M, Henry I, et al: Stent placement in the renal artery: Three-year experience with the Palmaz stent. J Vasc Radiol 7:343–350, 1996.

11. Hertz, SM, Holland GA, Baum RA, et al: Evaluation of renal artery stenosis by magnetic resonance angiography. Am J Surg 168:140–143, 1994.

12. Jacobson HR: Ischemic renal disease: An overlooked clinical entity? Kidney Int 34: 729–743, 1988.

13. Kohler TR, Zierler RE, Martin RL, et al: Noninvasive diagnosis of renal artery stenosis by ultrasonic duplex scanning. J Vasc Surg 4:450–456, 1986.

14. McNeil JW, String ST, Pfeiffer RB Jr: Concomitant renal endarterectomy and aortic reconstruction. J Vasc Surg 20:331–337, 1994.

15. Meier GH, Sumpio B, Setaro FJ, et al: Captopril renal scintigraphy: A new standard for predicting outcome after renal revascularization. J Vasc Surg 17:280–287, 1993.

16. Murray SP, Kent KC, Salvatierra O, Stoney RJ: Complex branch renovascular disease: Management options and late results. J Vasc Surg 20:338–346, 1994.

17. Novick AC, Zaki S, Goldfarb D, Hodge EE: Epidemiologic and clinical comparison of renal artery stenosis in black patients and white patients. J Vasc Surg 20:1–5, 1994.

18. Oskin TC, Hansen KJ, Deitch JS, et al: Chronic renal artery occlusion: Nephrectomy versus revascularization. J Vasc Surg 29:140–149, 1999.

19. Prince MR, Narasimham DL, Stanley JC, et al: Breath-hold 3D gadolinium enhanced MR angiography of the abdominal aorta and its major branches. Radiology 197: 785–792, 1995.

20. Sos TA, Pickering TG, Sniderman K, et al: Percutaneous transluminal renal angioplasty in renovascular hypertension due to atheroma or fibromuscular dysplasia. N Engl J Med 309:274–279, 1983.

21. Stanley JC. The evolution of surgery for renovascular occlusive disease. Cardiovasc Surg 2:195–202, 1994.

22. Stanley JC: Surgical treatment of renovascular hypertension. Am J Surg 174:102–110, 1997.

23. Stanley JC, Gewertz BL, Bove EL, et al: Arterial fibrodysplasia:histopathologic character and current etiologic concepts. Arch Surg 110:561–566, 1975.

24. Stanley JC, Gewertz BL, Fry WJ: Renal: systemic renin indices and renal vein renin ratios as prognostic indicators in remedial renovascular hypertension. J Surg Res 20: 149–155, 1976.

25. Stanley JC, Graham LM: Renovascular hypertension. In Miller TA (ed). Modern Surgical Care: Physiologic Foundations & Clinical Applications (2nd Ed). St. Louis, Quality Medical Publications, 1998, pp 918–924.

26. Stanley JC, Wakefield TW: Arterial fibrodysplasia. In Rutherford RB (ed). Vascular Surgery (5th Ed), Philadelphia, WB Saunders, 2000, pp 387–408.

27. Stanley JC, Whitehouse WM Jr, Graham LM, et al: Operative therapy of renovascular hypertension. Br J Surg 63(suppl):S63–S66, 1982.
28. Stoney RJ, Messina LM, Goldstone J, Reilly LM: Renal endarterectomy through the transected aorta: a new technique for combined aortorenal arteriosclerosis—a preliminary report. J Vasc Surg 19:224–233, 1989.
29. Tegtmeyer CJ, Selby JB, Hartwell GD, et al: Results and complications of angioplasty in fibromuscular disease. Circulation 83(suppl 2):I 155–I 161, 1991.
30. Thornbury TR, Stanley JC, Fryback DG: Hypertensive urogram: A nondiscriminatory test for renovascular hypertension. Am J Radiol 138:43–49, 1982.
31. National High Blood Pressure Education Program: 1995 update on the working group reports on chronic renal failure and renovascular hypertension. Arch Intern Med 156:1938–1947, 1996.

Carotid and Peripheral Vascular Disease

chapter

7

*Robert D. Brook, M.D.,
Henna Kalsi, M.D., and
Alan B. Weder, M.D.*

Atherosclerosis is a systemic disorder. Patients with symptoms that arise from one arterial bed are at high risk for atherosclerosis at other sites. Patients with coronary disease are at increased risk for carotid or peripheral vascular disease. This chapter reviews the diagnosis and management of atherosclerotic disease of the carotid and lower extremity vasculature.

Peripheral arterial disease (PAD) risk factors are identical to those for coronary artery disease, with tobacco smoking and diabetes mellitus[1,2] being particularly potent triggers for PAD[1,3]. Aggressive treatment of modifiable risk factors is the cornerstone of medical therapy for all atherosclerotic diseases (Table 1).[1,47] The roles of emerging factors, such as serum C-reactive protein, are being investigated with the hope of improving risk stratification and management of PAD[4].

Carotid Artery Disease

The incidence of carotid atherosclerotic disease increases with age. Carotid stenoses > 50% in diameter occur in < 1% of patients younger than age 50 years . However, it occurs in as many as 6% of the population over age 50 years.[5–7]

Carotid Artery Symptoms

Neurologic symptoms that arise from carotid disease are the result of ischemia in distal vessels, most commonly thromboembolism. The risk of transient ischemic attack (TIAs) and stroke increases with progressive severity of carotid artery narrowing.[5–7] However, even mild unstable stenoses can causing cerebrovascular events after ulceration, thrombus formation, and distal embolization. At the opposite end of the clinical

67

TABLE 1.   Treatment of Atherosclerosis Risk Factors in Peripheral Arterial and Carotid Disease

Risk Factor	Goals	Therapy
Tobacco smoking	Complete cessation	Counseling or drugs
Lipoproteins	LDL cholesterol < 100 mg/dl	Statin (first-line therapy)
	Non–HDL cholesterol < 130 mg/dl	Niacin, fibric acid, bile acid resin, ezetimibe, plant stanol (as needed to achieve goals)
Antiplatelet therapy	Use in all patients	Aspirin or clopidogrel (possible benefit for combination therapy in very high-risk patients)
BP	< 140/90 mmHg	ACE inhibitor (possible first-line therapy)
		Other drugs added to achieve goals
Diabetes mellitus	HbA1C < 7.0%	Metformin (first-line therapy if BMI > 27)
		Other drugs or insulin as needed
Emerging risk factors	Homocysteine, Lp(a), CRP	Uncertain benefits of treatment

ACE = angiotensin-converting enzyme; BB = beta-blocker; CAD = coronary artery disease; CRP = C-reactive protein; HDL = high-density lipoprotein; LDL = low-density lipoprotein; Lp(a) = lipoprotein(a).

spectrum, it is also possible for carotid atherosclerosis to slowly progress to complete occlusion in the absence of any symptoms because of the presence of adequate collateral circulation from the contralateral carotid artery or vertebrobasilar system.

Transient cerebral symptoms commonly last only several minutes. By definition, a TIA persists for < 24 hours. TIAs are generally of rapid onset, do not produce headaches, and manifest as either focal neurologic symptoms and signs or alterations in consciousness. Repeated TIAs usually have stereotyped symptoms. A neurologic deficit of longer duration that does not completely resolve is a stroke.[8]

Although carotid artery atherosclerosis can affect any vascular site in the brain, certain symptoms are particularly characteristic. Emboli to the ophthalmic artery, the first branch of internal carotid artery (ICA), produce a transient monocular visual loss called *amaurosis fugax*.[8] Ischemic events in the distribution of the middle cerebral artery produce unilateral localized neurologic findings, including mono- or hemiparesis or paresthesia. Ischemia may also produce significant aphasia if the dominant hemisphere is affected. As a whole, seven general syndrome categories of cerebral ischemia exist: the middle, anterior, and posterior cerebral artery syndromes; the vertebrobasilar and cerebellar artery strokes; lacunar strokes; and the carotid artery syndrome. Each has its own clinical presentation and set of symptoms and signs.

Diagnosis

The clinical presentation of a cerebrovascular event may provide valuable information that can lead to the localization of the site of cerebral injury and point to the particular arterial distribution that may require further evaluation. Auscultation of the neck vasculature can help to support the suspicion of carotid pathology; however, the absence of a carotid bruit on physical examination does not rule out the possibility of significant stenosis. The low sensitivity and specificity of carotid auscultation limit its value.

Although most commonly caused by carotid atherosclerosis or cardiac emboli,[5,7] ischemic strokes and TIAs can result from other diseases. Screening laboratory examinations should be undertaken to exclude predisposing conditions for patients at low risk for atherosclerosis (e.g., young patients) and those without identified sources of emboli. Especially important is evaluation for the presence of an underlying hypercoagulable state (e.g., anticardiolipin antibody, protein S and protein C deficiency, antithrombin III deficiency, activated protein C resistance). Folate and vitamin B12 deficiencies can contribute to hyperhomocysteinemia, which increases the risk of arterial thrombosis. Finally, consideration should be given to even less common causes of ischemic stroke (e.g., cerebral vasculitis or paradoxical emboli) in patients in whom atheroscloerotic disease has been ruled out.

Because of hemodynamic considerations, atherosclerosis usually begins at and is most severe in the distal carotid bulb and the first 2 cm of the ICA. It frequently arises from the posterior wall and extends inferiorly through the bulb and into the distal common carotid artery.[5-7] This region can be evaluated by several noninvasive techniques, thereby reducing the need for cerebral angiography, which has a minor risk of stroke.[9,12] Carotid duplex imaging (B-mode ultrasound images combined with pulsed Doppler spectral waveform analysis) is the most commonly used method for the detection and quantification of carotid disease. *Duplex examination is presently the screening test of choice for the majority of patients.*[5-7,9] Linear array high-frequency B-mode ultrasound assesses the various densities of the vasculature and surrounding tissues and produces a grayscale anatomical image. Blood appears black (echolucent), and tissues appear white (echogenic). The appearance of plaques depends on their densities, which, in turn, depends on the composition of the plaque: whereas lipid-rich lesions and areas are darker (hypoechoic), more calcified plaques appear bright white.[10] Pulsed Doppler spectral analysis of the peak systolic, end diastolic, and ratio of peak systolic ICA to common carotid velocity provides hemo-dynamic information that complements B-mode ultrasound imaging.[11] Often, the combined information provided by duplex carotid examina-tion is all that is required in order to determine the appropriate medical or surgical management (Fig. 1). At the University of Michigan Medical Center, duplex carotid study results are most frequently used, if ade-quate, in the decision-making process before surgery. Carotid magnetic resonance angiography (MRA) may enhance the management deci-sions[9] but is not routinely done at the authors' institution.

Other noninvasive imaging methodologies include MRA and com-puted tomography (CT) angiography.[9] These techniques are usually only required when a screening duplex evaluation is inadequate because of patient or examination problems, a high carotid bifurcation, suspected atherosclerosis in the intracranial cerebral vasculature, or an inability to identify the distal extent of an ICA plaque before planned surgery.[9–11] The authors' experience suggests that present MRA technology tends to over-estimate the degree of stenoses. In rare circumstances, the gold standard cerebral angiogram is required to determine the best course of action.

Medical Management

The presence of carotid disease is associated with an increased risk of arterial plaques in other vascular beds. Therefore, the initial manage-ment of patients with either symptomatic or asymptomatic carotid ath-erosclerosis is aggressive treatment of all risk factors in order to prevent not only strokes but other cardiovascular complications as well. The American Heart Association and National Stroke Association have pre-viously published guidelines for the prevention of stroke; interested readers are referred to these comprehensive reviews[14,15]. The manage-ment algorithms take into consideration many factors for deciding on the appropriate therapies, including whether the patient is symptomatic or asymptomatic, the degree of carotid stenosis, and the individual's short-term risk of stroke.

Standard contemporary therapy for patients with documented carotid disease includes antiplatelet therapy, control of hypertension, and use of antihyperlipidemic medications. *Antithrombotic therapy* with as-pirin and other antiplatelet agents (e.g., clopidogrel) reduces the risk of stroke among those with a history of TIA or stroke.[7] The optimal dosage of aspirin and the potential usefulness of combination antiplatelet ther-apies remain to be firmly established.[7] *However, 325 mg of aspirin daily is adequate for most patients.* The benefits of antiplatelet med-

Figure 1. *A,* B-mode image of a normal common carotid artery by vascular ultrasonography. *B,* Pulsed Doppler waveform analyses of a normal internal carotid artery. Peak systolic velocity is 60.6 cm/s (< 110 cm/s is considered normal in the vascular laboratory at the University of Michigan Hospital).

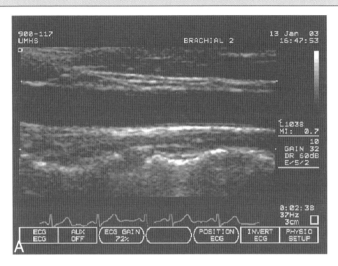

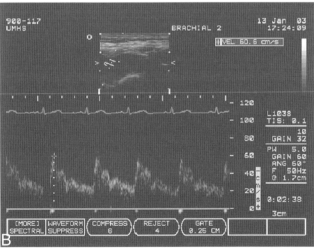

Peak ICA systolic velocity	ICA/Common carotid	ICA stenosis
< 100 cm/s	<1/8	normal to <40%
> 110 cm/s	<1.8	40–60%
> 130 cm/s	>1.8	60–80%
> 130 cm/s (diastolic >100 cm/s)	>1.8	60–80%

ications in the primary prevention of cerebrovascular disease and oral anticoagulants for primary or secondary prevention have not been demonstrated.[7,17,18]

Cholesterol-lowering therapy with an HMG CoA reductase inhibitor (statin) reduced the risk of stroke among high-risk patients in the large prospective Heart Protection Study.[19] Even patients with a previous stroke who initially had low-density lipoprotein (LDL) cholesterol at the recommended target of < 100 mg/dL before therapy had reduced stroke and cardiovascular disease outcomes. These results strongly argue in favor of initiating statin therapy in all patients with symptomatic carotid disease regardless of cholesterol level, unless contraindicated. It is possible that some of the cerebrovascular disease protection provided from statins is derived from vascular effects beyond cholesterol lowering.[20] Further uncertainty exists regarding the optimal LDL cholesterol goal to be targeted; however, achieving a level of at least < 100 mg/dL is currently the minimal requirement.

In addition to LDL cholesterol, further studies support raising high-density lipoprotein (HDL) cholesterol with medication to reduce the risk for stroke in those with established heart disease and an HDL cholesterol level < 40 mg/dL.[21] It is prudent at this point to try to raise HDL cholesterol pharmacologically, even in addition to LDL-lowering with statins, in patients with a low HDL cholesterol level and known cardiovascular disease.

In summary, the evidence to date supports the aggressive treatment of both LDL cholesterol (goal < 100 mg/dL) and HDL cholesterol (goal > 40 mg/dL) in patients with established heart disease and in those with a prior stroke to prevent cardiovascular and cerebrovascular events.[20]

Treatment of blood pressure (BP) reduces the risk of stroke in both primary and secondary prevention.[22–24] The goal should be to achieve a level of at least < 140/90 mmHg in all patients. Combinations of antihypertensive medications may be required to reach this level in many high-risk patients. The optimal BP goal still remains to be determined. However, certain patients require even further reduction, including diabetics, who should be treated to < 130/80 mmHg.

Recent results from the Perindopril Protection Against Recurrent Stroke Study (PROGRESS) demonstrated for the first time that aggressive BP reduction in patients with a previous cerebrovascular accident or TIA is both safe and beneficial.[23] The optimal antihypertensive agent to be prescribed in this population is still a matter of debate. Modern BP medications (e.g. angiotensin-converting enzyme [ACEs] inhibitors) are known to possess a variety of "BP-independent" pharmacologic effects upon the vasculature, as was demonstrated for carotid vessels in a substudy of the Heart Outcomes Prevention Study (HOPE).[25] In confirmation of this, the Losartan Intervention for Endpoints (LIFE) study demonstrated that the angiotensin receptor blocker (ARB) losartan was superior to atenolol in preventing strokes in hypertensive patients with left ventricular hypertrophy.[24] However, very recent results from ALLHAT (Antihypertensive and Lipid-Lowering Treatment to Prevent Heart Attack Trial) support, at least in the primary prevention of cerebrovascular disease, that a thiazide diuretic is at least as good as the newer BP medications.[22] *Therefore, the primary aim should be to aggressively treat hypertension in order to achieve the patient's BP target level, using the medication (or medications) required.* Whether the addition of an ACE inhibitor, an ARB, or both adds incremental cardiovascular or stroke risk reduction beyond BP lowering remains to be determined.

Revascularization Approaches

Symptomatic Carotid Stenosis

Carotid endarterectomy is beneficial in reducing cererbrovascular events for patients with symptomatic carotid stenosis $\geq$ 70%. Three large randomized trials comparing surgical and medical versus best medical management alone have been published. These trials are the North American Symptomatic Carotid Endarterectomy Trial (NASCET 1, 2, and 3), the European Carotid Surgery Trial (ECST), and the Veterans Affairs Cooperative Studies Program (VA).[26,27] For patients with high-grade symptomatic carotid stenoses, each trial showed significant relative and absolute stroke risk reductions for those randomized to surgery (Table 2).[28] No significant benefit, however, was demonstrated for patients with a symptomatic carotid stenosis < 50%. *Based on these studies and a recent meta-analyses,[29] a consensus exists that carotid endarterectomy is the best option for the prevention of recurrent events in*

TABLE 2. Randomized, Controlled Trials in Symptomatic Patients: CEA Plus Medical Therapy versus Medical Therapy Alone

Trial	Degree of Stenosis (%)	Patients (n)	Absolute Risk Reduction*	Relative Risk Reduction*	P
NASCET 1	> 70	659	17% at 1.5 years	65% at 1.5 years	< 0.001
ECST	> 60	778	9.6% at 2.7 years	44% at 2.7 years	< 0.001
VA	> 50	189	11.7% at 1 years	60.3% at 1 years	0.01
NASCET2	50–69	858	6.5% at 5 years	29.2% at 5 years	0.045
NASCET3	< 50	1368	3.8% at 5 years	20.3% at 5 years	0.16

* Absolute and relative risk reduction for stroke in symptomatic patients with carotid disease.

appropriate surgical candidates with symptomatic carotid stenosis ≥ 70% and is of marginal benefit for those with 50% to 69% stenoses.

It is important to note that the above studies used angiography to diagnose the extent of carotid narrowing. The methods used to calculate the percent stenosis differ between angiography and the most widely used screening test in the community, duplex ultrasound. In general, the degree of stenosis measured by duplex is overestimated by approximately 10% compared with angiography (Fig. 2). Therefore, when determined by duplex ultrasound, endarterectomy is clearly indicated in symptomatic patients with a ≥ 80% carotid stenosis (≥ 70% by angiography) and potentially beneficial in those with a 60% to 80% lesion (50% to 70% by angiography).

The benefits of endarterectomy for patients with moderate symptomatic carotid stenoses (50% to 70% by angiogram) are less than those seen for patients with more severe stenoses >70%.[30,31] Several factors determine the effectiveness of the surgery in these patients and must be

Figure 2. Determinations of percent carotid stenosis (ultrasound versus angiogram). The duplex examination overestimates the percent stenosis by approximately 10% compared with angiogram. The duplex study divides the minimal lumen diameter at the maximal stenosis by the width of the entire vessel at the site of plaque. The angiogram divides it by the lumen width at a distal disease-free segment in the internal carotid artery (ICA). ECA = external carotid artery, CCA = common carotid artery.

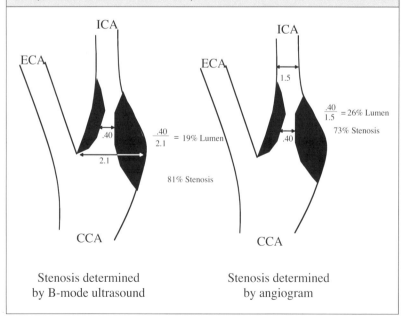

Stenosis determined
by B-mode ultrasound

Stenosis determined
by angiogram

considered when contemplating revascularization. These factors include gender, age, coexisting conditions, and the experience and skill of the surgeon.

Asymptomatic Carotid Stenosis

Although the risk is less than for symptomatic disease, asymptomatic carotid stenosis is a risk factor for cerebrovascular events. The rate of ipsilateral stroke is between 1% and 3% per year among patients with asymptomatic stenosis > 50%.[6,32].

Surgical treatment of high-degree asymptomatic carotid stenosis (> 70% by angiography) is beneficial. The correct approach to treatment of moderate stenoses is more controversial,[33,34] Table 3 summarizes the published data to date. *The consensus is that carotid endarterectomy is effective in asymptomatic patients with severe stenosis > 70% by angiogram (> 80% by duplex ultrasound) but only modestly effective and only for certain individuals with moderate lesions.* Other important factors to consider are that women benefited substantially less than men in the Asymptomatic Carotid Artery Study (ACAS) (reduction in risk, 66% in men vs. 17% in women), with a significantly higher rate of perioperative complications (1.7% in men vs. 3.6% in women). At present, the use of endarterectomy in asymptomatic disease of any severity requires access to an experienced surgeon with a low (< 3%) perioperative complication rate to be beneficial in reducing cerebrovascular events compared with medical therapy alone.

Percutaneous Interventions

Percutaneous angioplasty and *carotid artery stenting* are currently available at some centers. Endovascular treatment has the theoretical advantage of reducing the risk of surgical complications and allowing the inclusion of very high-risk patients who might otherwise not be candidates for revascularization. A review of the published studies regarding the effectiveness of endovascular treatment, however, suggests that

	Degree of Stenosis (%)	Patients (*n*)	Absolute Risk Reduction*	Relative Risk Reduction*	P
TABLE 3. Randomized Controlled Trials in Asymptomatic Patients: CEA Plus Medical Therapy versus Medical Therapy Alone					
Trial					
ACAS	> 60	1662	5.9% at 5 years	53% at 5 years	0.004
VA	> 50	444	4.7% at 4 years	50% at 4 years	0.056
CASANOVA	50–90	410	0.6% at 3 years	5.3% at 3 years	NS
* Absolute and relative risk reduction for stroke in asymptomatic patients with carotid disease.					

more research is required before it should be routinely offered. In the CAVATAS (Carotid and Vertebral Artery Transluminal Angioplasty Study),[36] endovascular treatment was similarly effective for stroke prevention with comparable risks to surgery.

As physicians performing carotid angioplasty plus stenting become more skilled and routinely use embolic protection devices, the risks and benefits may approach (or even exceed) those of expert surgeons performing carotid endarterectomy. More evidence is needed before widespread use of angioplasty and stenting can be recommended for patients with extracranial carotid stenosis. However, results from the recently completed SAPPHIRE study (presented at American Heart Association National Meeting in November 2002) are encouraging and support the notion that endovascular treatment may be superior to surgery in selected high-risk patients.

Peripheral Arterial Disease

Lower extremity PAD affects 8 to 12 million individuals in the United States,[37,38] and is most commonly caused by atherosclerotic disease of the aorta, iliac, and femoral arteries. Individuals with PAD are at an extremely high risk for cardiovascular mortality and have a reduced functional capacity and quality of life.[39,40] It is important for health care providers to identify this high-risk patient population in order to reduce the incidence of cardiovascular events and improve symptomatology. The following sections provide a practical algorithm for clinicians on the management PAD caused by atherosclerosis. More in-depth reviews on the standards for reporting lower extremity ischemia[41] and for the evaluation and management of PAD (TransAtlantic Inter-Society Consensus)[42] can be found in other publications.

Chronic Symptoms

The majority of patients with PAD are asymptomatic, and , 50% of patients with an abnormal ankle-brachial index (ABI) have classical symptoms.[39–43] The pain associated with chronic lower extremity ischemia is termed intermittent claudication (IC). It is traditionally described as a cramping discomfort in one or both legs that occurs with exertion, persists with continued activity, and rapidly resolves upon rest (< 5–10 minutes). When symptoms are narrowly defined as per the traditional Rose questionnaire, only 6% to 10% of patients with PAD are identified. Recent studies confirm that most individuals with PAD report lower extremity symptoms atypical of classical IC.[39,43]

When present, the location and degree of symptoms vary with the extent and levels of disease involvement. Pain most frequently localizes to the muscles of the calf,[37–42] because these muscles have a high metabolic demand and atherosclerosis is prevalent in the superficial femoral arteries. IC may also be localized to the buttocks and thighs, either in isolation or in addition to the calf. Symptoms tend to be reproducible, and patients can frequently quantify their exercise capacity in walking distance or time to the onset of symptoms.

Diagnosis of Chronic Disease

In order to enhance diagnostic sensitivity during the office visits of patients at risk for PAD, physicians should make frequent use of screening surveys, such as the San Diego Claudication Questionnaire,[44] and include a walking impairment history. It is important for clinicians to have a low threshold of suspicion for high-risk patients and to perform non-invasive screening tests when indicated (Table 4). Patients with atherosclerosis in other arterial sites (e.g., the coronary, carotid, or renal arteries) are at especially high risk for underlying PAD.[45] Other disease syndromes are associated with lower extremity pain and must be excluded during the diagnostic process (Table 5).

PAD can usually be confirmed or excluded by performing a noninvasive ankle-to-brachial systolic BP index (Fig. 3). Evaluation with an ABI measurement should be the first screening test in suspected PAD (see Table 4), because it has a very high degree of sensitivity and specificity, each approaching 95%. Most authorities define PAD by the pres-

---

TABLE 4. When to Suspect Peripheral Arterial Disease (Indications for an Ankle-Brachial Index)

- Increased age (asymptomatic individuals)
    - 50–69 years old plus a history of tobacco smoking or diabetes mellitus
    - ≥ 70 years old
- Leg pain with exertion
    - Positive screening history or survey results (e.g., San Diego questionnaire)
- Abnormal vascular or skin exam of lower extremities
    - Arterial skin ulcers
    - Thinned and dry skin; loss of hair and subcutaneous fat
    - Thickened, brittle nails
    - Absent peripheral pulses (1 pedal pulse may be absent in normal patients)
    - Muscle atrophy
    - Arterial bruits (aortic, iliac, popliteal)
    - Dependent leg rubor caused by chronically dilated arterioles
- Concomitant atherosclerotic disease
    - Carotid plaques, coronary artery disease, renal artery atherosclerosis
- Evaluation with an ABI may be indicated for enhancing cardiovascular risk stratification in patients with an intermediate global risk score (e.g., Framingham risk score between 10% and 20% event rate per 10 years)

TABLE 5. Differentiating Claudication of Peripheral Arterial Disease from other Causes of Lower Extremity Pain

Condition	Location	Characteristic
Intermittent claudication	Calf > thigh or buttocks	Cramping pain after same degree of exercise; rapid relief with rest No change with body position
Venous claudication	Entire leg thigh > calf	Tight bursting pain after exercise; slow relief with rest and with leg elevation; signs of edema and venous insufficiency present
Nerve root pain	Posterior leg radiation (common)	Sharp, lancinating pain immediately after exercise; slow relief; improves leaning forward; common with back problems; can occur at rest; associated parasethsias
Neuropathic pain	Dermatome distribution	Present at rest as well as exercise Relief with posture change that decreases pressure on peripheral nerve (Diabetic) painful neuropathy is usually in distal extremities
Baker's cyst	Behind knee	Pain at rest common; swelling and tenderness present
Hip arthritis	Hip, thigh, groin	Aching pain after variable usage; not rapidly relieved; may occur at rest; usually relieved with sitting when weight taken off hips and legs
Cord compression	Hips, thigh, buttocks (dermatome)	Pseudoclaudication Pain with upright posture alone; weakness > pain; relief with lumbar flexion; history of back problems;
Deep vein thrombosis	Calf usual	diffuse; leg swollen, red with pain at rest; history of trauma, immobility, hypercoagulablity
Compartment syndrome	Calves	Tight, bursting pain after extremes in exercise; hypertrophied calf muscles in athletes; slow relief with elevation of leg
Thrombangiitis obliterans (Buerger's disease)		Distal extremity ischemia in both hands and feet in smokers; ulcers;
Aortic coarctation		mild bilateral symptoms in young patients with hypertension
Takayasu's arteritis		Young women; pulseless upper arms; constitutional symptoms; fever

Figure 3. Measurement and interpretation of an ankle brachial index (ABI).

$$ABI = \frac{\text{Highest ankle pressure (dorsalis pedis vs. posterior tibialis)}}{\text{Highest arm pressure (left vs. right brachial)}}$$

> 1.3	Noncompressible (diabetes, renal failure) Rely on TBI or Doppler waveforms
0.91-1.3	Normal The UMMC-VL considers < 0.99 as abnormal
0.41-0.90	Mild-to-moderate PAD The UMMC-VL considers 0.50-0.80 as moderate and between 0.80-0.99 as mild PAD
0.0 – 0.40	Severe PAD The UMMC-VL considers < 0.50 as severe PAD

UMMC-VL = University of Michigan Medical Center Vascular Laboratory
TBI = Toe-brachial index (< 0.7 is abnormal)
Doppler waveforms: normal = triphasic, abnormal = biphasic or monophasic

ence of an ABI ≤ 0.90 to 0.95.[41–46] Patients with IC generally have an ABI between 0.4 and 0.9; lower values are associated with increasing disease severity and cardiovascular risk. Additional evaluations with segmental limb pressures, waveform analysis, and arterial duplex imaging can be used to localize disease anatomically after PAD has been diagnosed by an abnormal ABI. Further imaging studies with MRA and invasive arteriography are almost always reserved for planning a future intervention, because they are not required for diagnosis and provide no further information beyond ABI for medical management.

Exercise ABI testing should be performed on individuals with a normal resting ABI despite a high clinical suspicion for PAD. A normal test result usually rules out the presence of lower extremity arterial disease. On occasion, a falsely high normal ABI of > 1.2 to 1.3 can mask underlying PAD. Such situations are usually caused by concomitant diseases most commonly diabetes mellitus, which causes calcification of the media of the conduit arteries and prevents compression of the artery by the cuff. In this situation, a toe-brachial index of < 0.7 or an abnormal arterial wave-form analyses usually confirms the presence of underlying PAD.

Management of Chronic PAD

Patients are treated to relieve lower extremity symptoms, increase functional capacity and quality of life, prevent the progression of disease and ulcer formation, and preserve limb tissue (Fig. 4). Because most of the morbidity and mortality associated with PAD is from cardiac and cerebrovascular events,[40,47] aggressive modification of underlying atherosclerosis risk factors is a vitally important goal for all patients (refer back to Table 1).

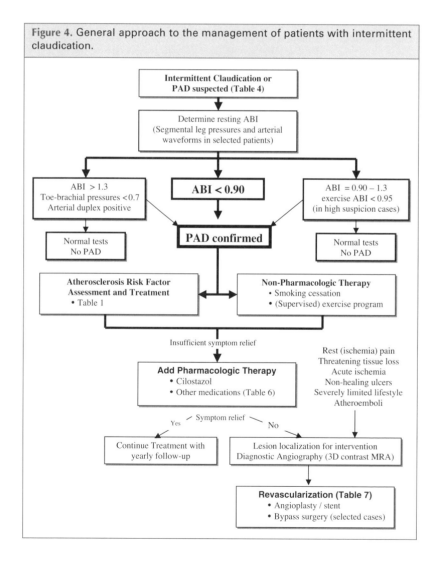

Figure 4. General approach to the management of patients with intermittent claudication.

The presence of an abnormal ABI of < 0.90 increases cardiovascular risk beyond estimates derived from traditional risk factors.[48] The diagnosis of PAD places individuals into the highest risk category (> 20% absolute risk for hard coronary events per 10 years) and is considered a coronary heart disease risk equivalent. Such patients should be treated with all the recommended risk reduction therapies afforded to post–myocardial infarction and coronary atherosclerosis patients unless contraindicated. The importance of evaluating and treating several emerging risk factors will be clarified by future studies.[49]

Specific Therapies

Exercise therapy is the primary modality to improve symptoms, functional capacity, and quality of life for PAD patients.[46] A meta-analysis of 10 studies on the effect of exercise on claudication confirms the beneficial effect on pain-free (139-m increase) and total walking (179-m increase) distance.[50] An exercise program, preferably a supervised rehabilitation program, should be the cornerstone of therapy for PAD patients.

Particular attention should be paid to complete tobacco smoking cessation.[1,3,46] Aspirin should be used in dosages between 81 and 325 mg daily in patients at high risk for cardiovascular events, including those with PAD.[51,52] The CAPRIE study (Clopidogrel Vs. Aspirin in Patients at Risk of Ischaemic Events) demonstrated a significant relative risk reduction of 23.8% for combined cardiovascular outcomes in PAD patients taking clopidogrel versus those taking aspirin.[53] Whether clopidogrel should be the first-line therapy instead of aspirin for these patients requires confirmation from addition studies. All patients with atherosclerosis, including those with PAD, are candidates for LDL-lowering treatment with statins. The British Heart Protection study confirmed the importance of this therapy in patients with PAD.[19] As for carotid disease, even patients with an initial LDL < 100 mg/dL benefited from therapy. Currently, the National Cholesterol Education Program (NCEP) III guidelines should be followed for dyslipidemia management in PAD patients, but it may be prudent to consider early statin usage in all patients with PAD, regardless of lipid values. Unfortunately, patients diagnosed with PAD commonly receive less intensive therapy and risk factor modification than individuals with established heart disease.[54]

Pharmacologic Therapy for Intermittent Claudication Symptoms

Several medications are available for the treatment of IC caused by PAD if nonpharmacologic therapy alone fails to be satisfactory (Table 6). Cilostazol is currently the mainstay of pharmacologic therapy for IC

TABLE 6. Medications for Peripheral Arterial Disease		
Medications	**Mechanism or Effect**	**Efficacy**
Cilostazol	FDA-approved for symptomatic claudication	Proven
	Type 3 phosphodiesterase inhibitor	Proven
	Vasodilatation, antiplatelet, improves lipoproteins	
Pentoxifylline	FDA-approved for symptomatic claudication relief	Marginal benefits
	Methylxanthine derivative	
	Increases RBC deformability, antiplatelet, reduces fibrinogen	
Prostaglandins*	PGI_2, Iloprost, Beraprost, PGE_1 vasodilatation, antiplatelet	Inconclusive
L-Carnitine	Skeletal muscle cofactor	Inconclusive
	Enhances muscle energy metabolism	
L-Arginine	Nitric oxide synthase substrate	Inconclusive
	Increases nitric oxide release	
Others*	Angiogenic growth factors, vasodilators, vitamin E, seratonin antagonists, chelation, ginkgo biloba, buflomedil, defibrotide, anticoagulants	Inconclusive

* = Investigational medications.
FDA = Food and Drug Aministration; RBC = red blood cell.

symptom relief. It is a type III phosphodiesterase inhibitor that increases intracellular cyclic adenosine monophosphate (cAMP) levels and promotes the release of prostaglandin I_2.[55] At the present time, cilostazol should be the first-line medication prescribed for symptomatic relief of IC when nonpharmacologic measures are unsatisfactory. Of all drugs investigated thus far, cilostazol demonstrates the most consistent symptom relief, improvement in walking time and distance, and enhancement of quality of life.[1,55,56] In a randomized, double-blind study, cilostazol (100 mg twice a day) produced a 51% increase in maximal walking distance and a 59% increase in pain-free walking distance.[57] Cilostazol is superior to the methylxanthine derivative pentoxifylline in reducing IC.[58] At the recommended dosage of 100 mg twice a day, cilostazol is generally well tolerated and the side effects are usually mild.[57,56] The most commonly reported adverse reactions include gastrointestinal symptoms in 44%, headaches in 20%, and palpitations in 17% of patients. Cilostazol is contraindicated for patients with congestive heart failure of any severity or an ejection fraction of < 40%. The other medications listed in Table 6 are either investigational or have not yet been proven to be more effective than cilostazol for the treatment of chronic IC.

Revascularization

When combined lifestyle and medical therapies are not successful in adequately improving symptoms, revascularization of the affected limb should be considered (see Fig. 4). Firm indications for revascularization are progression from IC to rest pain or tissue ischemia (ABI usually < 0.20), threatened loss of a limb, acute arterial obstruction, and recalcitrant skin ulcers.[59] Revascularization may be appropriate in selected cases of lifestyle-limiting IC, such as those that are disabling or that significantly interfere with quality of life or occupational performance.

After revascularization has been deemed appropriate by clinical criteria and feasible by subsequent imaging studies (MRA or angiogram), the optimal method to achieve the desired results (surgical vs. percutaneous) needs to be considered on an individual basis. In general, long-term patency rates are lower for femoropopliteal reconstructions than for aorta-iliac procedures; infrapopliteal bypasses have even lower long-term durability. Establishing good inflow to the affected vessel by proximal revascularization is critical for achieving optimal results in distal procedures.[60] Improving inflow with angioplasty or stenting of proximal aorta-iliac lesions often improves clinical complaints related to claudication and obviates the need for reconstruction of distal lesions.

The rationale for endovascular approaches is the desire to avoid the operative risk associated with surgical revascularization, shorten recovery times, and decrease medical costs. Indications for percutaneous techniques are generally similar to those for operative intervention, and the choice between approaches is often dictated by factors such as the location, length, severity of disease, and overall medical status of the patient (Table 7). In general, percutaneous intervention (with or without stenting) provides similar long-term patency rates to surgery for aorta-iliac disease in selected patients. However, it appears to be inferior for lesions distal to the inguinal ligament.[61] Referral to a vascular surgeon for traditional revascularization should be made for patients who have failed therapy or who are not candidates for percutaneous therapies.

Conclusions

The presence of PAD or symptomatic carotid disease markedly increases cardiovascular risk. Early identification of these high-risk patients and aggressive medical treatment provide health benefits far in excess of improvement in symptoms alone. Management of atherosclerosis risk factors, lifestyle interventions, and pharmacologic treatment improve functional capacity and quality of life, slows the progression of disease, and ultimately reduces overall mortality. Surgical or percuta-

TABLE 7. Factors that Determine the Revascularization Approach	
Variables Favoring Angioplasty	**Variables Favoring Surgery**

PAD of the aorto-iliac region
Short occlusions
  < 5 cm in the iliac artery
  < 10 cm in the superficial femoral artery
  < 2 cm in the tibial artery
Stenoses that are uncovered after occlusions
  are treated with thrombolysis
High-risk surgical candidates
Improve inflow to lower leg lesions
  (or hybrid procedures)
	PAD below the inguinal ligament (any
	  lesion location)
	Long occlusions
	  > 5 cm in the iliac artery
	  > 10 cm in the superficial femoral artery
	  > 2 cm in the superficial femoral artery
	Stenoses adjacent to aneurysms
	Lesions causing atheromatous embolism
	Lesions not amenable to angioplasty or
	  stenting
	Failed angioplasty

PAD = peripheral arterial disease	

neous revascularizations are treatment options available for appropriate candidate individuals for both carotid and lower extremity PAD. The effectiveness of new treatments for PAD, such as various angiogenic growth factors,[62] must be evaluated in future investigations.

References

1. Hiatt WR: Medical treatment of peripheral arterial disease and claudication. N Engl J Med 344:1608–1621, 2001.
2. Hughson WG, Mann JL, Garrod A: Intermittent claudication: Prevalence and risk factors. Br Med J 1:1379–1381, 1978.
3. Kannel WB, Shurleff D: The Framingham Study: Cigarettes and the development of intermittent claudication. Geriatrics 28:61–68, 1973.
4. Ridker PM, Stampfer MJ, Rifai N: Novel risk factors for systemic atherosclerosis. JAMA 285:2481–2485, 2001.
5. Sacco, RL: Extracranial carotid stenosis. N Engl J Med 345:1113–1118, 2001.
6. Goldstein LB, Adams R, Becker K, et al: Primary prevention of ischemic stroke: A statement for healthcare professionals from the Stroke Council of the American Heart Association. Stroke 32:280–299, 2001.
7. Straus SE, Majumdar SR, McAlister FA: New evidence for stroke prevention. JAMA 288:1388–1395, 2002.
8. Johnston SC: Transient ischemic attack. N Engl J Med 347:1687–1692, 2002.
9. Johnston DCC, Goldstein LB: Clinical carotid endarterectomy decision making: Non-invasive vascular imaging versus angiography. Neurology 56:1009–1015, 2001.
10. Zwiebel WJ: Ultrasound assessment of carotid plaque. Introduction to Vascular Ultrasonography, 4th ed. Philadelphia, W.B. Saunders Company, 2000, pp 125–135.
11. Zwiebel WJ. Doppler evaluation of carotid stenosis. Introduction to Vascular Ultrasonography, 4th ed. Philadelphia, W.B. Saunders Company, 2000, pp 125–135.
12. Timsit SG, Sacco RL, Mohr JP, et al: Early clinical differentiation of cerebral infarction from severe atherosclerotic stenosis and cardioembolism. Stroke 23:486–491,1992.
13. Silvestrini M, Vernieri F, Pasqualetti P, et al : Impaired cerebral vasoreactivity and

risk of stroke in patients with asymptomatic carotid stenosis. JAMA 283:2122–2127, 2000.

14. Moore WS, Barnett HJM, Beebe HG, et al: Guidelines for carotid endarterectomy: A multidisciplinary consensus statement from the Ad Hoc Committee, American Heart Association. Circulation 91:566–579, 1995.

15. Gorelick PB, Sacco RL, Smith DB, et al: Prevention of a first stroke: A review of guidelines and a multidisciplinary consensus statement from the National Stroke Association. JAMA 281:1112–1120, 1999.

16. Albers GW, Hart RG, Lutsep HL, et al: Supplement to the guidelines for the management of transient ischemic attacks: A statement from the Ad Hoc Committee on Guidelines for the Management of Transient Ischemic Attacks, Stroke Council, American Heart Association. Stroke 30:2502–2511, 1999.

17. Albers GW, Amarenco P, Easton JD, et al: Antithrombotic and thrombolytic therapy for ischemic stroke. Chest 119(suppl):300S–320S, 2001.

18. Mohr JP, Thompson JLP, Lazar RM, et al: A comparison of warfarin and aspirin for the prevention of recurrent ischemic stroke. N Engl J Med 345:1444–1451, 2001.

19. Heart Protection Study Collaborative Group: MRC/BHF heart protection study of cholesterol lowering with simvastatin in 20 536 high-risk individuals: A randomized placebo-controlled trial. Lancet 360:7–22, 2002.

20. Gorelick PB: Stroke prevention therapy beyond antithrombotics: Unifying mechanisms in ischemic stroke pathogenesis and implications for therapy. Stroke 33: 862–875, 2002.

21. Rubins HB, Davenport J, Babikian V, et al: Reduction in stroke with gemfibrozil in men with coronary heart disease and low HDL cholesterol. The veterans affairs HDL intervention trial (VA-HIT). Circulation 103:2828–2833, 2001.

22. Officers and Coordinators for the ALLHAT Collaborative Research Group: Major outcomes in high-risk hypertensive patients randomized to angiotensin-converting enzyme inhibitor or calcium channel blocker vs diuretic. The antihypertensive and lipid-lowering treatment to prevent heart attack trial (ALLHAT). JAMA 288:2981–2997, 2002.

23. PROGRESS Collaborative Group: Randomised trial of a perindopril-based blood-pressure-lowering regimen among 6105 individuals with previous stroke or transient ischaemic attack. Lancet 358:1033–1041, 2001.

24. Dahlof B, Devereux RB, Kjeldsen SE, et al: Cardiovascular morbidity and mortality in the Losartan Intervention for Endpoint reduction in hypertension study (LIFE): A randomised trial against atenolol. Lancet 359:995–1003, 2002.

25. Lonn E, Yusuf S, Dzavik V, et al: Effects of ramipril and vitamin E on atherosclerosis: The Study to Evaluate Carotid Ultrasound changes in patients treated with Ramipril and vitamin E (SECURE). Circulation 103:919–925, 2001.

26. North American Symptomatic Carotid Endarterectomy Trial Collaborators: Beneficial effect of carotid endarterectomy in symptomatic patients with high-grade carotid stenosis. N Engl J Med 325:445–453, 1991.

27. Mayberg MR, Wilson SE, Yatsu F, et al: Carotid endarterectomy and prevention of cerebral ischemia in symptomatic carotid stenosis. JAMA 266:3289–3294, 1991.

28. Rothwell PM, Gutnikov SA, Eliasziw M, et al: Overall results of a pooled analysis of individual patient data from trials of endarterectomy for symptomatic carotid stenosis. Stroke 32:327–327, 2001.

29. Rothwell PM, Eliasziw M, Gutnikov SA, et al: Analysis of pooled data from the randomised controlled trials of endarterectomy for symptomatic carotid stenosis. Lancet 361:107–116, 2003.

30. Barnett HJM, Taylor DW, Eliasziw M, et al: Benefit of carotid endarterectomy in patients with symptomatic moderate or severe stenosis. N Engl J Med 339:1415–1425,1998.

31. ECST Collaborative Group: Randomised trial of endarterectomy for recently symptomatic carotid stenosis: Final results of the MRC European Carotid Surgery Trial (ECST). Lancet 351:1379–1387, 1998.

32. Norris JW, Zhu CZ, Bornstein NM, Chambers BR: Vascular risks of asymptomatic carotid stenosis. Stroke 22:1485–1490, 1991.

33. The CASANOVA Study Group: Carotid surgery versus medical therapy in asymptomatic carotid stenosis. Stroke 22:1229–1235, 1991.

34. Executive Committee for the Asymptomatic Carotid Atherosclerosis Study: Endarterectomy for asymptomatic carotid artery stenosis. JAMA 273:1421–1428, 1995.

35. Goldstein LB, Samsa GP, Matchar DB, Oddone EZ: Multicenter review of preoperative risk factors for endarterectomy for asymptomatic carotid artery stenosis. Stroke 29:750–753, 1998.

36. CAVATAS Investigators: Endovascular versus surgical treatment in patients with carotid stenosis in the Carotid and Vertebral Artery Transluminal Angioplasty Study (CAVATAS): A randomised trial. Lancet 357:1729–1737, 2001.

37. Criqui MH, Fronek A, Barrett-Connor E, et al: The prevalence of peripheral arterial disease in a defined population. Circulation 71:510–555, 1985.

38. Criqui MH, Denenberg JO, Langer RD, Fronek A: The epidemiology of peripheral arterial disease: importance of identifying the population at risk. Vasc Med 2:221–226, 1997.

39. McDermott MM, Greenland P, Liu K, et al: Leg symptoms in peripheral arterial disease. JAMA 286:1599–1606, 2001.

40. Criqui MH, Langer RD, Fronek A, et al: Mortality over a period of 10 years in patients with peripheral arterial disease. N Engl J Med 326:381–386, 1992.

41. Rutherford RB, Baker JD, Ernst C, et al: Recommended standards for reports dealing with lower extremity ischemia: Revised version. J Vasc Surg 26:517–538, 1997.

42. Clinical Evaluation of Intermittent Claudication. J Vasc Surg 31,S56–S74, 2000.

43. McDermott MM, Mehta S, Greenland P: Exertional leg symptoms other than intermittent claudication are common in peripheral arterial disease. Arch Intern Med 159:387–92, 1999.

44. Hiatt WR, Hirsch AT, Regensteiner J: Peripheral Arterial Disease. 2000, pp 57–79.

45. Zierler RE, Bergelin RO, Polissar NL, et al: Carotid and lower extremity arterial disease in patients with renal artery atherosclerosis Arch Intern Med 158:761–767, 1998.

46. Criqui MH, Denenberg JO, Bird CE, et al: The correlation between symptoms and non-invasive test results in patients referred for peripheral arterial disease testing. Vasc Med 1:65–71, 1996.

47. Criqui MH: Systemic atherosclerosis risk and the mandate for intervention in atherosclerotic peripheral arterial disease. Am J Cardiol 88:43J–47J, 2001.

48. Greenland P, Abrams J, et al: Prevention converence v. beyond secondary prevention: Identifying the high-risk patient for primary prevention: noninvasive tests of atherosclerotic burden: Writing Group III. Circulation 101:E16–22, 2000.

49. Ridker PM, Stampfer MJ, Rifai N: Novel risk factors for systemic atherosclerosis: A comparison of C-reactive protein, fibrinogen, homocysteine, lipoprotein(1), and standard cholesterol screening as predictors of peripheral arterial disease. JAMA 285:2481–2485, 2001.

50. Girolami, B, Bernardi E, et al: Treatment if intermittent claudication with physical training, smoking cessation, pentoxifylline, or nafronyl. Arch Intern Med 159:337–345, 1999.

51. Smith SC Jr, Blair SN, Bonow RO, et al: AHA/ACC guidelines for preventing heart attack and death in patients with atherosclerotic cardiovascular disease: 2001 update. Circulation 104:1577–1579, 2001.

52. Sachdev GP, Ohlrogge KD, Johnson CL: Review of the Fifth American College of Chest Physicians Consensus Conference on Antithrombotic Therapy: Outpatient management for adults. Am J Health Syst Pharm 56:1505–1514, 1999.

53. CAPRIE Steering Committee: A randomised, blinded, trial of clopidogrel versus aspirin in patients at risk of ischaemic events (CAPRIE). Lancet 348:1329–1339, 1996.

54. Hirsch AT, Criqui MH, Treat-Jacobson D, et al: Preripheral arterial disease detection, awareness, and treatment in primary care. JAMA 286:1317–1324, 2002.

55. Eberhardt, RT, Coffman JD: Drug treatment of peripheral vascular disease. Heart Disease 2:62–47, 2000.

56. Dawson DL, Cutler BS, Meissner MH, Strandness E Jr: Cilostazol has Benificial Effects in Treatment of Intermittent Claudication. Circulation 98:678–686, 1998.

57. Beebe HG, Dawson DL, Cutler BS, et al: A new pharmacological treatment for intermittent claudication: Results of a randomized, multicenter trial. Arch Intern Med 159:2041–2050, 1999.

58. Dawson DL, Cutler BS, Hiatt WR, et al: A comparison of cilostazol and pentoxifylline for treating intermittent claudication. Am J Med 109:523–530, 2000.

59. Matsi PJ, Manninen HI, Suhonen MT, et al: Chronic critical lower-limb ischemia: prospective trial of angioplasty with 1–36 months follow-up. Radiology 188:381–387, 1993.

60. Eagleton, MJ, Illig KA, Green RM, et al: Impact of inflow reconstruction on infrainguinal bypass. J Vasc Surg 26:928–936, 1997.

61. Garasic JM, Creager MA: Percutaneous interventions for lower-extremity peripheral atherosclerotic disease. Rev Cardiovasc Med 2:120–125, 2001.

62. Lederman RJ, Mendelsohn FO, Anderson RD, et al: for the TRAFFIC investigators: Therapeutic angiogenesis with recombinant fibroblast growth factor-2 for intermittent claudication (the TRAFFIC study): A randomised trial. Lancet 359:2053–2058, 2002.

SECTION III

Screening and Diagnosis of Selected
Secondary Causes of Hypertension

chapter
8

Sleep Apnea: The Not So Silent Epidemic

Narayana S. Murali, M.D., Anna Svatikova, and Virend K. Somers, M.D., Ph.D.

Sleep has cognitive, reparative, and restorative properties essential to health and well-being. It is increasingly evident that disordered sleep, sleep apnea in particular, may have significant physiologic and pathologic implications for the cardiovascular system.

Sleep apnea syndromes comprise two related disorders, obstructive sleep apnea (OSA) and central sleep apnea (CSA). Repetitive partial (hypopnea) or complete (apnea) cessation of breathing during sleep can be caused by obstructive, central, or mixed mechanisms. An apneic episode is generally defined as cessation of airflow for at least 10 seconds regardless of the oxygen saturation. Hypopnea is defined as 30% or more reduction in airflow or thoracoabdominal excursion with at least a 4% decrease in arterial oxygen saturation or arousal.[18,31,35] The apnea-hypopnea index (AHI) or respiratory disturbance index (RDI) is the average number of apneas and hypopneas that occur per hour of sleep.

Obstructive apneas occur because of loss of patency of the upper airway, resulting in partial or complete occlusion of the airway during inspiration. CSA is a result of loss of the central respiratory drive. CSA can occur in normal subjects at higher altitudes, and in those with pathologic conditions such as heart failure or central neural disturbance. OSA has been increasingly implicated in the pathophysiology of hypertension[7,13,15] and is the primary focus of this review.

Prevalence of Obstructive Sleep Apnea

The prevalence of OSA in the general U.S. population is estimated to be close to 2 % in women and 4% in men (AHI $\geq$ 5 events per hour and daytime somnolence).[40] It has a similar prevalence estimate in other countries.[11,16,22,23] Twenty-four percent of men and 9% of women between the ages 30 and 60 years have significant apnea.[40] Prevalence in elderly individuals may be even higher. An estimated 2% to 3% of children have OSA with substantial variability, depending on ethnicity and other demographic characteristics.[30]

Evidence Linking OSA to Hypertension

Evidence to suggest that sleep-disordered breathing may be independently associated with high blood pressure (BP) was provided by the Sleep Heart Health Study, from cross-sectional data on 6132 subjects.[21] The odds of hypertension appeared to rise with increasing AHI in a dose-response fashion. The prospective Wisconsin Sleep Cohort Study persuasively demonstrated this association.[25] In a sample of 709 people followed over a period of 4 years, there was a threefold increase in the odds ratio of developing new hypertension if the baseline AHI was 15 or more events per hour (Fig. 1). In both of those epidemiologic studies,[21,25] the relationship between OSA and BP persisted even after adjusting for a variety of confounding variables, including age, gender, body mass index, tobacco, alcohol use, and baseline hypertension status.

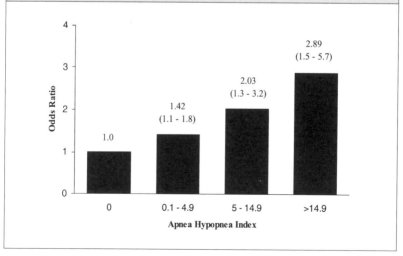

Figure 1. Association of hypertension with apnea hypopnea index (AHI) adjusted for baseline hypertension, body mass index (BMI), and waist and neck circumference. (Adapted from Peppard PE, Young T, Palta M, Skatrud J: Prospective study of the association between sleep-disordered breathing and hypertension. N Engl J Med 2000, 342:1378–1384.)

Acute Effects of Obstructive Sleep Apnea

Apneic events elicit a breadth of stressful stimuli, including hypoxemia, carbon dioxide retention,[3] and marked negative swings in intrathoracic pressure,[24,34] which increase afterload and myocardial wall stress.[9,37,28] Responses to the apneic events include chemoreflex activation with consequent sympathetic activation and increases in BP (Fig. 2),[32] which overwhelm the normal cardiovascular physiologic response to sleep.[33] Overall during sleep, neither BP nor sympathetic activity decline in severe OSA patients,[32] in contrast to findings in healthy subjects. For reasons that are not well understood, high sympathetic activity and high BPs during sleep carry over into daytime wakefulness so that even when OSA patients are normoxic, awake, and breathing normally, they have a heightened sympathetic drive and higher BPs.[4,32]

Potential Mechanisms Linking Obstructive Sleep Apnea to Hypertension

High sympathetic activity to peripheral blood vessels is likely to explain higher daytime BP in OSA patients. The reasons for the increased sympathetic drive are unclear but may be associated with increased

Figure 2. A patient with sleep apnea on CPAP therapy during REM sleep. The *arrow* indicates onset of obstruction with reduction in CPAP and consequent increase in SNA and BP. (From Somers VK, Dyken ME, Clary MP, Abboud FM: Sympathetic neural mechanisms in obstructive sleep apnea. J Clin Invest 1995, 96:1897–1904; with permission.)

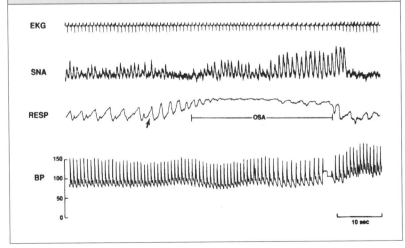

chemoreflex gain. Application of 100% oxygen to OSA patients results in significant reductions in sympathetic activity, BP, and heart rate (Fig. 3).[20] Patients with OSA who are normotensive and free of other overt cardiovascular diseases have clear abnormalities in daytime cardiovascular variability. They have faster heart rates, decreased heart rate variability, and increased BP variability, even during normoxic daytime wakefulness.[19] These abnormalities in variability may be associated with an increased likelihood of future cardiovascular disease, including hypertension.[8,36,38]

Other mechanisms that may induce higher daytime BPs include vasoactive substances such as endothelin. Endothelin levels are increased in response to untreated sleep apnea and are decreased after treatment

Figure 3. Recordings of MSNA in a patient with OSA during administration of 100% oxygen (*top*) and room air (*bottom*). MSNA, MAP, and HR decrease during administration of 100% oxygen but do not change with administration of room air. (From Narkiewicz K, van de Borne PJ, Montano N, et al: Contribution of tonic chemoreflex activation to sympathetic activity and blood pressure in patients with obstructive sleep apnea. Circulation 1998, 97:943–945; with permission.)

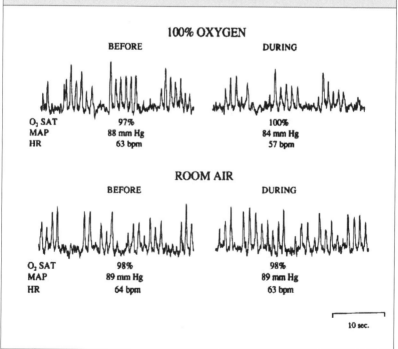

with continuous positive airway pressure (CPAP) therapy.[27] Prolonged vasoconstriction secondary to increased endothelin, as well as trophic effects of endothelin on blood vessels, may contribute to sustained hypertension.

OSA appears to be an independent cause of endothelial dysfunction. Both nitric oxide levels[12] and the vasodilator response to nitric oxide stimulation are blunted in sleep apneics.[14] The impaired endothelial function may be a consequence of the repetitive nocturnal hypoxemia and surges in BP.

Characteristics of Hypertensive Patients with Sleep Apnea

Although the possibility of sleep apnea should be entertained in all hypertensive patients, the index of suspicion should be particularly high in several subgroups of patients. Patients with obesity and daytime somnolence who also have hypertension are likely to have sleep apnea. The likelihood is further increased if there is a history of witnessed apneas (i.e., the spouse or bed partner has noted cessation of breathing during sleep in the patient). Because of the acute pressor responses to apnea and consequent increased nocturnal pressures, OSA patients also exhibit a nondipper diurnal BP pattern in that they often do not manifest the appropriate BP fall during sleep. Indeed, in a population of nondipper hypertensive patients, a substantial percentage were noted to have significant sleep apnea.[29] Sleep apnea should also be suspected in patients with resistant hypertension. Treatment of the sleep apnea often potentiates the antihypertensive effect of drug therapy.

Treatment of Sleep Apnea

In obese patients, weight loss is very effective at attenuating the severity of sleep apnea. Patients often have a predominant or significant positional component to their apnea because sleep apnea is worst when they lie on their backs. Simple maneuvers such as a pouch of tennis balls sewn into the back of the night shirt may prevent sleeping on the back and encourage patients to sleep on their sides. Avoidance of sleep deprivation is also helpful because sleep deprivation may worsen apnea severity.

The use of CPAP to overcome airway obstruction has already been referred to earlier. Other mechanical approaches include mandibular devices, which are substantially less effective. Surgical approaches, including uvulopalatopharyngoplasties, are also not yet proven to be effective. However, in patients with anatomical abnormalities of the mandible and upper airway, there may be a more clear indication for surgical intervention. Although tracheostomy is a very effective treatment for intractable and life threatening sleep apnea, it is often a last resort and should be considered when refractory to or noncompliant with CPAP.

Effects of Treatment of Sleep Apnea on Blood Pressure

Although treating normotensive patients with sleep apnea with CPAP does not appear to substantially affect BP levels, more clear results are evident in hypertensive patients. In a randomized study comparing appropriate CPAP treatment of OSA with subtherapeutic CPAP, patients receiving appropriate treatment showed a small but significant reduction in daytime BP.[26] These results have been supported further by other recent data that show declines in BP after various durations of nocturnal CPAP treatment (Fig. 4).[1,2,5,6,10,39]

Summary

OSA has been linked to a number of cardiovascular disorders. Presently, the most compelling evidence suggests that it is etiologically

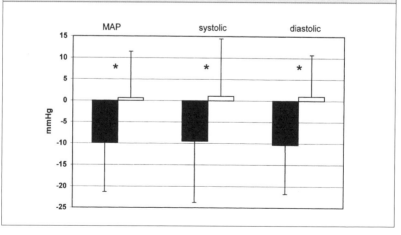

Figure 4. Change in mean arterial pressure (MAP), systolic and diastolic blood pressure (mm Hg) with effective (*closed bars*) and subtherapeutic (*open bars*) nocturnal continuous positive airway pressure (nCPAP) treatment. Both nocturnal and daytime blood pressures were lower after effective compared to subtherapeutic CPAP. *$P<0.05$ (From Becker HF, Jerrentrup A, Ploch T, et al: Effect of nasal continuous positive airway pressure treatment on blood pressure in patients with obstructive sleep apnea. Circulation 2003, 107:68–73; with permission.)

associated with hypertension. Not only does untreated sleep apnea increase the likelihood of new "essential" hypertension[25] but also treatment of OSA is accompanied by lower daytime BPs, even in patients with relatively mild hypertension.[2,26] In patients with resistant hypertension, OSA should be suspected and treated, because treatment of the apnea may often result in significant decreases in daytime BP and improved overall BP control.

If OSA indeed has an etiologic role in events such as stroke, myocardial infarction, heart failure, and renal failure, which are all also consequences of hypertension, it may well be that treating the OSA may decrease the potential effects of hypertension in leading to these disease conditions.

Acknowledgments

Dr. Somers is supported by National Institute of Health grants HL 65176, HL 61560, HL 70302, and General Cardiovascular Research Center grant M01-RR00585. We appreciate the expert secretarial assistance of Debra Pfeifer.

References

1. Akashiba T, Kurashina K, Minemura H, et al: Daytime hypertension and the effects of short-term nasal continuous positive airway pressure treatment in obstructive sleep apnea syndrome. Intern Med 1995, 34:528–533.

2. Becker HF, Jerrentrup A, Ploch T, et al: Effect of nasal continuous positive airway pressure treatment on blood pressure in patients with obstructive sleep apnea. Circulation 2003, 107:68–73.

3. Bradley TD, Rutherford R, Lue F, et al: Role of diffuse airway obstruction in the hypercapnia of obstructive sleep apnea. Am Rev Respir Dis 1986, 134:920–924.

4. Carlson JT, Hedner J, Elam M, et al: Augmented resting sympathetic activity in awake patients with obstructive sleep apnea. Chest 1993, 103:1763–1768.

5. Dimsdale JE, Loredo JS, Profant J: Effect of continuous positive airway pressure on blood pressure: a placebo trial. Hypertension 2000, 35:144–147.

6. Faccenda JF, Mackay TW, Boon NA, Douglas NJ: Randomized placebo-controlled trial of continuous positive airway pressure on blood pressure in the sleep apnea-hypopnea syndrome. Am J Respir Crit Care Med 2001, 163:344–348.

7. Fletcher EC, DeBehnke RD, Lovoi MS, Gorin AB: Undiagnosed sleep apnea in patients with essential hypertension. Ann Int Med 1985, 103:190–195.

8. Frattola A, Parati G, Cuspidi C, et al: Prognostic value of 24-hour blood pressure variability. J Hypertens 1993, 11:1133–1137.

9. Hall MJ, Ando S, Floras JS, et al: Magnitude and time course of hemodynamic responses to Mueller maneuvers in patients with congestive heart failure. J Appl Physiol 1998, 85:1476–1484.

10. Hla KM, Skatrud JB, Finn L, et al: The effect of correction of sleep-disordered breathing on BP in untreated hypertension. Chest 2002, 122:1125–1132.

11. Hui DS, Choy DK, Wong LK, et al: Prevalence of sleep-disordered breathing and continuous positive airway pressure compliance: results in Chinese patients with first-ever ischemic stroke. Chest 2002, 122:852–860.

12. Ip MS, Lam B, Chan LY, et al: Circulating nitric oxide is suppressed in obstructive sleep apnea and is reversed by nasal continuous positive airway pressure. Am J Respir Crit Care Med 2000, 62:2166–2171.

13. Kales A, Cadieux RJ, Shaw LC, et al: Sleep apnoea in a hypertensive population. Lancet 1984, ii:1005–1008.

14. Kato M, Roberts-Thomson P, Phillips BG, et al: Impairment of endothelium-dependent vasodilation of resistance vessels in patients with obstructive sleep apnea. Circulation 2000, 102:2607–2610.

15. Lavie P, Ben-Yosef R, Rubin AE: Prevalence of sleep apnea syndrome among patients with essential hypertension. Am J Cardiol 1985, 55:1019–1022.

16. Marin JM, Gascon JM, Carrizo S, Gispert J: Prevalence of sleep apnoea syndrome in the Spanish adult population. Int J Epidemiol 1997, 26:381–386.

17. Mark AL: Regulation of sympathetic nerve activity in mild human hypertension. J Hypertens 1990, 8(suppl):67–75.

18. Meoli AL, Casey KR, Clark RW, et al: Hypopnea in sleep-disordered breathing in adults. Sleep 2001, 24:469–470.

19. Narkiewicz K, Montano N, Cogliati C, et al: Altered cardiovascular variability in obstructive sleep apnea. Circulation 1998, 98:1071–1077.

20. Narkiewicz K, van de Borne PJ, Montano N, et al: Contribution of tonic chemoreflex activation to sympathetic activity and blood pressure in patients with obstructive sleep apnea. Circulation 1998, 97:943–945.

21. Nieto FJ, Young TB, Lind BK, et al: Association of sleep-disordered breathing, sleep apnea, and hypertension in a large community-based study. Sleep Heart Health Study. JAMA 2000, 283:1829–1836.

22. Ohayon MM, Guilleminault C, Priest RG, Caulet M: Snoring and breathing pauses during sleep: telephone interview survey of a United Kingdom population sample. Br Med J 1997, 314:860–863.

23. Olson LG, King MT, Hensley MJ, Saunders NA: A community study of snoring and sleep-disordered breathing. Prevalence. Am J Respir Crit Care Med 1995, 152:711–716.

24. Parish JM, Shepard JW Jr: Cardiovascular effects of sleep disorders. Chest 1990, 97:1220–1226.

25. Peppard PE, Young T, Palta M, Skatrud J: Prospective study of the association between sleep-disordered breathing and hypertension. N Engl J Med 2000, 342:1378–1384.

26. Pepperell JC, Ramdassingh-Dow S, Crosthwaite N, et al: Ambulatory blood pressure after therapeutic and subtherapeutic nasal continuous positive airway pressure for obstructive sleep apnoea: a randomised parallel trial. Lancet 2002, 359:204–210.

27. Phillips BG, Narkiewicz K, Pesek CA, et al: Effects of obstructive sleep apnea on endothelin-1 and blood pressure. J Hypertens 1999, 17:61–66.

28. Pinsky MR: Sleeping with the enemy: the heart in obstructive sleep apnea. Chest 2002, 121:1022–1024.

29. Portaluppi F, Provini F, Cortelli P, et al: Undiagnosed sleep-disordered breathing among male nondippers with essential hypertension. J Hypertens 1997, 15:1227–1233.

30. Redline S, et al: Epidemiology and genetics of sleep disordered breathing. In Sleep Symposium, Washington DC, 2002.

31. Sleep-related breathing disorders in adults: recommendations for syndrome defini-

tion and measurement techniques in clinical research. The Report of an American Academy of Sleep Medicine Task Force. In Sleep 1999, 667–689.

32. Somers VK, Dyken ME, Clary MP, Abboud FM: Sympathetic neural mechanisms in obstructive sleep apnea. J Clin Invest 1995, 96:1897–1904.

33. Somers VK, Dyken ME, Mark AL, Abboud FM: Sympathetic-nerve activity during sleep in normal subjects. N Engl J Med 1993, 328:303–307.

34. Stoohs R, Guilleminault C: Cardiovascular changes associated with obstructive sleep apnea syndrome. J Appl Physiol 1992, 72:583–589.

35. Strollo PJ Jr, Rogers RM: Obstructive sleep apnea. N Engl J Med 1996, 334:99–104.

36. Task Force of the European Society of Cardiology and the North American Society of Pacing and Electrophysiology: Heart rate variability: standards of measurements, physiological interpretation, and clinical use. Circulation 1996, 93:1043–1065.

37. Tkacova R, Rankin F, Fitzgerald FS, et al: Effects of continuous positive airway pressure on obstructive sleep apnea and left ventricular afterload in patients with heart failure. Circulation 1998, 98:2269–227.

38. Van Vliet BN, Hu L, Scott T, et al: Cardiac hypertrophy and telemetered blood pressure 6 wk after baroreceptor denervation in normotensive rats. Am J Physiol 1996, 271:R1759-R1769.

39. Wilcox I, Grunstein RR, Hedner JA, et al: Effect of nasal continuous positive airway pressure during sleep on 24-hour blood pressure in obstructive sleep apnea. Sleep 1993, 16:539–544.

40. Young T, Palta M, Dempsey J, et al: The occurrence of sleep-disordered breathing among middle-aged adults. N Engl J Med 1993, 328:1230–1235.

HOT TOPICS

Primary Aldosteronism

Marion Wofford, M.D., MPH

chapter 9

Primary aldosteronism (PA) has been the subject of much interest and debate for the past decade. Previously thought to be very rare, this disorder is the most common endocrine cause of secondary hypertension. Consideration of its occurrence among the hypertensive population and the use of an effective screening test have led to much higher prevalence estimates among hypertensive patients.

Jerome Conn first described PA in 1955 as a syndrome associated with hypokalemia, hypertension, high aldsoterone, and suppressed renin levels.[1] Although Conn later recognized that patients with PA could be normokalemic,[2] the search for patients with Conn's syndrome was usually limited to hypertensive patients with hypokalemia. A case series published in 1977 from the Mayo Clinic reported a prevalence of 0.01% among patients screened for PA, supporting the understanding that PA was quite rare.[3]

In 1994 Gordon, et al. reported an incidence of PA of 8.5% among patients previously diagnosed with essential hypertension.[4] Lim et al. reported a PA prevalence of 9.2% among patients seen in a hypertension clinic.[5] Screening for PA among patients with treatment-resistant hypertension has led to enhanced detection and provide opportunities to improve blood pressure (BP) control.

Screening Tests

The plasma aldosterone (ng/dL) to plasma renin activity (ng/mL/h) is the preferred method for screening test for PA. Hiramatsu et al. first proposed this method of screening for PA as a more sensitive test than a random aldosterone level.[6] The normal response to increased renin is enhanced aldosterone production. In PA, the plasma renin and aldosterone change inversely—that is, a high aldosterone level in the presence of a suppressed plasma renin indicates that the production of aldosterone is independent of the formation of renin as in PA. The result of these tests may suggest other forms of hypertension related to renin and aldosterone release. For example, an elevation of both hormones with a ratio < 10 may result from forms of secondary aldosteronism such as renovascular hypertension. If both hormones are suppressed, endocrinopathies that result from alternative forms of excess mineralocorticoids (e.g., apparent mineralocorticoid excess [AME] or Cushing's syndrome) are possible.[7]

Screening using the aldosterone-to-renin ratio (ARR) is best if performed in the early morning. Although postural changes and the use of antihypertensive medications may alter the ratio, it is considered acceptable to perform seated measures in patients taking antihypertensive agents. Spironolactone significantly increases aldosterone levels, so this medication must be held for at least 6 weeks before screening.[7] Amiloride or triamterene may be used in place of spironolactone during screening and diagnosis in patients with high suspicion for PA. Angiotensin-converting enzyme (ACE) inhibitors can elevate plasma renin levels. Therefore, a suppressed renin level while patients are taking ACE inhibitors provides additional evidence of autonomous aldosterone secretion. Beta-blockers, calcium channel blockers, angiotensin receptor blockers, and diuretics may all effect the ARR. Although medication use should be taken into consideration when interpreting the ARR, discontinuation of these antihypertensive drugs in patients with moderate to severe hypertension is potentially dangerous. Stopping antihypertensive drugs is not recommended or necessary in screening for PA.[7–9]

Wineberger and Fineberg found that an ARR of > 30 combined with a plasma aldosterone level > 20 ng/dL had a sensitivity and specificity of 90% for the diagnosis of PA.[10] Young proposed that an ARR of > 20 with a plasma aldosterone level of 15 ng/dL was consistent with a positive test result for PA.[7] A suppressed renin and an elevated aldosterone level are critical to the recognition of PA. Although there is no consensus on the absolute values consistent with a positive screening test result for PA, an ARR > 20 and a plasma aldosterone level ≥ 15 ng/dL in hypertensive patients should be followed with a repeat ARR and then confirmatory tests.

Confirmatory Tests

Confirmatory testing to detect autonomous production of aldosterone should be done after a positive screening test result. There is no consensus on the best procedure for diagnosis of PA, but several strategies have been recommended. Each is based on detecting nonsuppressable aldosterone production.

A saline infusion should cause renin suppression and subsequent aldosterone reduction. After infusion of 2 L of normal saline, a plasma aldosterone level > 10 ng/dL is consistent with PA.[11]

An alternative procedure is oral salt loading for 3 days, which should result in low renin and low aldosterone levels in patients with primary hypertension. The risk of increasing daily sodium intake in hypertensive patients must be considered. After a 3-day high salt intake, a 24-hour urine for aldosterone, sodium, and potassium is collected. Sodium excretion of > 200 mEq confirms adequate sodium intake and urinary secretion of aldosterone > 14 μg/24 hours confirms autonomous aldosterone secretion.[11]

The captopril suppression test is an effective confirmatory test that may be used in ambulatory patients in whom salt loading is considered a high risk. After administration of a single dose of captopril, the aldosterone level should decrease in patients with normal ARRs. In patients with autonomous production of aldosterone, captopril should have no effect on the level of this hormone.[12]

Imaging

High-resolution computed tomography (CT) may reveal a solitary adenoma or evidence of unilateral or bilateral adrenal hyperplasia. In many patients with biochemical evidence of PA, imaging may reveal normal-appearing adrenal glands. For patients with large adenomas (> 1 cm), surgical resection may be considered.[12] Adenomas > 2.5 to 3.0 cm should be resected because they may be related to primary or metastatic carcinomas.

Subtypes of Primary Aldosteronism

The determination of subtypes of PA is based on anatomic and physiologic responses and may impact management decisions. Patients with aldosterone-producing adenomas (APAs) or unilateral adrenal hyperplasia may be treated surgically, but those with idiopathic hyperplasia (IHA) or glucocorticoid-remediable aldosteronism (GRA) are managed pharmacologically.[7]

In general, whereas patients with APA have more severe hypertension and hypokalemia, those with IHA typically have milder hypertension and may be normokalemic. In young patients with a unilateral adenoma > 1 cm, an adrenalectomy may be the best option. In older patients, use of potassium-sparing diuretics may be preferred.[7] Given the high prevalence of benign adrenal "incidentalomas," adrenal vein sampling should be considered before surgery to determine the functionality of an adenoma. This procedure, although technically difficult and often not readily available, may be used to distinguish between unilateral and bilateral disease when CT imaging reveals hyperplasia.[14] Patients with IHA, which affects the

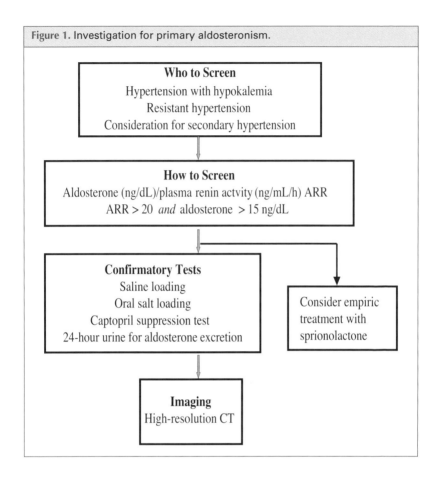

Figure 1. Investigation for primary aldosteronism.

adrenal glands bilaterally, should be managed with potassium-sparing diuretics in combination with other antihypertensive therapy as needed.

Genetic analysis is needed to confirm the diagnosis of GRA, which is caused by an autosomal dominant mutation. This disorder should be suspected in patients with a family history of PA, in those with PA diagnosed in the first 3 decades of life, and in patients with a family history of strokes at an early age.[15] A low dose of dexamethasone decreases aldosterone, improves BP control, and may be useful for long-term management.

Practical Considerations

Primary aldosterone is much more common than previously thought and appears to have prevalence rates among hypertensive patients as high as 10% to 15%. Given the number of patients with hypertension in the United States and around the world, screening for this disorder may result in identifying many patients who could benefit from the use of potassium-sparing diuretics. A random ARR can be obtained on patients, despite use of most anithypertensive medications. This simple test should be considered in patients who require multiple BP-lowering drugs or in whom the family history or biochemical profile suggests PA.

Although the confirmatory tests, subtype analysis, and long-term management are debated among hypertension specialists, some advocate a therapeutic trial of spironolactone in patients suspected to have PA. A favorable BP response has been observed in patients in whom the actual diagnosis and subtype may not be clear.[16] A strategy of screening and initiation of spironolactone may be reasonable for patients in whom further diagnostic tests cannot be arranged. Although this strategy does not lead to the diagnosis of PA, it may result in a reduction of morbidity and mortality in patients with poorly controlled hypertension.

References

1. Conn JW: Primary aldosteronism, a new clinical syndrome. J Lab Clin Med 45:3–17, 1955.
2. Conn JW: Plasma renin activity in primary aldosteronism. JAMA 90:222–225, 1964.
3. Tucker RM, Labarthe DR: Frequency of surgical treatment of hypertension in adults at the May Clinic from 1973 to 1975. Mayo Clin Proc 52:549–555, 1977.
4. Gordon RD, Stowasser M, Tunny IJ, et al: High incidence of primary aldosteronism in 199 patients referred with hypertension. Clin Exp Pharmacol Physiol. 21:315–318, 1994.
5. Lim PO, Dow E, Brennan G, et al: High prevalence of primary aldosteronism in the Tayside hypertension clinic population. J Hum Hypertens 14:311–315, 2000.
6. Hiramatsu K, Yamada T, Yukimura Y, et al: A screening test to identify aldosterone-producing adenoma by measuring plasma renin activity. Results in hypertensive patients. Arch Intern Med 141:1589–1593, 1981.
7. Young WF Jr: Primary aldosteronism: management issues. Ann N Y Acad Sci 970:61–76, 2002.
8. Gallay BJ, Ahmad S, Xu L, et al: Screening for primary aldosteronism without discontinuing hypertensive medications: plasma aldosterone-renin ratio. Am J Kidney Dis 37:699–705, 2001.
9. Mulatero P, Rabbia F, Milan A, et al: Drug effects on aldosterone/plasma renin activity ratio in primary aldosteronism. Hypertension. 40:897–902, 2002.
10. Weinberger MH, Fineberg NS: The diagnosis of primary aldosteronism and separation of two major subtypes. Arch Intern Med 153:2125, 1993.
11. Holland OB, Brown H, Kuhnert L, et al: Further evaluation of saline infusion for the diagnosis of primary aldosteronism. Hypertension 6:717, 1984.
12. Agharazii M, Douville P, Grose JH, Lebel M: Captopril suppression versus salt loading in confirming primary aldosteronism. Hypertension 37:1440, 2001.
13. Kloos RT, Gross MD, Francis IR, et al: Incidentally discovered adrenal masses. Endocr Rev 16:460–484, 1995.

14. Rossi GP, Sacchetto A, Chiesura-Corona M, et al: Identification of the etiology of primary aldosteronism with adrenal vein sampling in patients with equivocal computed tomography and magnetic resonance findings: results in 104 consecutive cases. J Clin Endocrinol Metab 86:1083, 2001.
15. Williams GH, Dluhy RG: Glucocorticoid-remediable aldosteronism. J Endocrinol Invest 18:512–517, 1995.
16. Lim PO, Jung RT, MacDonald TM: Is aldosterone the missing link in refractory hypertension? Aldosterone-to-renin ratio as a marker of inappropriate aldosterone activity. J Hum Hypertens 16:153–158, 2002.

SECTION IV
Management of Hypertension:
Goals and Objectives

chapter
10

Treating to Goal Blood Pressure

William J. Elliott, M.D., Ph.D.

Hypertension has been recognized as a major contributor to the risk of adverse cardiovascular events (stroke, heart attack, and death) for more than a century.[1] For the past 50 years, effective drug therapies have been available to treat patients with this disorder, but only in the past 35 years have data from clinical trials *proven* the benefits of these therapies in reducing the rates of stroke and heart attack. In 1967, there was little argument about the benefits of treatment seen in the first Veterans Administration (VA) Cooperative study.[2] Investigators in this study enrolled 143 U.S. military veterans with supine diastolic blood pressure (BP) between 115 and 129 mm Hg after 6 days of bedrest and low-sodium hospital food. Investigators gave active drug treatment to half of the participants and placebo to the other half. The study was stopped prematurely because there was such a major improvement in prognosis (0 vs. 4 deaths, 1 vs. 27 hospitalizations in therapy vs. placebo, respectively) that statistics were not even needed or included in the paper describing the results.

Current Antihypertensive Drug Therapies

Clinical trials against placebo have now demonstrated the benefits of antihypertensive drug therapy, as summarized in meta-analyses, which show an approximate 38% reduction in stroke, 16% reduction in heart attack, 51% reduction in heart failure, 21% reduction in cardiovascular death, and 35% reduction in left ventricular hypertrophy (LVH).[3–5] Antihypertensive drug therapy is beneficial in reducing adverse cardiovascular and renal events in large studies and may contribute to reduction in stroke and heart disease deaths in the U.S. population.[6]

105

Hypertension Control in the United States

Some improvements in the awareness, treatment, and control of hypertension have been documented in the series of National Health and Nutritional Evaluation Surveys (NHANES). In the 1991 to 1994 survey, BP control rates declined for the first time. Using the standard for BP control in the United States since 1977, only 27.4% of adults between the ages of 18 and 74 have "controlled hypertension" (< 140 mm Hg systolic and < 90 mm Hg diastolic).[1,7] Inclusion into the calculation of individuals age 75 years and older makes the percentage controlled even lower because many older individuals have "isolated systolic hypertension," which often requires more drug therapy.[8] In more recent data from NHANES IV (1999–2001), 31% of 18- to 74-year-old Americans had controlled hypertension. Thus, on average, fewer than one in three hypertensive people in the United States have "controlled hypertension."

Achieving Blood Pressure Goals

There are obviously many reasons for the large proportion of uncontrolled hypertensives in the United States. The cost of medications and medical follow-up are important. The high rates at which patients discontinue taking medications over a year also contribute.[9,10] Evidence indicates that physicians play an important role as well.[8,11] Many physicians appear to be unwilling to intensify antihypertensive drug therapy, even when presented with a hypertensive patient whose BP is consistently higher than goal.

BP is considered a simple "vital sign" that is to be recorded at each medical encounter. Because BP is frequently measured, is usually recorded in every office note, and is perhaps more legible than other notations written by physicians, it has become a "quality of care indicator" for many managed care organizations. These entities must report the results of their own surveys of their "covered lives" to national authorities if they wish to keep their Medicare certification. Many physicians' offices are having their charts audited to assess the prevalence of "controlled hypertension" in their offices and are receiving negative feedback if the proportion is lower than 50%, which was the goal in *Healthy People 2000*.[12]

Currently Recommended Blood Pressure Targets

Since the late 1970s, the goal BP for the majority of patients with hypertension has been less than 140/90 mm Hg. Physicians' attention was originally focused more on the diastolic number because it was intrinsically less variable than the systolic and was the better predictor of death

TABLE 1. Currently Recommended Blood Pressure Targets for Various Groups of Hypertensive Patients

Group	BP goal, mm Hg	Recommended by	Based on
Uncomplicated hypertensives	< 140/90	JNC VI[1]	HOT Study[21]
Diabetic hypertensives	< 130/80	American Diabetes Association[22] National Kidney Foundation[23] British Hypertension Society[24]	UKPDS 38,[20] HOT Diabetic Substudy[21]
Hypertensives with proteinuria > 1 g/day	< 125/75*	National Kidney Foundation[23]	MDRD[17]
Hypertensives with renal impairment	< 130/80	National Kidney Foundation[23]	AASK[19]

* This recommendation may soon be revised to < 130/80 mm Hg based on the results of the second randomization in the AASK study.

in databases from insurance companies in the 1920 to 1950s. Only recently was it recognized that the majority of men who underwent "insurance physicals" were typically in their mid-20s, and the majority of the hypertensive people in the United States were about 4 decades older. This and much epidemiologic and clinical trial data on the benefits of treating "isolated systolic hypertension"[13] led to a refocusing of attention on systolic BP, which is currently estimated to be uncontrolled (i.e., ≥ 140 mm Hg) in about 82% of older American hypertensives who are not controlled.[8]

It was only in the Sixth Report of the Joint National Committee (JNC) on Prevention, Detection, Evaluation, and Treatment of High Blood Pressure that the expert panel recommend an even lower goal for higher-risk patients, including especially diabetics and those with renal impairment (see Table 1 for even more current BP goals set out by other more recent expert panels). JNC VI recommended a target BP of less than 130/85 mm Hg for diabetic patients and less than 125/75 mm Hg for patients with renal impairment and more than 1 gram of proteinuria per day.[1]

Clinical Benefits of Achieving these Targets

Most clinical trials in hypertension are directed toward proving the benefits of a certain treatment strategy in large numbers of patients. Because it is generally difficult to have large numbers of patients *achieve* specific levels of control (for *any* parameter, including BP, serum low-density lipoprotein cholesterol level, or glycosylated hemoglobin value), few clinical trials have attempted to randomize patients to different target levels of BP as their primary intervention. A notable exception is the Hypertension Optimal Treatment (HOT) Study, discussed in detail later in this chapter.

Much of our information about the clinical results achieved according to intensity of treatment (or in our case, the benefits of achieving a specific target BP) comes from *post-hoc* analyses of data gathered to answer other questions. There is justifiable concern about any conclusion drawn from such analyses because these are not the primary outcome measures of randomized clinical trials, analyzed according to the proper "intent-to-treat" principle. *Post-hoc*, and especially "on-treatment," analyses[14] can lead to skewed and even incorrect conclusions, because of expectation bias or indication bias, and their interpretation is always a matter for some discussion.[15] Nonetheless, these analyses often offer interesting (and often useful) insights about the benefits of actually achieving certain target BPs.

Perhaps one of the most impressive examples of such a *post-hoc* analysis was published recently, more than 10 years *after* the primary results of the Systolic Hypertension in the Elderly Program (SHEP).[16] The risk of stroke according to on-treatment BP during follow-up was calculated for people who received either placebo or active treatment (Fig. 1). In SHEP, the BP goal for the entire study was a systolic BP less than 160 mm Hg or at least a 20 mm Hg–decline from baseline. A systolic BP of lower than 160, achieved by 3162 of the 4763 enrolled patients, reduced the risk of stroke by 33% (95% confidence interval [CI]: 11%–49%). The 2335 patients who maintained systolic BP below 150 mm Hg did even better, with a 38% reduction in stroke risk (95% CI: 18% to 53%). Unfortunately, only 1356 patients achieved systolic BP lower than 140 mm Hg, which limited the statistical power of the comparison; the 22% reduction in stroke risk was not statistically significant (95% CI: -7% to 43%). These data should *not* be interpreted that achieving a goal systolic BP of less than 140 is not as effective as a higher goal because of the smaller numbers of patients that achieved the lower target.

One of the first American studies to *randomize* patients to different BP goals was named Modification of Diet in Renal Disease because its primary purpose was to see if lower intake of dietary protein would have a beneficial effect on the progression of renal impairment, as had been seen in smaller, earlier studies, particularly from Australia. Fortunately, the investigators also wished to see if a lower-than-usual BP goal would also slow renal disease progression.[17] Therefore, all 585 subjects enrolled in this study (who had baseline glomerular filtration rates [GFR] between 13 and 55 mL/min/1.73 m^2) were randomized *twice* (in a two-by-two factorial design): once to different levels of dietary protein intake

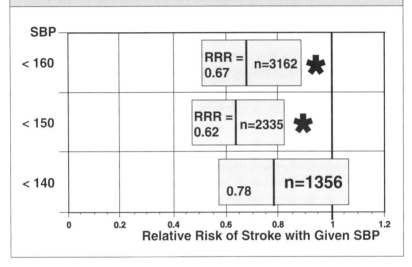

Figure 1. Relative risk reduction (RRR) for stroke, the primary endpoint, according to average in-trial systolic blood pressure (SBP) in the Systolic Hypertension in the Elderly Program. The goal SBP for the patients in this study was < 160 mm Hg systolic, or a decrease from initial SBP of at least 20 mm Hg. The average baseline BP was 170/77 mm Hg. The number of patients who achieved each SBP goal (*y axis*) is shown in the *right* of each bar; each bar corresponds to the 95% confidence limits for the point estimate (*dark vertical lines*). *Denotes $P < 0.05$. (Adapted from Perry HM Jr, Davis BR, Price TR, et al: Effect of treating isolated systolic hypertension on the risk of developing various types and subtypes of stroke: the Systolic Hypertension in the Elderly Program (SHEP). JAMA 2000, 284:465–471.)

and once to different BP targets (mean arterial pressure < 107 or < 92 mm Hg, corresponding to usual BPs of < 140/90 or 125/75 mm Hg). Many were disappointed in the final results of the study because there were no significant differences in progression of renal disease, hospitalization, or death between randomized groups for either intervention.[17] Furthermore, the achieved mean arterial pressures in the two randomized groups turned out to be quite similar (93.0 ± 7.3 vs. 97.7 ± 7.7 mm Hg).[18] However, when data from both goal BP groups were pooled and statistical adjustments made, each 1–mm Hg increase in mean arterial pressure was associated with a significant 35% increase in the risk of hospitalization for cardiovascular disease.[18] This was the primary evidence on which JNC VI recommended a target BP of less than 125/75 mm Hg for patients with more than 1 gram of proteinuria per day.

The most recent data about an appropriate BP goal in nondiabetic patients with renal disease comes from the African American Study on Kidney disease and hypertension (AASK).[19] The first randomization in this study was to different antihypertensive drugs, of which amlodipine was found to be the poorest choice. Those randomized to the lowest BP goal (mean arterial pressure < 92 or BP < 125/75 mm Hg) did not fare better than those at a more modest goal in terms of losing renal function.

Another trial in the United Kingdom examined the effects in type 2 diabetics of different initial antihypertensive drug therapy (captopril vs. atenolol), as well as two different BP goals. While patients randomized to atenolol vs. captopril had similar outcomes,[20] the 758 patients randomized to the lower BP goal fared much better than the 390 randomized to the higher goal. They had 24% fewer diabetes-related endpoints (the primary endpoint, which included amputations, $P = 0.0046$), 32% fewer deaths related to diabetes ($P = 0.019$), 44% reduction in stroke ($P = 0.013$), and 37% reduction in microvascular endpoints (including retinal hemorrhages requiring photocoagulation, $P = 0.0092$). These data strongly support the clinical benefit associated with a lower-than-usual BP for diabetic hypertensives. The absolute numbers, however, must be interpreted in the context of the time the study was done. In 1985 in the United Kingdom, a BP target of 150/85 mm Hg was considered "tight BP control." Then, as now, most of Europe considered the threshold for BP treatment to be 160/95 mm Hg. The unfortunate individuals who were randomized to "less tight" BP control were recommended to achieve less than 180/105 mm Hg. The physicians and patients in this study achieved lower BPs than the (now alarming) targets set for them, however; they achieved a mean BP during follow-up of 144/82 mm Hg and 154/87 mm Hg in the two randomized groups. Although it is difficult to be certain of the generalizability of these conclusions from the United Kingdom to the United States, the results can be manipulated to support the JNC VI recommendation for American diabetics. One must first assume that Americans with uncomplicated hypertension should have a BP target of less than 140/90 mm Hg (which has been recommended since JNC I) and then accept that the UKPDS 38 data show a significant benefit in type 2 diabetics treated to a lower goal. If the achieved BP difference (10/5 mm Hg) in the two groups in UKPDS 38 is subtracted from the usual target BP (140/90 mm Hg), one gets exactly the recommendation from JNC VI for diabetics' BP target (i.e., 130/85 mm Hg).

HOT[21] included 1501 diabetic patients who were randomized (in the larger trial discussed later) to one of three diastolic BP goals: 80 mm Hg or less, 85 mm Hg or less, or 90 mm Hg or less. After 3.8 years of follow-up, there was a 51% reduction in the primary cardiovascular endpoints for those randomized to a diastolic BP of 80 mm Hg or less compared with those with diastolic BP target of 90 mm Hg or less (Fig. 2). Even when other endpoints were compared (e.g., silent myocardial infarction, car-

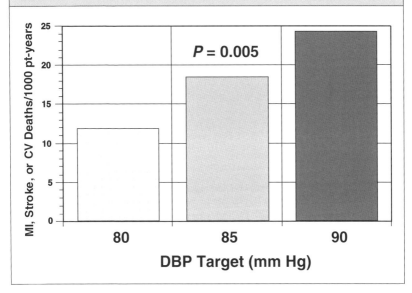

Figure 2. Results of intent-to-treat analysis of major cardiovascular events (the primary endpoint) for the 1501 diabetic subjects enrolled in the Hypertension Optimal Treatment (HOT) Study. The subjects randomized to the lowest diastolic blood pressure (DBP) goal ($\leq$ 80 mm Hg) had a 51% reduction in the incidence of myocardial infarction (MI), stroke, or cardiovascular death. (Adapted from Hansson L, Zanchetti A, Julius S, et al., on behalf of the HOT Study Group. Effects of intensive blood pressure lowering and low-dose aspirin in patients with hypertension: principal results of the Hypertension Optimal Treatment (HOT) randomised trial. Lancet 1998, 351:1755–1762.)

diovascular death), the group randomized to the lowest diastolic BP had the best prognosis. These data have caused the American Diabetes Association,[22] National Kidney Foundation,[23] British Hypertension Society,[24] and Canadian Consensus Conference on Hypertension to recommend the BP target of less than 130/80 mm Hg for *all* diabetics (see Table 1).

HOT[21] was organized primarily to address the question of whether a lower BP goal would increase the risk of cardiovascular events (the so-called "J-shaped curve"). Many patients and physicians are aware that very low BPs are associated not only with many symptoms but also with a higher risk of cardiovascular events (in several epidemiologic and some cohort studies). This risk associated with achieving a very low BP during treatment is often taught to medical students in the context of hypertensive emergencies, in which the major contributor to adverse outcomes is decreasing the BP too low too quickly.

In the HOT study, 18790 hypertensive patients from 26 countries were enrolled and randomized to one of three different diastolic BP targets: 80 mm Hg or less, 85 mm Hg or less, or 90 mm Hg or less.[21] After 3.8 years of follow-up, there were only small differences (~2 mm Hg, rather than the expected 5 mm Hg) between the achieved BPs. However, decreases from baseline BP (during placebo run-in: 169.6/105.4 mm Hg) were impressive: 29.9/24.3, 28.0/22.3, or 26.2/20.3 mm Hg, respectively, in the three randomized groups. The optimum BP to prevent the major cardiovascular events was 138.5/82.6 mm Hg, and there was no significant increase in risk with lower BPs. Because these results were somewhat confounded by the difficulty in keeping BPs at the original target and because many patients randomized to the highest goal BP actually achieved a much lower BP during the study, the results of the "actual on-treatment" analyses are of great interest (Fig. 3).[25] These results confirm and extend the graphs of the primary publication,[21] but their interpretation is open to question. Even if it is true that a lower BP target is safe, many economists and policymakers have argued that it is wasteful of scarce medical resources (i.e., drugs and doctor visits) to treat to a lower BP goal than needed to minimize cardiovascular events.[26] These arguments support the original recommendations of America's

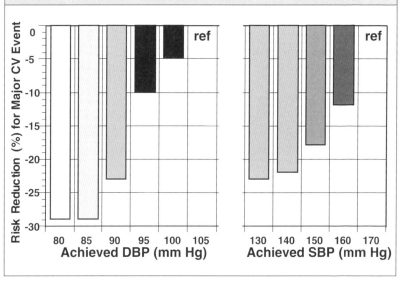

Figure 3. Major cardiovascular event risk reduction in the Hypertension Optimal Treatment (HOT) Study, according to average level of achieved diastolic blood pressure (DBP, *left panel,* relative to 105 mm Hg) and systolic blood pressure (SBP, *right panel,* relative to 170 mm Hg). (Adapted from Hansson L: The Hypertension Optimal Treatment study and the importance of lowering blood pressure. J Hypertension 1999, 17(suppl 1):9–13.)

Figure 4. Results of a meta-analysis of all three clinical trials comparing a more intensive with a less intensive regimen for treating hypertension. The more intensive regimen (the definition of which varies across studies) was significantly better at preventing major cardiovascular events, stroke, and coronary heart disease events but showed only a nonsignificant trend toward prevention of heart failure, cardiovascular mortality, or all-cause mortality. The point estimates are given as *vertical bars* and in Arabic numbers to the right of the vertical bars; the limits of the *horizontal bars* are the 95% confidence intervals for the effect size in the meta-analysis. (Adapted from Blood Pressure Lowering Treatment Trialists' Collaborative: Effects of ACE-inhibitors, calcium antagonists, and other blood-pressure-lowering drugs: Results of prospectively designed overviews of randomised trials. Lancet 2000, 356:1955–1964.)

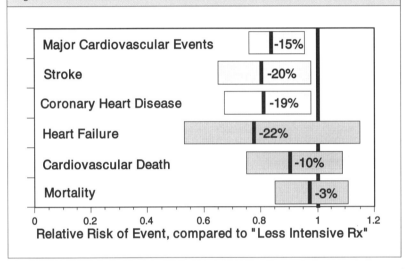

Expert Panels on hypertension since 1977 and suggest that less than 140/90 mm Hg is an appropriate goal BP for all patients with uncomplicated hypertension.

Data from all three clinical trials in hypertension that studied a more- or less-intensive treatment regimen were pooled in a meta-analysis by the BP Lowering Treatment Trialists' Collaborative[5] (Fig. 4). The more intensive regimen was better at preventing stroke (20%), coronary heart disease (19%), and major cardiovascular events (15%). These conclusions may change as more large studies are completed and after data from them are included in the Trialists' next meta-analysis.

Economic Benefits of Achieving these Targets

According to the American Heart Association, approximately $50.3 billion will be spent on hypertension in the United States in 2003.[27] This sum must be compared with the $351.8 billion that will be spent on cardiovascular disease, of which about 77% pays for indirect costs and hospital and nursing home admissions. Because hypertension-related adverse events (i.e., stroke, heart attack, heart failure, and renal failure[28]) are so expensive (see Table 2), it has been estimated that improving the hypertension control rates from the current 31% to even 50% (as recommended in *Healthy People 2000*, but lower the 60% recommended by *Healthy People 2010*), would result in a $120 billion savings to the national treasury. Perhaps the easiest way to do this is to be more judicious in the use of antihypertensive drug therapy ($17.8 billion in 2003). Put another way, by more effectively using our antihypertensive drugs, the return on investment would be about 750%, which is far better than the annual return of nearly every stock or other investment in the marketplace.

Two recent publications go beyond economic speculation about what might happen if BP were better controlled. One of these was a formal cost-effectiveness analysis of the UKPDS study. Despite the fact that the diabetics in the tight BP control group had higher costs (about double for antihypertensive drugs but about the same for healthcare provider visits), they had an overall cost savings of £1049 per year of extended life without diabetic complications and an overall cost savings of £720 per year of extended life.[29] Despite changing many baseline assumptions in sensitivity analyses, the conclusion remained that more intensive treatment of hypertension in type 2 diabetics more than paid for itself by decreasing hospital costs and costs associated with eye and renal complications of diabetes. We reached a very similar conclusion using epidemiologic data from the entire United States, coupled with recent clinical trial results. For American diabetics beginning at age 60 years, a BP goal of less than 130/85 mm Hg saves $3070 per year of extended life as compared with leaving the BP target at less than 140/90 mm Hg.[30] These economic benefits are again realized because the higher cost of treatment (≤ $414 annually) is more than offset in the next

TABLE 2. HCFA Estimates of Cost of Hypertension-related Adverse Clinical Events, 2001		
Event	**Direct Medical Cost/Event**	**Annual Treatment Cost**
Renal transplant	Variable	$49,096
Dialysis	Variable	$45,286
Nonfatal myocardial infarction	$11,273	$9600
Nonfatal stroke	$5955	$26,100 (based on $40,000/year in nursing home)
Heart failure	$5501	$10,500

Data adapted from the American Heart Association's Heart & Stroke Facts, Statistical Supplement[27] and the 2001 Report of the United States Renal Data Systems[28]

few years by savings on stroke, heart failure, heart attack, and end-stage renal disease (ESRD).

Who "Wins" When Blood Pressure Targets Are Achieved?

Achieving BP targets should be seen as a true "win-win-win" situation. The patient benefits from a longer life, free of cardiovascular complications that would have occurred earlier if BP had not been controlled. The physician benefits from the gratitude of the patient; increased self-esteem in good performance; and increased clinical revenue from the increased number of visits, both to intensify therapy and beyond the time that the patient would have otherwise succumbed to the cardiovascular event. Additionally, the health care plan benefits because overall money is saved when BP is controlled, with less hospitalization, nursing home placement, and ESRD. Even apart from the human costs, all of these hypertension-related adverse events are vastly more expensive than effectively treating patients with hypertension, particularly when the patient is at high absolute cardiovascular risk (e.g., by virtue of age or comorbidities).

Key Points

- ∞ The goal BP for patients with uncomplicated hypertension is less than 140/90 mm Hg, but for those with diabetes or renal impairment it should be lower (< 130/80 mm Hg).
- ∞ Although only 27.4% of American hypertensives were below goal in 1991 to 1994, recent public health initiatives have slightly improved this poor showing to 31%.
- ∞ Achieving goal BP is important for patients, who will suffer fewer cardiovascular and renal problems than if their BP remained uncontrolled.
- ∞ Physicians benefit from achieving goal BP in their patients, and this is being monitored in many managed care plans by chart audits in doctors' offices.
- ∞ Health care plans will benefit from patients' achieving goal BP because it will save money overall.
- ∞ The increase in pharmacy fees and physician visits will likely be offset by fewer expensive hospitalizations, nursing home admissions, and dialysis and renal transplantation.
- ∞ Treating to goal BP is important because it has tangible (human, clinical, and economic) benefits for all involved parties in health care.

References

1. The sixth report of the Joint National Committee on Prevention, Detection, Evaluation, and Treatment of High Blood Pressure (JNC VI): Arch Intern Med 1997, 157:2413–2446.

2. Veterans Administration Cooperative Study Group on Antihypertensive Agents: Effects of treatment on morbidity in hypertension: Results in patients with diastolic blood pressure averaging 115 through 129 mm Hg. JAMA 1967, 202:1028–1034.

3. Moser M, Hebert PR: Prevention of disease progression, left ventricular hypertrophy and congestive heart failure in hypertension treatment trials. J Am Coll Cardiol 1996, 27:1214–1218.

4. Psaty BM, Smith NL, Siscovick DS, et al. Health outcomes associated with antihypertensive therapies used as first-line agents: A systematic review and meta-analysis. JAMA 1997, 277:739–745.

5. Blood Pressure Lowering Treatment Trialists' Collaborative: Effects of ACE-inhibitors, calcium antagonists, and other blood-pressure-lowering drugs: Results of prospectively designed overviews of randomised trials. Lancet 2000, 356:1955–1964.

6. Hoyert DL, Kochanek KD, Murphy SL: Deaths: final data for 1997. National Vital Statistics Reports, 47, June 30, 1999.

7. Burt VL, Whelton PK, Roccella EJ, et al: Prevalence of hypertension in the U.S. adult population: Results from the Third National Health and Nutritional Examination survey, 1988–91. Hypertension 1995, 25:305–313.

8. Hyman DJ, Pavlik VN: Characteristics of patients with uncontrolled hypertension in the United States. N Engl J Med 2001, 345:479–486.

9. Jones JK, Gorkin L, Lian JF, et al: Discontinuation of and changes in treatment after start of new courses of antihypertensive drugs: A study of a United Kingdom population. BMJ 1995, 311:293–296.

10. Bloom BS: Continuation of initial antihypertensive medication after one year of therapy. Clin Ther 1998, 20:671–681.

11. Berlowitz DR, Ash AS, Hickey C, et al: Inadequate management of blood pressure in a hypertensive population. N Engl J Med 1998, 339:1967–1963.

12. Institute of Medicine: Healthy People 2000: Citizens Chart the Course. Washington, DC: National Academy Press, 1990.

13. Staessen JA, Gasowski J, Wang JG, et al: Risks of untreated and treated isolated systolic hypertension in the elderly: meta-analysis of outcome trials. Lancet 2000, 355:865–872.

14. Elliott WJ: Glucose and cholesterol elevations during thiazide therapy: intention-to-treat vs. actual on-therapy experience. Am J Med 1995, 99:261–269.

15. Gibaldi M, Sullivan S: Intention-to-treat analysis in randomized clinical trials: who gets counted? J Clin Pharmacol 1997, 37:667–672.

16. Perry HM Jr, Davis BR, Price TR, et al: Effect of treating isolated systolic hypertension on the risk of developing various types and subtypes of stroke: The Systolic Hypertension in the Elderly Program (SHEP). JAMA 2000, 284:465–471.

17. Klahr S, Levey AS, Beck GJ, et al: The effects of dietary protein restriction and blood-pressure control on the progression of chronic renal disease: modification of Diet in Renal Disease Study Group. N Engl J Med 1994, 330:877–884.

18. Lazarus JM, Bourgoignie JJ, Buckalew VM, et al., for the Modification of Diet in Renal Disease Study Group: Achievement and safety of a low blood pressure goal in chronic renal disease: the Modification of Diet in Renal Disease Study Group. Hypertension 1997, 29:641–650.

19. Agodoa LY, Appel L, Bakris GL, et al: African American Study of Kidney Disease and Hypertension (AASK) Study Group: Effect of ramipril vs. amlodipine on renal out-

comes in hypertensive nephrosclerosis: a randomized controlled trial. JAMA 2001, 285:2719–2728. (*See also reference 32*)

20. Turner R, Holman R, Stratton I, et al., for the United Kingdom Prospective Diabetes Study Group: Tight blood pressure control and risk of macrovascular and microvascular complications in type 2 diabetes: UKPDS 38. BMJ 1998, 317:707–713.

21. Hansson L, Zanchetti A, Julius S, et al., on behalf of the HOT Study Group. Effects of intensive blood pressure lowering and low-dose aspirin in patients with hypertension: principal results of the Hypertension Optimal Treatment (HOT) randomised trial. Lancet 1998, 351:1755–1762.

22. American Diabetes Association: Clinical practice recommendations, 2001. Diabetes Care 2001, 24(suppl. 1):1–133. (*See also reference 33*)

23. Bakris GL, Williams M, Dworkin L, et al., for the National Kidney Foundation Hypertension and Diabetes Executive Committee Working Group: Preserving renal function in adults with hypertension and diabetes: a consensus approach. Am J Kidney Dis 2000, 35:646–661.

24. Ramsay LE, Williams B, Johnston GD, et al: British Hypertension Society Guidelines for hypertension management 1999: summary. Br Med J 1999, 319:630–635.

25. Hansson L: The Hypertension Optimal Treatment study and the importance of lowering blood pressure. J Hypertension 1999, 17(suppl 1):9–13.

26. Kaplan N: J-curve not burned off by HOT Study: Hypertension Optimal Treatment [editorial]. Lancet 1998, 351:1748–1749.

27. American Heart Association's Heart & Stroke Facts, Statistical Supplement. Dallas, TX: American Heart Association, 2003, p. 40.

28. United States Renal Data System: USRDS 2001 Annual Data Report. National Institutes of Health, National Institute of Diabetes and Digestive and Kidney Disease, Bethesda, MD, July 31, 2001. Also found on the Internet at: www.usrds.org/adr_2001.htm, accessed 06 SEP 01 at 19:28 CDT.

29. Raikou M, Gray A, Briggs A, et al: Cost-effectiveness analysis of improved blood pressure control in hypertensive patients with type 2 diabetes: UKPDS 40. U.K. Prospective Diabetes Study Group. Br Med J 1998, 317:720–726.

30. Elliott WJ, Weir DR, Black HR: Cost-effectiveness of the lower treatment goal (of JNC VI) in hypertensive diabetics. Arch Intern Med 2000, 160:1277–1283.

31. Conlin PR, Gerth WC, Fox J, et al: Four-year persistence patterns among patients initiating therapy with the angiotensin II receptor antagonist losartan versus other antihypertensive drug classes. Clin Ther 2001, 23:1999–2010.

32. Wright JT Jr., Bakris GL, Greene T, et al: Effect of blood pressure lowering and antihypertensive drug class on progression of hypertensive kidney disease: Results from the AASK Trial. JAMA 2002, 288:2421–2431.

33. American Diabetes Association: Treatment of hypertension in adults with diabetes. Diabetes Care 2003, 26 (Suppl 1):S80–S83.

High Normal Blood Pressure

Stevo Julius M.D., Sc.D.

chapter

11

Definition

High normal blood pressure (HNBP) is the gray zone between clearly normal and clearly elevated BP levels. The Joint National Committee VI[1] defines HNBP as systolic BP between 130 and 139 mmHg or diastolic BP between 85 and 89 mmHg. In a previous report, the Ann Arbor group[2] used the term "borderline hypertension" to describe a similar population of subjects who had repeated BP determinations on three different days and whose BP readings exceeded 140 or 90 mmHg at least once and was below those values at least once. The average BP in these individuals was 145.5/87.8 mmHg, and their self-determined BP at home was 131.1/84.2 mmHg.

Both definitions have limitations. The word "normal" in the JNC definition is a misnomer because the cardiovascular prognosis of these patients is poorer than in subjects with optimal or ideal BP readings. The term "hypertension" in "borderline hypertension" has the potential of negatively affecting an individual's employment and insurance classifications. Probably the most appropriate and innocuous term for these subjects is "borderline BP elevation," a term that proved too lengthy to be accepted in clinical practice. The latest term, "pre-hypertension," coined in the recent JNC VII report, encompasses BP values of 120–139/80–89, or between optimal and stage 1 hypertension. Regardless of the specific term and BP values, the clinical considerations are generally similar.

Clinical Importance

Epidemiologic studies show that even in the normotensive range, with the exception of extremely low BP values, a higher BP reading is associated with a poorer prognosis. This association is linear and because that line does not provide a convenient break point to separate sick from normal people, every BP classification is arbitrary. However, the definition of hypertension can be defended on the basis of the BP distribution

119

in the general population (the cut point of ≥ 140 or 90 mmHg is close to 2 standard deviations above the population mean BP) and on the basis of excessive cardiovascular mortality (relative risk for men adjusted for other known risk factors of 2.33, i.e., 130% excessive risk compared with "optimal" (< 120 and < 80 mmHg) BP.[3]

Why then bother with defining yet another category of marginal BP elevation? There are four reasons:

- Cardiovascular prognosis
- Abnormal cardiovascular physiology and metabolism
- Public health impact
- Nonlinearity of future BP and mortality trends

Cardiovascular Prognosis

Figure 1 is adapted from the impressive follow-up of a large cohort of men ($n = 347,978$) screened for the MRFIT study.[3] In the short term, the cardiovascular prognosis in the two groups was not much different. But with passage of time, the group with HNBP accrued substantially more coronary heart disease (CHD) deaths than the optimal BP group. Cumulative percentage rates for strokes in the same population were much lower in absolute terms, but the difference between the two groups after 15 years of observation was dramatic (0.24 for HNBP vs. 0.1 for optimal BP, a relative excess risk of 140%). Even when the comparison is made

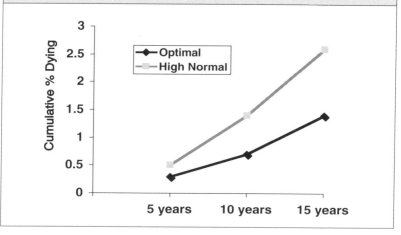

Figure 1. A comparison of the cumulative incidence of CHD deaths in a group with optimal BP and in subjects with high normal BP. Data from persons screened for the MRFIT study. (Adapted from Neaton JD, Kuller L, Stamler J, et al: Impact of systolic and diastolic blood pressure on cardiovascular mortality. In Laragh JH, Brenner BM (eds): Hypertension: Pathophysiology, Diagnosis and Management, 2nd ed. New York, Raven Press, 1995, pp 127–144.)

between the HNBP and the normal but not optimal BP group (120–129/80–84 mmHg), cardiovascular mortality in the HNBP group is excessive (2.6% vs. 1.9%).

Abnormal Cardiovascular Physiology and Metabolic Abnormalities

Besides a slightly higher BP, subjects with HNBP exhibit a number of other physiologic abnormalities. In enumerating these abnormalities, we will rely on our previous work, which used the definition of borderline hypertension instead of the contemporary definition of HNBP. As shown above, the average BP of the borderline group is rather similar to the BP range presently defined as HNBP.

Subjects with borderline hypertension consistently show signs of a hyperkinetic circulation: their heart rates are faster and cardiac outputs higher than control subjects.[4] An elevation of heart rate and cardiac output was found also in the Tecumseh epidemiologic study among subjects who were unaware of their slight BP elevation.[5] The faster heart rate is associated with higher plasma norepinephrine[5,6] and renin[6] values. It is frequently assumed that the elevated heart rate and BP in these individuals may be a transient response to the stress of examination. However, the Tecumseh study records[5] show that individuals who exhibited a fast heart rate in the third decade of life had higher BP readings and tachycardia as children and young adults. Thus, a faster heart rate seems to be a lifelong characteristic of these subjects. Furthermore, a fast heart rate is a strong predictor of future sustained hypertension.[7–10] It is hard to conceive of a mechanism whereby a transient tachycardia might have such a long-term effect.

The association of the hyperkinetic circulation and elevated plasma norepinephrine level strongly suggest that both the higher BP and hyperkinetic circulation might be consequences of sympathetic overactivity in subjects with HNBP. This concept is supported by experimental evidence that the faster heart rate and cardiac output are normalized after a blockade of cardiac autonomic nervous system receptors. Moreover, complete blockade of parasympathetic as well as sympathetic alpha and beta receptors abolish the BP elevation in these subjects.[6] The elevation of plasma renin can be explained in the context of sympathetic overactivity: stimulation of renal beta adrenoreceptors increases renin secretion. Increased hematocrit and decrease plasma volume values have been described in patients with borderline hypertension.[11] These abnormalities can also be attributed to the enhanced sympathetic tone. Infusion of alpha-adrenergic agonists elicits an instant decrease of plasma volume in normal volunteers[12] because of an enhanced constriction of postcapillary venules, which, in turn, increases the capillary filtration pressure.

The enhanced sympathetic tone in men (similar work in women has not been performed) with marginal BP elevation might be a primary[13] or a secondary phenomenon related to metabolic abnormalities.[14] However, within the context of this presentation, the evidence of a widespread sympathetic overactivity is presented only to underscore that in HNBP, a slightly higher BP is associated with multiple other physiologic abnormalities. Thus, the state of HNBP is not just a matter of a *different quantity* of BP but also a state of *qualitative* changes in underlying pathophysiology.

Subjects with HNBP are also distinctly different from normotensive individuals in regards to a very important anthropometric characteristic: body weight. In all studies published by the Ann Arbor group, subjects with borderline hypertension were between 22[2] and 27[15] pounds heavier than control subjects. Because their height was normal, the higher body weight in subjects with borderline hypertension was entirely caused by being overweight. In the Tecumseh study, the average percentage over ideal body weight in borderline hypertension was 30.1% compared with 13.6% in the normotensive population. The waist-to-hip ratio, plasma insulin, glucose, insulin-to-glucose ratio, cholesterol, and triglyceride levels were also significantly elevated in patients with borderline hypertension; high-density lipoprotein cholesterol was significantly lower.[15]

Needless to say, all metabolic abnormalities cited above aggravate the coronary risk in subjects with HNBP. Although less well appreciated, elevated hematocrit level[16,17] and tachycardia[18] are also strong coronary risk factors. This early constellation of an excessive nonhypertensive risk combined with mild BP elevation is clinically relevant and will be discussed later.

Public Health Impact

HNBP is a very frequent condition. Among 347,978 subjects screened for the MRFIT study,[3] 79,308 (22.8%) had high normal systolic BP values. The relative risk of coronary deaths was 66% higher than in subjects whose systolic BP was < 120 mmHg (optimal blood pressure, according to JNC VI). Whereas this risk is much less than the 242% excess risk seen in patients with stage 2 systolic hypertension (systolic BP, 160–179 mmHg), only 13,321 subjects followed in the MRFIT cohort had stage 2 readings. As Figure 2 shows, among people with higher BP values after 15 years of observation, a much larger portion of total cumulative coronary deaths accrued in the category of HNBP than in stage 2 hypertension. In other words, an individual's risk is much higher in stage 2 systolic hypertension than in the HNBP group. Because of a large number of cases with marginal BP elevation, the impact of HNBP on public health is larger.

Figure 2. Cumulative coronary heart disease deaths over 15 years among men with HNBP screened for the MRFIT study. Note that the impact of 9-mmHg BP range in the HNBP group is only 29% below the impact of the 19-mmHg BP range in the stage 1 hypertension. The deaths in the HNBP group far exceed the deaths seen in all subjects whose BP was ≥ 160 mmHg. (Adapted from Neaton JD, Kuller L, Stamler J, et al: Impact of systolic and diastolic blood pressure on cardiovascular mortality. In Laragh JH, Brenner BM (eds): Hypertension: Pathophysiology, Diagnosis and Management, 2nd ed. New York, Raven Press, 1995, pp 127–144.)

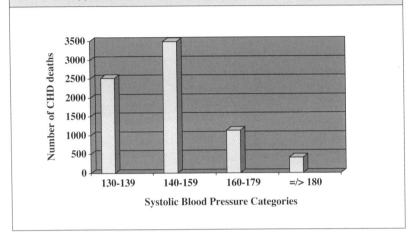

Nonlinearity of Blood Pressure and Mortality Trends

Patients with hypertension have higher BP values throughout their entire lifespan. We analyzed previous records of subjects who, at an average age of 31 years, were either deemed normotensive or having borderline hypertension.[16] Subjects with borderline hypertension had significantly higher BP readings already at age 6 years and again at age 21 years. However, the BP difference between the two groups increased dramatically between ages 21 and 31 years because of a steep increase of the diastolic BP (from ~ 75 mmHg to ~ 94 mmHg) in patients with borderline hypertension. In other words, BP in the borderline hypertension group "took off" sometime in the third decade of life and "crossed the border" in the fourth decade. Whereas longitudinal data in untreated patients are hard to come by, there is no doubt that if it were left unmanaged, hypertension would feed on itself and the BP would continue to increase in a precipitous fashion. This self-acceleration of hypertension is most likely caused by an enhanced vasoconstriction in patients with hypertension. Infusion of norepinephrine into brachial arteries[19,20] and of angiotensin 2[21] elicits an excessive increase of vascular resistance in stage 1 hypertension. Because an excessive response was observed both to norepinephrine and angiotensin, this nonspecific abnormality is more likely related to altered properties of arteries than to a hypersensitivity of vascular receptors. The underlying mechanism of arteriolar hyperresponsiveness in hypertension reflects in part vascular hypertrophy that evolves since the early stages of hypertension. An abnormal compensatory vasodilation, possibly related to endothelial dysfunction, may also play a role in the enhanced vascular responses in the early phases of hypertension.

Among patients with HNBP (see Fig. 1), the increase in cumulative CHD mortality was moderate between 5 and 10 years of observation; however, between 10 and 15 years, the increase was quite steep. This nonlinear acceleration of mortality might partly reflect the expected increase of BP in untreated patients with hypertension. However, a prolonged BP elevation also negatively affects the function and structure of the cardiovascular system, a process that is further accelerated by metabolic and neurohormonal abnormalities associated with HNBP (Fig. 3). Whereas the figure shows the nonlinearity of cardiovascular events, it also differentiates an early phase of reversibility of underlying pathology versus a later irreversible phase. Treatment in that later phase can positively affect cardiovascular *events* but cannot fully reverse the underlying *vascular damage*. These differences in cardiovascular physiology and pathology should affect the clinical management of patients with hypertension.

Clinical Implications

In many ways, the treatment of hypertension is an ideal topic for investigation. The consequences of high BP (e.g., strokes, myocardial infarctions, heart failure, sudden deaths, and renal failure) are easily enumerated, and the effect of the treatment on BP can be determined with a reasonable precision. Consequently, the treatment of essential hypertension is rooted in the evidence from numerous well-designed studies showing how many "hard endpoints" can be avoided by a certain degree of BP reduction. For practical reasons, such trials must be finished within a reasonable time, usually 5 to 6 years of follow-up after the enrollment into the study. To show the effect of treatment, it is necessary to enroll patients in whom one can expect a sufficient number of endpoints within that time frame. Consequently, almost all trials have been performed in patients in whom hypertension is complicated by signs of cardiovascular disease or by high-risk factors for atherosclerosis. Even studies investigating "mild hypertension" have been performed in elderly patients with somewhat higher risk[21] or had a design that beclouded the interpretation[22] of findings.

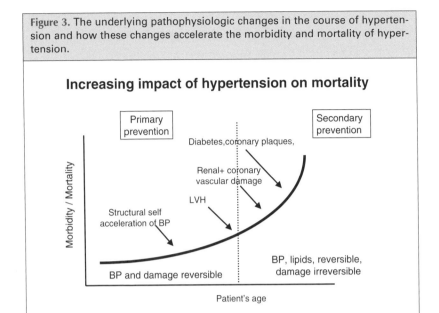

Figure 3. The underlying pathophysiologic changes in the course of hypertension and how these changes accelerate the morbidity and mortality of hypertension.

Nevertheless, the JNC VI[1] correctly identified HNBP as an area of interest and developed an acceptable management scheme for such patients. The committee suggested that patients with HNBP be stratified by the presence or absence of risk factors. Only patients with diabetes, heart failure, or renal insufficiency are selected for antihypertensive treatment. In all other patients with HNBP, lifestyle modification is suggested, and the patients should be recalled annually for repeat BP measurement. This scheme provides a good beginning. However, it does not evaluate the efficacy of lifestyle management and does not provide a good scheme for BP determination.

Regarding lifestyle modification, research has provided the proof of principle that a **rigorous DASH diet**[23] can effectively lower BP. However, in this particular study, a large supportive staff of physicians and a dietitian in addition to in-hospital food preparation were required to achieve a relatively short-term BP lowering. Whereas the DASH diet sets a good goal for individual patients, the efficacy of this diet as a measure to manage HNBP in the general population has not been evaluated.

Weight loss is clearly associated with significant BP reduction and should be suggested as a good goal for individual patients. However, long-term weight reduction is hard to achieve, and most patients eventually regain the weight.[24]

Physical exercise is probably the most practical measure for longer-term BP control. Although the topic has not been specifically investigated in patients with HNBP, it has been demonstrated that systematic physical exercise reduces BP in patients with hypertension.[25] Surprisingly, no drastic measures are required to garner the full BP-lowering effect of exercise. Exercising three times a week for half an hour is sufficient. All types of dynamic (as opposed to isometric) exercise are equally effective as long as they steadily increase the subject's heart rate to around 130 bpm throughout the exercise periods. In addition to lowering BP, physical exercise is also helpful in improving insulin sensitivity and glucose control. Finally, regular physical exercise is an important component in efforts to reduce body weight.

The JNC VI suggests an annual BP follow-up in patients who have not been selected for treatment; however, in my opinion, this is inadequate. Sporadic BP measurements are not sufficient to evaluate time-related BP trends in individual patients. Thus, if a patient at the annual reexamination shows high BP values, then further BP measurements at different days are required to determine whether the BP is constantly elevated. We find that self-measurement of BP at home is practical way to obtain good average BP readings in patients with marginal hypertension.[2] Self-measurement BP cuffs are now widely available, and obtaining repeated BP readings (i.e., twice a day over 7 days) before clinic visits is very helpful in assessing the BP trends in an individual. Annual measurements of plasma lipids and blood glucose and, when indicated, usage of lipid-lowering drugs must also be components of the management of patients with HNBP.

Finally, if BP treatment is indicated, diuretic or beta-blocking agents should not be the first drugs of choice in patients with HNBP because both negatively affect the glucose and lipid metabolism. It is important to point out that the ALLHAT study investigated patients with complicated hypertension, and its results are not applicable to milder forms of hypertension.[26] In complicated hypertension, because of the high risk of BP-related cardiovascular events, lowering BP outweighs all other considerations. However, it is important to note that blood glucose levels in the diuretic arm of the ALLHAT study were significantly elevated and that this group showed a significant excess of new-onset diabetes. On the other hand, angiotensin-converting enzyme inhibitors[27] and angiotensin II receptor antagonists[28] decrease the rates of new-onset diabetes. It would make absolutely no sense to treat a patient with HNBP with diuretics or beta-blocking agents and trade the BP improvement for a substantial long-term worsening of the metabolic profile.

References

1. Joint National Committee on Prevention, Detection, Evaluation, and Treatment of High Blood Pressure: The Sixth Report of the Joint National Committee on Prevention, Detection, Evaluation, and Treatment of High Blood Pressure. Arch Intern Med 157:2413–2446, 1997.
2. Julius S, Ellis CN, Pascual AV, et al: Home blood pressure determination: Value in borderline ("labile") hypertension. JAMA 229:663–666, 1974.
3. Neaton JD, Kuller L, Stamler J, et al: Impact of systolic and diastolic blood pressure on cardiovascular mortality. In Laragh JH, Brenner BM (eds): Hypertension: Pathophysiology, Diagnosis and Management, 2nd ed. New York, Raven Press, 1995, pp 127–144.
4. Julius S, Pascual AV, London R: Role of parasympathetic inhibition in the hyperkinetic type of borderline hypertension. Circulation 44:413–418, 1971.
5. Julius S, Krause L, Schork NJ, Mejia AD, et al: Hyperkinetic borderline hypertension in Tecumseh, Michigan. J Hypertension 9:77–84, 1991.
6. Esler M, Julius S, Zweifler A, et al: Mild high-renin essential hypertension: Neurogenic human hypertension? N Engl J Med 296:405–411, 1977.
7. Levy RL, White PD, Stroud WD, Hillman CC: Transient tachycardia: prognostic significance alone and in association with transient hypertension. JAMA 129:585–588, 1945.
8. Kahn HA, Medalie JH, Neufeld HN: The incidence of hypertension and associated factors: the Israel ischemic heart disease study. Am Heart J 84:171–182, 1972.
9. Stamler J, Berkson DM, Dyer A, et al: Relationship of multiple variables to blood pressure—findings from four Chicago epidemiologic studies. In Paul O (ed): Epidemiology and Control of Hypertension. Miami, Symposia Specialists, 1975, pp 307–352.
10. Garrison RJ, Kannel WB, Stokes J III: Incidence and precursors of hypertension in young adults. Prev Med 16:235–251, 1987.
11. Julius S, Pascual A, Reilly K, London R: Abnormalities of plasma volume in borderline hypertension. Arch Intern Med 127:116–119, 1971.
12. Cohn JN: Relationship of plasma volume changes to resistance and capacitance vessel effects of sympathomimetic amines and angiotensin in man. Clin Sci 30:267–278, 1966.
13. Julius S: Sympathetic hyperactivity and coronary risk in hypertension. Hypertension 21:886–893, 1993.
14. Landsberg L: Diet, obesity and hypertension: An hypothesis involving insulin, the sympathetic nervous system, and adaptive thermogenesis. Quarterly J Med 61:1081–1090, 1986.
15. Julius S, Jamerson K, Mejia A, et al: The association of borderline hypertension with target organ changes and higher coronary risk. Tecumseh Blood Pressure Study. JAMA 264:354–358, 1990.
16. Cirillo M, Laurenzi M, Trevisan M, Stamler J: Hematocrit, blood pressure, and hypertension. The Gubbio Population Study. Hypertension 20:319–326, 1992.
17. Sorlie PD, Garcia-Palmieri MR, Costas R Jr., Havlik RJ: Hematocrit and risk of coronary heart disease: The Puerto Rico Health Program. Am Heart J 101:456–461, 1981.
18. Palatini P, Julius S: Heart rate and the cardiovascular risk. J Hypertens 15:1–15, 1997.
19. Sivertsson R, Olander R: Aspects of the nature of the increased vascular resistance and increased "reactivity" to noradrenaline in hypertensive subjects. Life Sci 7(part 1):1291–1297, 1968.

20. Egan B, Panis R, Hinderliter A, et al: Mechanism of increased alpha-adrenergic vaso-constriction in human essential hypertension. J Clin Invest 80:812–817, 1987.

21. Anonymous: The Australian Therapeutic Trial in Mild Hypertension. Lancet 1: 1261–1267, 1980.

22. Hypertension Detection and Follow-up Program Cooperative Group: Five-year findings of the hypertension detection and follow-up program. (JAMA 1979;242:2562–71) JAMA;277(2):157–66, 1997.

23. Vollmer WM, Sacks FM, Ard J, et al: DASH—Sodium Trial Collaborative Research Group: Effects of diet and sodium intake on blood pressure: subgroup analysis of the DASH—sodium trial. Annals of Intern Med 135:1019–1028, 2001.

24. Kassirer JP, Angell M: Losing weight—An ill-fated New Year's Resolution. New Engl J Med 338:52–54, 1998.

25. Puddey IB, Cox K: Exercise lowers blood pressure—sometimes? Or did Pheidippides have hypertension? J Hypertension 13:1229–1233, 1995.

26. Officers and Coordinators for the ALLHAT Collaborative Research Group: Major Outcomes in High-Risk Hypertensive Patients Randomized to Angiotensin-Converting Enzyme Inhibitor or Calcium Channel Blocker vs Diuretic: The Antihypertensive and Lipid-Lowering Treatment to Prevent Heart Attack Trial (ALLHAT) JAMA 288:2981–2997, 2002.

27. Hansson L, Lindholm LH, Niskanen L, et al: for the Captopril Prevention Project (CAPPP) study group: Effect of angiotensin-converting-enzyme inhibition compared with conventional therapy on cardiovascular morbidity and mortality in hypertension: The Captopril Prevention Project randomized trial. Lancet 353: 611–616, 1999.

28. Dahlöf B, Devereux RB, Kjeldsen SE, Julius S, et al: for the LIFE study group: Cardiovascular morbidity and mortality in the Losartan Intervention For Endpoint reduction in hypertension study (LIFE): A randomized trial against atenolol. Lancet 359:996–1003, 2002.

Patient-related Barriers to Hypertension Control

Miyong Kim, R.N., Ph.D.,
Martha Hill, R.N., Ph.D., and
Hwayum Lee, R.N., M.P.H.

Only about half of the individuals diagnosed with high blood pressure (BP) are undergoing treatment, and half of those being treated are not receiving treatment adequate to control their BP. Estimates of controlled BP among identified patients with high BP have typically ranged from 20% to 30% in the United States. Barriers to care and control of cardiovascular risk factors, especially high BP, are well recognized and exist at the patient, provider, and organizational levels. Effective care and control of high BP cannot be achieved in the absence of adequate treatment regimens and compliance with treatment regimen recommendations. In a critical review conducted by Rogers and Bullman in 1995,[10] noncompliance rates with prescribed therapeutic regimens ranged from 30% to 60%, and at least 50% of the patients for whom drugs were prescribed failed to receive full benefit because of inadequate compliance. These high noncompliance rates in high BP treatment have multiple implications at the individual and societal levels. They jeopardize patients' health and well-being, produce suboptimal health outcomes, lead to inefficient use of health resources, and result in costly therapy for the complications of untreated or inadequately treated high BP.

Although the magnitude and impact of the noncompliance with high BP treatment regimens are well recognized, the current literature lacks practical information about patient-related barriers to treatment. It has been recognized that the lack of compliance of patients with their treatment regimen is a clearly multifaceted issue. Along with the traditional barriers related to low socioeconomic status (e.g., income, education, lack of education, time available), individuals' social and cultural background (e.g., attitude, knowledge and beliefs about high BP and health in general) also influence their level of compliance with the recommended HBP treatment regimen. Moreover, an individual's particular characteristics (or predisposing factors) and circumstances can create additional barriers to achieving adequate control of high BP. For example, lifestyle-related risk factors such as smoking, alcohol or illicit drug abuse, sedentary lifestyle, and salty or fast food–dominant diets are all very important factors that influence an individual's level of compliance. Furthermore, for many individuals with high BP, other existing comorbidities such as other chronic illness (e.g., diabetes mellitus, renal disease, asthma) have an impact on the management of their high BP. In addition, their level of health literacy, including effective communication with health care providers as well as accessibility to the health care system and relevant health information are critical elements that affect hypertension control.

Identification of barriers to compliance with high BP care and treatment is essential if targeted strategies to overcome these barriers are to be effective. Successful BP control programs identify and address relevant barriers among target populations and subgroups. This chapter explores the various types of patient-related barriers to hypertension control.

Socioeconomic Barriers

Although adhering to BP treatment recommendations is an undisputedly difficult task for many people, those with low socioeconomic status face relatively more strenuous challenges. The problems they encounter are numerous and complex because these individuals often do not have access to continuous BP care as a result of high levels of unemployment, low educational attainment and income, lack of health insurance, and a feeling of social isolation. Social isolation has also been posited as a significant contributor to noncompliance among 80% of inner-city minorities with uncontrolled hypertension.

Those who face social isolation are less likely to be informed consumers. With access to the Internet, many Americans who have a home computer are able to obtain the breadth of health information desired. However, many inner-city minorities do not have the means to possess computer systems for their homes, and some may not be able to understand the material because of their reading levels. Despite the efforts to improve health literacy, those with low education level and those whose first language is other than English suffer from lack of accessible, easy-to-understand health information.

Lack of accessibility to care is a well-recognized problem that adversely affects BP control. Physical, logistical, structural and economic factors (e.g., inconvenient locations and appointment times, absence of convenient transportation, long waiting times, lack of continuity of providers, follow-up appointments not being made for participants, lack

TABLE 1. Patient-Related Barriers

Low socioeconomic status–related barriers
Lack of access to health care
Lack of access to health-promoting facilities
Lack of access to fresh, healthy foods
Low health literacy
Social isolation

Sociocultural-related barriers
Attitude toward health
Knowledge of high BP
Beliefs in treatment of high BP
Patient–provider communication
Lack of familial or social support
Salty or fast food diet

Predisposing individual–related barriers
Comorbidity (e.g., diabetes mellitus, renal disease, asthma)
Lifestyle-related risk factors (e.g., smoking, alcohol or illicit drug use)
Mental health (e.g., depression)
Life priorities (e.g., family or business responsibilities)
Forgetfulness

of health insurance) have all been shown to be associated with low rates of entry into and continuation in health care and therefore with achieving inadequate BP control.

Studies have shown that less active persons have 30% to 50% greater risk of having high BP and that for those with mild high BP, exercise and weight loss helped in reducing and managing their BP. However, contributing factors such as lack of opportunities (places), time, resources, and motivation limit these individuals from obtaining leisure activities. In addition, low socioeconomic status also plays a role in the availability or affordability of healthy foods. Compared with suburban areas, urban settings have fewer stores that carry fresh fruits and vegetables and meats. Because of these decreased activity options and food choices, it may also decrease the chances for those living in low socioeconomic level to have successful weight loss and management of their high BP.

Sociocultural Barriers

Attitudes, knowledge, and beliefs, including perceptions about the severity or susceptibility of high BP and about the risks and benefits of treatments, are important influences on participation in BP care and adherence to BP treatment. There are significantly different beliefs about the causes and prevention of cardiovascular diseases (CVDs) and different perceptions about HBP care and treatment within and among ethnic groups. Studies comparing health behaviors across several ethnic groups, in particular between African Americans and White Americans, have indicated that the specific attitudes, beliefs, and concerns that are characteristic of these ethnic groups influence BP control. Some frequently cited myths from African American communities include "HBP medication-associated impotence" and "high BP medication addiction." Members of certain ethnic groups that subscribe to a strong fatalistic notion of health have a tendency to believe there is very little they can do to prevent or control any disease, including high BP. Other common misconceptions about the nature of high BP include the belief that high BP must have symptoms; it is acceptable to stop taking the medication when a BP crisis is over (or symptoms subside); high BP is a natural part of the aging process; and high BP medications are toxic and may cause damage to vital organs and expedite the aging process. One of the major barriers for the patients who believe in these myths is the lack of understanding of the nature of high BP and its links to CVD, stroke, and renal complications. Having high BP is often *not* thought of as being "deadly" as having HIV or a tumor; these patients simply do not realize that there are more deaths from coronary heart disease each year than from cancer and AIDS combined. These misconceptions stemming from lack of knowledge clearly belie the seriousness of hypertension and the importance of controlling BP. Patients who were not aware that their target systolic BP should be ≤ 140 mmHg were more likely to have higher BP readings and be less likely to take their medication, adopt healthy lifestyles changes or see their health care providers.

Other factors that stem from various cultural practices may also prevent some ethnic groups from successfully controlling their BP. For example, various ethnic groups have difficulty with physician–patient communication or relationships. Asians, for example, have great respect for their physicians and would rarely question or discuss their care regimen with their care provider because such behavior would be considered rude or impolite. Consequently, some Asian patients who anticipate or experience complications from their medical regimen adjust their medication dosages on their own. They skip doses or take less than the prescribed dose, behaviors that lead to uncontrolled high BP. In addition, some Asians do not have much faith in the "Western" treatment of high BP and may resort to herbal medication or combine Western medication and herbal remedies without any professional consultation. Other ethnic groups, such as African Americans, have reported being wary of the regimens their physicians may prescribe. Their skepticism of the medical system hinders them from visiting physicians until they are symptomatic and very sick, which, in turn, results in the later diagnosis of high BP.

A lack of social support from family and friends is another major factor associated with uncontrolled high BP and with low rates of awareness and adherence to treatment recommendations. Many socioeconomically disadvantaged groups or individuals, especially those who reside in urban settings, live by themselves without an adequate level of social support or social integration. Social integration, social support, and material resources, all measures of social ties, have been associated with more positive health status and better control of high BP. Researchers suggest that socially isolated individuals often experience real or perceived barriers to health care access and are probably less likely to communicate with health care professionals.

Another important cultural influence on BP management may be the diet the individual grew up eating. Studies have shown that a high-sodium diet contributes to HBP; however, people from certain cultures, such as Asian Americans, are more accustomed to preparing foods with high sodium, and many urban blacks tend to buy more processed foods or dine at fast food restaurants.

Individual Barriers

Predisposing individual barriers include individuals' comorbidities, lifestyle-related health risk behaviors, and circumstances that also affect how the patients maintain their high BP regimen. Because many patients with high BP have other chronic illnesses such as diabetes or lifestyle-related risk factors, it is important to assess and understand the challenges associated with the management of multiple risk factors. In particular, people with many chronic health problems are prone to suffer from depression, which often creates a vicious cycle of poor mental health to poor physical health outcomes. Furthermore, a recent study of hypertensive urban blacks found that depression was a significant correlate of alcohol and illicit drug use, which were strongly associated with high BP adherence behaviors.

Other individual barriers are related to the life priorities of the individual and his or her level of individual responsibility. Aside from old age, having a busy schedule filled with appointments or having to travel a lot (for work or while on vacation) may contribute to individuals' forgetting to take their medications. Several recent studies have suggested that "forgetfulness" is a common barrier for patients. For some, as have been shown with many minority women, their obligation to family responsibilities makes them more susceptible to their being less compliant with their BP management. Therefore, when looking at their lifestyles, it is also important to consider whether they have a daily routine for taking their medications. Incorporating the taking of BP medication into their daily routine may prompt them and help them to control their BP.

Overcoming Patient-related Barriers

In order to break down the patient-related barriers in any and all interventions, it is imperative to include the other two major players, health care providers and the organizations or systems involved (see figure). There must be an equal effort from all three levels if high BP is to be successfully controlled and managed. It has been acknowledged by patients that they identify their provider as the primary source of information on hypertension, a finding that emphasizes the importance of patient–provider communication.

Factors that may influence patients' compliance with controlling their BP include their level of knowledge, perception of their health and the benefits of treatment, and level of social support. Models that guide research into BP control include the health education model or health belief model, cognitive appraisal, and self-efficacy. Many of these models implicitly include some measure of psychological barriers, including perceived difficulty of adhering to preventive and/or treatment behaviors. Also, assessing patients' level of readiness is important for maintaining their motivation and making behavioral changes, such as reducing sodium intake or increasing physical activity level.

According to the self-efficacy model, social persuasion may influence patients by strengthening their beliefs that they have what it takes to succeed. Currently, an intervention is being tested in Baltimore, Maryland, in which self-help hypertension workshops are provided for 6 weeks, with 4 months of monthly follow-up. These workshops have been able to empower patients by providing education and building knowledge

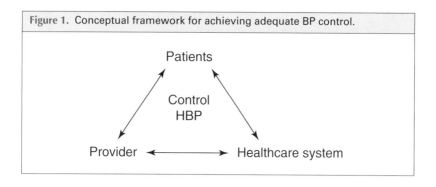

Figure 1. Conceptual framework for achieving adequate BP control.

about hypertension and its management and by providing skills such as tips on improving patient–provider communications. Thus far, the participants have deemed the self-help workshops as being valuable in their increasing level of knowledge on hypertension, changing their eating habits, and receiving social support from the group and their families.

Other possible interventions come from studies on African Americans with high BP, in which culturally sensitive, community-based education programs using lay health workers from their own culture offer an important approach to this problem. These programs have been shown to be effective in supplementing providers' detection, treatment, and follow-up of traditionally known as "hard-to-reach" populations such as urban African Americans.

Conclusions

Identifying and understanding the barriers to BP care and treatment is essential for planning intervention strategies, especially for high-risk populations that include elderly and low socioeconomic or underserved ethnic minority groups. Effective care and control of high BP cannot be achieved without understanding individual family and community health behaviors because these factors are not only part of the high BP problem but also constitute a major part of the solution. This chapter identified patient-related barriers and some strategies to overcome these barriers to high BP care and treatment. The next logical step will be implementing those strategies into practice because compliance is not an individual issue but is an organizational and provider issue as well. A 1992 American Heart Association Medical and Scientific Statement stated that future research and practice "must put greater emphasis on identifying and correcting environmental factors, including the access and utilization of health services relevant to the prevention and treatment of cardiovascular risk factors."

References

1. Cramer JA: Effect of partial compliance on cardiovascular medication effectiveness. Heart 88:203–206, 2002.
2. Dezii CM. Medication noncompliance: What is the problem? Managed Care 9(suppl)8–14, 2000.
3. Douglas JG, Ferdinand KC, Bakris GL, Sowers JR: Barriers to blood pressure control in African Americans. Postgrad Med 112:51–2, 55, 59–62, 2002.
4. Hill MN, Bone LR, Kim MT, et al: Barriers to hypertension care and control in young urban black men. Am J Hypertens 12:951–958, 1999.
5. Kim MT, Kim KB, Juon HS, Hill MN: Prevalence and factors associated with high blood pressure in Korean Americans. Ethn Dis 10:364–374, 2000.

6. Kim MT, Han HR, Hill MN, et al: Depression, substance use, adherence behaviors, and blood pressure control in urban hypertensive black men. Ann Behav Med 51: 309–316, 2003.
7. Knight E, Bohn RL, Wang PS, et al: Predictors of uncontrolled hypertension in ambulatory patients. Hypertension 38:809–814, 2001.
8. Nuesch R, Schroeder K, Dieterle T, et al: Relation between insufficient response to antihypertensive treatment and poor compliance with treatment: A prospective case-control study. Br Med J 323:142–146, 2001.
9. Patel RP, Taylor SD: Factors affecting medication adherence in hypertensive patients. Ann Pharmacother 36:40–45, 2002.
10. Rogers PG, Bullman WR: Prescription medication compliance: A review of the baseline of knowledge. A report of the National Council on Patent Information and Education. J Pharm Epidemiol 2:3, 1995.
11. Rose LE, Kim MT, Dennison CR, Hill MN: The contexts of adherence for African Americans with high blood pressure. J Adv Nurs 32:587–594, 2000.
12. Svensson S, Kjellgren KI, Ahlner J, Saljo R. Reasons for adherence with antihypertensive medication. Int J Cardiol 76:157–163, 2000.
13. The sixth report of the Joint National Committee on Prevention, Detection, Evaluation, and Treatment of High Blood Pressure. Arch Intern Med 157:2413–2446, 1997.
14. Wang PS, Bohn RL, Knight E, et al: Noncompliance with antihypertensive medications. J Gen Intern Med 17:504–511, 2002.

Hypertension Control: Focus On Providers

David Hyman, M.D., MPH

chapter

13

Many physicians have heard the frequently cited data that about 25% of persons with high blood pressure (BP) are unaware of it and that many of the aware are untreated such that only about 50% of all persons with hypertension are being treated. Only about 50% of treated hypertensives are controlled, so that overall BP control to less than 140/90 mm Hg is only about 27%.[1] These numbers suggest the health care system collectively is not doing a good job overall. Most physicians would probably attribute this to a failure of the system to provide access to care, the high cost of medications, drug side effects, or a failure of patients to comply with monitoring or treatment.

However, on closer examination, the situation appears quite different. The proportion of persons with hypertension who have controlled BP in the United States is twice the rate of Canada and better than in Western Europe.[2] Our impression of poor performance centers on not appreciating the BP criteria upon which the often-quoted statistics are based; rather, the data comes from the National Health and Nutrition Examination Survey III (NHANES III; Fig. 1). The definition of hypertension is having a systolic BP greater than 140 mm Hg *or* diastolic BP greater than 90 mm Hg, and the definition of control requires systolic BP less than 140 mm Hg *and* diastolic BP less than 90 mm Hg. There is no age modification of these criteria. Accordingly, a 65-year-old patient on medication with a BP of 142/78 mm Hg would be "treated, but uncontrolled." The characteristics of uncontrolled hypertensives in the U.S. population are known (Tables 1 and 2).[3] The majority have diastolic BPs less than 90 mmHg, have physician access and insurance, and tend to be older adults. Although lack of health care access is still a major problem for a segment of the population, it does not explain a large part of the lack of control. *Lack of systolic BP control in patients under care is the main issue.*

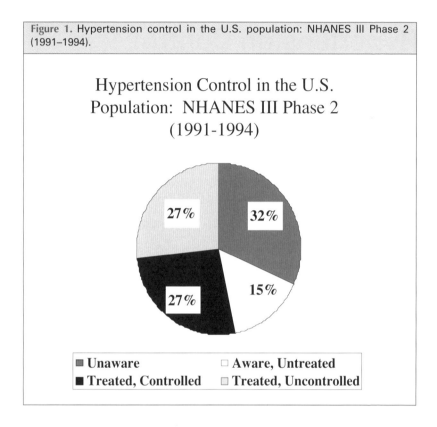

Figure 1. Hypertension control in the U.S. population: NHANES III Phase 2 (1991–1994).

Former Control of Blood Pressure

Widespread efforts to treat hypertension only date from the 1960s, and they received a large impetus from the *Recommendations for a National Blood Pressure Program Data Base for Effective Antihypertensive Therapy: Report of Task Force I*, which was published in 1973,[4] and the first report of the Joint National Committee (JNC) of Detection, Evaluation, and Treatment of High Blood Pressure, which was published in 1977.[5] For pathophysiological reasons, the leading hypertension experts in the mid-20th century focused on controlling diastolic BP. The widely disseminated "stepped-care" approach promulgated in JNC I was based on diastolic BP criteria, as were the modifications of the treatment algorithm published in JNC II (1980) JNC III (1984) JNC IV (1988).[6–8] As of JNC IV, the treatment of diastolic BP in the 90 to 94 mm Hg was still not clearly endorsed as the standard. JNC V (1992)[6–9] quietly gave equal footing to SBP, yet this was hardly noted in the medical community, which was more concerned with debating the report's suggestion that thiazide diuretics (HCTZ) and β-blockers be restored to first-line agent status. JNC

TABLE 1. Distribution of Healthcare Access Variables by Hypertensive Classification*

Factor	Hypertension	Unaware of Condition	Uncontrolled Hypertension		Total	Treated, Controlled Hypertension
			Acknowledged, Untreated Hypertension	Treated, Uncontrolled Hypertension		
Mean age, years	38.14 ± 0.31	58.31 ± 0.64	55.34 ± 0.68	64.85 ± 0.59	60.08 ± 0.44	58.64 ± 0.65
Male gender, %	47.49 ± 0.52	58.70 ± 1.35	54.36 ± 2.92	40.76 ± 1.73	51.15 ± 1.22	37.69 ± 1.72
High school graduation, %	76.31 ± 1.00	66.06 ± 1.66	67.17 ± 2.11	58.37 ± 2.14	63.46 ± 1.50	65.61 ± 2.46
Family income, %						
< $20,000/y	27.08 ± 1.02	37.72 ± 2.56	38.34 ± 2.34	42.23 ± 2.02	39.51 ± 1.86	39.18 ± 2.46
$20,000–$50,000/yr	47.44 ± 0.83	44.15 ± 2.23	48.46 ± 2.55	40.40 ± 1.70	43.67 ± 1.56	39.32 ± 2.00
> $50,000/y	25.47 ± 1.36	18.13 ± 1.70	13.20 ± 149	17.37 ± 1.84	16.82 ± 1.24	21.00 ± 2.61
Has health insurance	85.69 ± 0.95	90.16 ± 1.32	89.50 ± 2.04	95.72 ± 0.66	92.09 ± 0.81	93.50 ± 1.12
Has a usual source of care, %	74.94 ± 0.93	79.22 ± 1.88	80.38 ± 2.63	97.05 ± 0.58	86.05 ± 1.06	95.20 ± 0.71
Use of health care						
• Visited physician ≥1 time in past 12 mo, %	75.90 ± 0.63	71.70 ± 1.80	72.52 ± 2.69	96.00 ± 0.62	80.84 ± 1.08	96.73 ± 0.93
• No. of visits to physician in past 12 mo	3.47 ± 0.08	3.04 ± 0.18	3.52 ± 0.30	6.13 ± 0.23	4.28 ± 0.13	6.26 ± 0.25
Time since last BP, %						
< 6 mo	59.43 ± 0.92	60.11 ± 1.46	62.33 ± 4.00	88.79 ± .91	72.39 ± 1.05	89.57 ± 1.46
6–12 mo	18.21 ± 0.66	14.89 ± 1.26	12.40 ± 2.17	7.98 ± .78	11.71 ± 0.79	8.25 ± 1.17
1–4 yr	18.58 ± 0.64	19.32 ± 1.59	23.60 ± 3.71	3.19 ± .65	13.05 ± 0.96	2.13 ± 0.66
≥ 5 yr	3.91 ± 0.26	5.69 ± 0.70	1.68 ± 0.55	0.04 ± .03	2.86 ± 0.33	—
Lifestyle						
Current smoking, %	29.07 ± 0.83	22.80 ± 1.70	26.08 ± 1.72	16.32 ± 1.70	21.12 ± 1.11	18.80 ± 1.55

*Plus-minus values are mean ± SE.
From Hyman P: Characteristics of patients with uncontrolled hypertension in the United States. New Engl J Med 345:479–486, 2001; with permission.

Age Group	Hypertension Present but Subject Unaware of It		Acknowledged, Untreated Hypertension		Treated, Uncontrolled Hypertension	
	Mean Blood Pressure, mm Hg	SBP ≥ 140 mm Hg and DBP < 90 mm Hg, %	Mean Blood Pressure, mm Hg	SBP ≥ 140 mm Hg and DBP < 90 mm Hg, %	Mean Blood Pressure, mm Hg	SBP ≥ 140 mm Hg and DBP < 90 mm Hg, %
25–44 y	138/91	51.9 ± 7.4	141/94	25.1 ± 7.9	147/95	29.1 ± 7.9
45–64 y	148/86	69.4 ± 3.3	152/89	53.5 ± 4.8	150/87	66.1 ± 2.8
> 65 yr	153/77	91.1 ± 1.1	160/81	81.5 ± 2.7	159/78	87.6 ± 1.3
All subjects	148/83	78.8 ± 2.0	151/88	59.1 ± 2.7	155/82	76.9 ± 1.5

TABLE 2. Blood Pressure Levels in Uncontrolled Hypertensives by Age*

*Plus-minus values are means ± SE. DBP = diastolic blood pressure; SBP = systolic blood pressure.
From Hyman P: Characteristics of patients with uncontrolled hypertension in the United States. New Engl J Med 345:479–486, 2001; with permission.

VI (1996)[1] gave more official status to systolic BP, with the issuance of a JNC clinical advisory statement in 2000 that recommended that systolic BP receive predominant status in hypertension management decision.[10] Even lower BPs are now recommended for patients with diabetes, renal insufficiency, and congestive heart failure. It is beyond the scope of this chapter to discuss the evidence for, achievability of, or outcomes with these lower goals. Over the course of the last decades of the 20th century, hypertension control improved dramatically using the older, higher standards. Based on the old standard of 160/95 mm Hg or greater, hypertension awareness had increased to 89% and control had increased to 64% by 1988 to 1991.[11] By comparison, only 16% of patients with hypertension were controlled to less than 160/95 mm Hg in 1971 to 1974.

Noncompliance with the Latest Blood Pressure Control Criteria

It is clear that many physicians have simply not accepted the BP treatment threshold of systolic BP less than 140 mm Hg and diastolic BP less than 90 mm Hg recommended by the JNC. With regard to diastolic BP, a physician survey in the mid-1990s showed that almost one third of primary care physicians would not start drug therapy for persistent diastolic BP of 90 to 94 mm Hg in a patient with uncomplicated hypertension.[12] In the same survey, few physicians reported being willing to start antihypertensive drugs for systolic BP between 140 and 160 mm Hg if diastolic BP control was "satisfactory." Most physicians would not intensify therapy in a treated patient who had persistently mildly elevated systolic BPs. Several studies of physician behavior documented that physicians rarely intensify drug therapy when systolic BP remains above 140 mm Hg but diastolic BP is less than 90 mm Hg.[13-15] Diastolic BP is the target most physicians have used, and target diastolic BP is often achieved. A key factor in achieving "better" BP goals is for physicians to decide that it should happen and proceed accordingly.

Physician Factors That May Interfere With Achieving Desired Targets

Drug Side Effects

The public and many physicians have firmly linked to antihypertensive medications to a high frequency of intolerable or least very troublesome side effects. The evidence contradicts this notion. In a randomized, double-blind trial, most modern classes of antihypertensive agents had discontinuation rates the same as placebo.[16] This includes diuretics and β-blockers as well as angiotensin-converting enzyme (ACE) inhibitors and calcium channel blockers. *Placebo had a 2-year discontinuation rate of 13% compared with 12% with active antihypertensive agents.* It is well established that combination therapy for resistant hypertension is more successful when diuretics are included,[17] but this class has received an undeserved bad reputation for side effects in many quarters. β-blockers also have acquired a largely unjustified reputation for side effects.[18] Although various classes of medications clearly have specific side effects, overattribution of human symptoms to BP medications can limit patient compliance and physician willingness to intensify drug therapy. This issue will take on even more importance as patients need multiple drugs to achieve lower and lower goals. Physicians may have to resist the immediate temptation to attribute side effects to drugs and strive to convince patients to persist with prescribed treatment.

Drug Costs

For certain patients, drug costs can be a major barrier to long-term adherence. Patients with prescription coverage are more likely to continue therapy. There is a huge range in cost of antihypertensive drugs. Generic diuretics are available for pennies a day, with the largest component of the cost often being the $5 to $6 fixed costs for a pharmacy to fill a prescription. Writing prescriptions for 200 pills at a time can minimize this component of cost, especially for inexpensive generic compounds. Generic β-blockers are also in the pennies-per-day-range. Generic ACE inhibitors are cheaper than brand name ones but still cost more than $30 per month at this time. Physicians need to gently inquire about patients' ability to pay and be sensitive to it. For patients of limited financial means who must have expensive drugs, many manufactures have patient assistance programs to which patients can be directed.

Polypharmacy

Many patients take multiple drugs. The average age of a treated hypertensive patient is 59 years. It is typical to see patients taking two or three antihhypertensive agents, two or three antidiabetic drugs, and a statin as well as a cyclooxygenase-2, proton pump inhibitor, selective serotonin inhibitor, and others. Frequently at least some prescription are generated by multiple providers. Studies from several parts of the world found a discordance in 25% to 75% of cases between which medications were being taken by patients and what was recorded in the medical record in patients on polypharmacy.

Surprisingly, despite conventional wisdom, the mere presence of polypharmacy may not be a barrier to compliance.[19] Although it may not always be possible to eliminate polypharmacy, it is critical to physically review the patient's medications and determine if they are actually taking the necessary antihypertensive agents and to be aware if they are taking other medications that may interfere with the antihypertensive agents.

Measurement and Monitoring Interval

BP is variable. If physicians hope to achieve specified target BPs, they must take a reasonable number of measurements over time to determine how the BP is running. Most physicians still use office BPs, yet the randomized trials that have clearly demonstrated the morbidity and mortality benefits of treating hypertension have used clinic BPs. The appointment frequency for patients with hypertension is highly variable among physicians.[20–22] If a patient with a BP somewhat above target is told to recheck in 6 months, it is quite possible that little action will ever be taken. Physicians and their office staff are also imprecise on how BP is measured. Physicians' staff frequently do not adhere to American Heart Association standards on correct BP cuff size.[23] Physicians selectively recheck BPs that are above their treatment threshold more than those that are just below it.[24] By regression to the mean, the higher values are likely to be somewhat lower on repeated measurement, which provides a potential bias to intensifying treatment.

Key Points

- ∞ Lack of insurance, limited access to health care, cost of medications, and adverse effects of treatment contribute to the high rates of uncontrolled hypertension in the United States.
- ∞ Most patients with uncontrolled hypertension are older Americans with regular access to health care.
- ∞ Evidence suggests that reluctance of physicians to initiate treatment in patients with isolated systolic hypertension or to intensify treatment when the systolic BP remains greater than 140 mm Hg but the diastolic BP is less than 90 mm Hg comprises a major barrier to higher control rates.
- ∞ Significant improvement in the national control rates for hypertension will require changes in physician attitudes and behaviors in managing patients with isolated systolic BP elevations.

References

1. Joint National Committee on Prevention, Detection, Evaluation, and Treatment of High Blood Pressure: The sixth report of the Joint National Committee on Prevention, Detection, Evaluation, and Treatment of High Blood Pressure. Arch Intern Med 1997, 157:2413–2446.

2. Joffres MR, Hamet P, MacLean DR, et al: Distribution of blood pressure and hypertension in Canada and the United States. Am J Hypertens 2001, 14(11 pt 1):1099–1105.

3. Hyman DJ, Pavlik VN: Characteristics of patients with uncontrolled hypertension in the United States. N Engl J Med 2001, 345:479–486.

4. Perry HC: Recommendations for a National High Blood Pressure Program Data Base for Effective Antihypertensive Therapy: report of Task Force I. Bethesda, Maryland: US Dept of Health, Education, and Welfare; 1973. Report No.: DHEW publication No. (NIH) 75–593.

5. Joint National Committee on Detection, Evaluation and Treatment of High Blood Pressure: Report of the Joint National Committee on Detection, Evaluation, and Treatment of High Blood Pressure. JAMA 1977, 237:255–261.

6. Joint National Committee on Detection, Evaluation, and Treatment of High Blood Pressure: The 1980 Report of the Joint National Committee on Detection, Evaluation, and Treatment of high Blood Pressure. Arch Intern Med 1980, 140:1280–1285.

7. Joint National Committee on Detection, Evaluation, and Treatment of High Blood Pressure: The 1984 Report of the Joint National Committee on Detection, Evaluation, and Treatment of High Blood Pressure. Arch Intern Med 1984, 1045–1057.

8. Joint National Committee on Detection, Evaluation, and Treatment of High Blood Pressure: The 1988 Report of the Joint National Committee on Detection, Evaluation, and Treatment of High Blood Pressure. Arch Intern Med 1988, 148:1023–1038.

9. Joint National Committee on Detection, Evaluation, and Treatment of High Blood Pressure: The fifth report of the Joint National Committee on Detection, Evaluation, and Treatment of High Blood Pressure. Arch Intern Med 1993, 152:154–183.

10. Izzo JJ, Levy D, Black H: Clinical advisory statement: important of systolic blood pressure in older Americans. Hypertension 2000, 35:1021–1024.

11. Burt VL, Cutler JA, Higgins M, et al: Trends in the prevalence, awareness, treatment, and control of hypertension in the adult US population. Hypertension 1995, 26:60–69.

12. Hyman D, Pavlik V: Self-reported hypertension treatment practices among primary care physicians: blood pressure thresholds, drug choices, and the role of guidelines and evidence-based medicine. Arch Intern Med 2000, 160:2281–2286.

13. Berlowitz D, Ash A, Hickey R, et al: Inadequate management of blood pressure in a hypertensive population. N Engl J Med 1998, 339:1957–1963.

14. Hyman D, Pavlik V, Vallbona C: Physician role in lack of awareness and control of hypertension. Clin Hypertens 2000, 2:324–330.

15. Lapuerta P, L'Italien G: Awareness, treatment and control of systolic blood pressure in the United States. Am J Hypertension 1999, 12(pt 2):92.

16. Preston RA, Materson BJ, Reda DJ, Williams DW: Placebo-associated blood pressure response and adverse effects in the treatment of hypertension: observations from a Department of Veterans Affairs Cooperative Study. Arch Intern Med 2000, 160:1449–1454.

17. Yakovlevitch M, Black HR: Resistant hypertension in a tertiary care clinic. Arch Intern Med 1991, 151:1786–1792.

18. Ko DT, Hebert PR, Coffey CS, et al: Beta-blocker therapy and symptoms of depression, fatigue, and sexual dysfunction. JAMA 2002, 288:351–357.

19. Shalansky SJ, Levy AR: Effect of number of medications on cardiovascular therapy adherence. Ann Pharmacother 2002, 36:1532–1539.

20. Schwartz LM, Woloshin S, Wasson JH, et al: Setting the revisit interval in primary care. J Gen Intern Med 1999, 14:230–235.

21. Petitti DB, Grumbach K: Variation in physicians' recommendations about revisit interval for three common conditions. J Fam Pract 1993, 37:235–240.

22. Parchman ML, Bisonni RS, Lawler FH: Hypertension management: relationship between visit interval and control. Fam Pract Res J 1993, 13:225–231.

23. Manning DM, Kuchirka C, Kaminski J: Miscuffing: inappropriate blood pressure cuff application. Circulation 1983, 68:763–766.

24. Pavlik VN, Hyman DJ, Vallbona C, Grim CE: Selective physician blood pressure remeasurement in the office setting may contribute to poor hypertension control. Am J Hypertens 2002, 15(4, part 2):81.

Culturally Congruent Medical Care

B. Waine Kong, Ph.D., J.D., and Stephanie Kong, M.D.

chapter

14

Communication disconnects are evident in numerous clinical situations when physicians and patients have different beliefs and values. The challenge is to bridge the cultural divide and ensure that meaningful clinical exchanges occur. With the increasing diversity of American society, doctors' offices, clinics, and hospitals are advised to be culturally and linguistically versed. Cultural diversity has significant implications for patient outcomes, health care costs, health care delivery, and public policy. To the extent that barriers exist to effective communication and relationships, our efforts to optimize care for our citizens will continue to be hindered.

Racial Differences in Medical Care

Culture shapes individual behaviors and values for both caregiver and patient, and also impacts health care outcomes. The lack of diversity in the physician workforce (most are white men) suggests that there is a need to address the potential negative impact this may have on health care outcomes in minorities.[1] On a long-term basis, we may be obligated to develop a physician workforce resembling the racial, ethnic, and gender profiles of the people we serve. In other words, we need to start planning now for a medical profession that looks like America will in 2050.[2]

In today's America, most African-American patients receive care from non–African-American providers because fewer than 3% of U.S. physicians are African American. Although African-American physicians are more likely to provide care to minority populations, practice in underserved areas, and serve patients from their own ethnic groups, imbalances in the racial composition of American physicians exacerbates health access and delivery problems in both minority and low socioeconomic patient populations.

The persistent segregation of the health delivery system along race, economic, and class lines has created an African-American health crisis.[3] This African-American health crisis is characterized by inequities and

147

inequalities endemic to each structural component of the health system. Our current health delivery system is 375 years old, and significant race- and class-based health outcomes and health status disparities are just as old.[4] According to the American Medical Association (AMA), the profession must be aggressive in confronting and addressing the related and underlying issues that contribute to the existence of minority health disparities. The AMA has adopted a policy of "zero tolerance" toward racially or culturally biased disparities in care, including but not limited to identifying and correcting overt or subliminal racial, ethnic, and cultural bias.

In the February 25, 1999, issue of the *New England Journal of Medicine,* the authors of the article "The effect of race and sex on physicians' recommendations for cardiac catherization" found that "the race and sex of a patient influence the recommendations of physicians [on managing chest pain] independently of other factors." Actors representing each of the possible combinations of race, gender, and age were videotaped portraying patients with similar symptoms, emotions, types of dress, and insurance coverage. As we all know now, the race and gender of the patient affected the physicians' decisions about whether to refer patients with chest pain for cardiac catherization. The conclusion of the authors was that although they could not assess the form of bias, the bias represented by the study did represent overt prejudice on the part of physicians and, at the very least, was a result of subconscious perceptions. The authors also concluded that the negative outcomes from such perceptions could be reduced with a culturally competent physician workforce and a profession that better reflects our diverse population.

Another example was associated with physicians working for the Tenet Hospital system in Atlanta, Georgia. In September 1999, three radiologists employed by the Diagnostic Imaging Specialists of Atlanta and working at Atlanta Medical Center (a Tenet Hospital) finished dictating their notes and spoke informally with each other, not knowing that one of their tape recorders was recording. On the tape that was subsequently sent to the medical transcriber, one of the doctors complained about a noncompliant patient, saying: "You can take the nigger out of the ghetto; you can't take the ghetto out of the nigger." A second doctor responds, "They ain't middle class black people, they are like low-class white, white trash, mirror images of the same behavior." When contacted, the president of Diagnostic Imaging Specialists said, "The comments were not directed to or about any specific individual or patient. The conversation did not take place in the presence of any patient or other individual except those involved in the conversation."[15]

Were these racially insensitive comments a reflection of cultural biases, and could these biases affect patient care? This question is at the heart of the controversy surrounding the need for cultural competency within the physician workforce. Because of the selection process, special training, and the oath they take, are physicians more humanistic toward and accepting of diverse patients they encounter? Or are they just as likely to be influenced by ethnic, racial, and gender differences of their patient base? Is good science and good medicine all that matters? Does it matter that patients may not receive medical care from providers who are members of their own ethnic group? As underscored by the landmark Task Force study commissioned in 1986 by then Secretary of Health Margaret Heckler, minority Americans suffer disproportionately and die prematurely from chronic and catastrophic illnesses. Although great strides have been made in the area of infant mortality, immunizations, cardiac disorders, and other chronic disease, minority ethnic subgroups still do not enjoy the quality and quantity of life as their white counterparts. To the extent that physicians play a role in this disparity, their participation in activities to increase their cultural sensitivity and competence is necessary and urgent.

Awareness of the Role of Culture in Affecting Health Outcomes

Case Study 1

Mrs. Jones is a 53-year-old-black head of household. She is the primary caregiver for her 13-year-old grandson and 15-year-old granddaughter. When asked why she had so many pill bottles, she replied, "I've had a lot of illness, and every time I see a doctor, they give me another pill bottle. I really prefer to stay home until I get better by taking anything I can because every time I see a doctor, they want me to fill out a different form to collect money. I can't read or write and feel embarrassed to ask for help; to ask them to fill out the forms for me. They might get upset or they might say, 'That lazy lady. She never learned to read.' That's how I feel."

To the extent that physicians have patients like Mrs. Jones in their practice, to be effective, they must structure their practices to respond to patients who cannot adequately communicate other than orally. It is unclear what parts of physicians' medical school and clinical training have prepared them for a "Mrs. Jones." In response to the inadequacies of medical school curricula in preparing physicians to be culturally responsive, the federal government and private foundations have launched mandates for the development of innovative approaches to multicultural training of physicians. The Pew Health Professions Commission, specifically seeking to give direction to health professions education for the twenty-first century, states: "Cultural sensitivity must be a part of the educational experiences that touches the life of every medical and health professional student."[5] This emphasis on cultural specific or sensitive care is recent and, when confronted with this issue, physicians may ponder, "What is culture, and why is culture relevant in a clinical practice setting?"

Culture can be defined as "the integrated pattern of human behavior that includes thought, communications, actions, customs, beliefs, values and institutions of a racial, ethnic, religious or social group."[6] The fact that the majority of physicians in this country are white compared with the increasing cultural, racial, and ethnic diversity of the United States should compel medical practitioners to develop respectful techniques to negotiate the implications of the diversity in their clinical practice. The lack of a homogenous practice may create unintentional barriers to effective clinical information exchange between physicians and patients and create nonfinancial barriers that operate at the level of the physician–patient relationship.[7]

Under the best of circumstances, the relationship between a physician and patient is dynamic and can easily be compromised by the added weight of the various sociocultural mismatches between patients and providers, including the providers' lack of knowledge regarding the patients' health beliefs and life experiences and providers' unintentional and intentional processes of racism, classism, homophobia, and sexism.[8–10] As illustrated in the next example, cultural beliefs and practices influence the ability of both the patient and physician to arrive at an appropriate treatment option.

Case Study 2

A 58-year-old Mexican American man concerned about urinary retention and symptoms of prostatism arrives at a physician's office. When the physician is ready to perform the digital rectal examination, the patient adamantly refuses it because it will violate his moral integrity. The challenge for physicians with a diverse population of patients is to be able to convince their patients of the value and need for the specific procedures and interventions being proposed. Cultural congruence becomes a tool that practitioners can use to positively influence the decisions made by and on behalf of their patients. Cultural congruence in clinical practice setting is best defined not as a discrete endpoint but as a commitment and active engagement in a lifelong process that individuals enter into on an ongoing basis with patients, communities, colleagues, and themselves.[11] It is a process that requires humility in how physicians bring into check the power imbalances that exist in the dynamics of physician–patient communication by using patient-focused interviewing and care.[12,13]

National standards for culturally and linguistically appropriate health care services, based on key laws, regulations, contracts, and standards currently in use by federal and state agencies, now exist. These standards are predicated on the fact that culture and language have considerable impact on how patients access and respond to health care services. The 14 standards promulgate equal access to quality health care can be maximized if organizations and providers[14]:

1. Promote and support the attitudes, behaviors, knowledge, and skills necessary for staff to work respectfully and effectively with patients and each other in a culturally diverse work environment.
2. Have a comprehensive management strategy to address culturally and linguistically appropriate services, including strategic goals, plans, policies, procedures, and designated staff responsible for implementation.
3. Use formal mechanisms for community and consumer involvement in the design and execution of service delivery, including planning, policymaking, operations, evaluation, training, and (as appropriate) treatment planning.
4. Develop and implement a strategy to recruit, retain, and promote qualified, diverse, and culturally competent administrative, clinical, and support staff that are trained and qualified to address the needs of the racial and ethnic communities being served.
5. Require and arrange for ongoing education and training for administrative, clinical, and support staff in culturally and linguistically competent service delivery.
6. Provide all clients with limited English proficiency (LEP) access to bilingual staff or interpretation services.
7. Provide oral and written notices, including translated signage at key points of contact, to clients in their primary language informing them of their right to receive no-cost interpreter services.
8. Translate and make available signage and commonly used written patient educational materials and other materials for members of the predominant language groups in service areas.
9. Ensure that interpreters and bilingual staff can demonstrate bilingual proficiency and receive training that includes the skills and ethics of interpreting and knowledge in both languages of the terms and concepts relevant to clinical or nonclinical encounters. Family or friends are not considered adequate substitutes because they usually lack these abilities.
10. Ensure that the clients' primary spoken language and self-identifies regarding race or ethnicity are included in the health care organization's management information system as well as any patient records used to provider staff.

11. Use a variety of methods to collect and use accurate demographic, cultural, epidemiologic, and clinical outcome data for racial and ethnic groups in the service area and become informed about the ethnic or cultural needs, resources, and assets of the surrounding community.

12. Undertake ongoing organizational self-assessments of cultural and linguistic competence and integrate measures of access, satisfaction, quality, and outcomes for culturally and linguistically appropriate services (CLAS) into other organizational internal audits and performance improvement programs.

13. Develop structures and procedures to address cross-cultural ethical and legal conflicts in health care delivery and complaints or grievances by patients and staff members about unfair culturally insensitive or discriminatory treatment, difficulty in accessing services, or denial of services.

14. Prepare an annual progress report documenting the organizations' progress with implementing CLAS standards, including information on programs, staffing, and resources.

Cultural competence has progressed from the concept of providing interpreter services to one of providing an opportunity for communication that takes into consideration patients' and providers' belief systems, stereotypes, and prejudices. Physicians should look within themselves and, when necessary, address personal barriers that will eliminate social injustice and cultural insensitivity in their practices.

Practical Guidance in Developing Cultural Sensitivity

Self assessment
Various self-assessment tools provided by the Office of Minority Health allow participating physicians to explore issues of prejudice and bias without judgment by others.

Culturation
Learn more about the communities from which your patient population arises. The Association advocates discussions with community leaders, traditional healers, and patients. Learn more about the demographics, traditional health and illness beliefs, home remedies, health resources, neighborhood centers, and rituals and beliefs surrounding death and dying.

Personnel
Hire staff that reflect the community from which your patients come. Place more emphasis on creating a culturally congruent staff as opposed to just focusing on hiring a multilingual staff.

Active interaction with patients
Encourage patients and their families to provide feedback concerning the quality of interaction with the physician and office staff, especially staff in the reception area and nursing staff.

Outcome data
Maintain an active knowledge base concerning disease outcomes by race and ethnicity, especially the ethnicity represented in your practice.

The disconcerting issue is that African Americans are still suffering disproportionately from acute and chronic health conditions. After 30 years of Medicaid and Medicare, African-American and other minority patients are still not receiving the same level of care as their white counterparts and are suffering higher rates of mortality and morbidity because of it. The physician community often prides itself with delivering the same relevant, quality care irrespective to payment source; this does not hold true for ethnic minorities. Because incongruent patient–doctor relationships have been shown to adversely impact the quality of care, physicians should be motivated to increase their ability to communicate more effectively with their increasingly diverse patient populations.

References

1. Finishing the Bridge to Diversity; Association of American Medical Colleges. President's Address: Plenary Session of the 107th Annual Meeting of the Association of American Medical Colleges, November 1996.
2. Diversity in Medical Education: Report of the Board of Trustees. American Medical Association; Board of Trustees Report 15-A-99.
3. Byrd WM, Clayton LA: An American Health Dilemma.
4. Byrd WM, Clayton LA: America's Dual Health Crisis in Black and White.
5. Pew Health professions Commission. Critical challenges: Revitalizing the Health Professions for the Twenty-First Century. San Francisco, UCSF Center for the Health Profession, 1995.
6. Uhlman M: Cultural savvy is coming to health care. Philadelphia, Philadelphia Inquirer. April 12, 1998, B1, B4.
7. Tervalon M, Murray-Garcia J: Cultural humility versus cultural competence: A critical distinction in defining physician training outcomes in multicultural education. Journal of Health Care for the Poor and Underserved. 9, 1998.
8. Borkman JM, Neher JA: A developmental model of ethnosensitivity in family practice training. Fam Med 23:212–217, 1991.
9. Pinderhughes E: Understanding Race, Ethnicity and Power. The Key to Efficacy in Clinical Practice. New York, Free Press, 1989.
10. Kavanagh K, Kennedy P: Promoting Cultural Diversity: Strategies for Health Care Professionals. Newbury Park, CA, Sage, 1992.
11. Borkan JM, Neher JA: A developmental model of ethnosensitivity in family practice training. Fam Med 23:212–217, 1991.
12. Smith RC, Hoppe RB: The patient's story: Integrating the patient and physician centered approaches to interviewing. Ann Intern Med 115:470–477, 1991.
13. Ventres W, Gordon P: Communication strategies in caring for the underserved. J Health Care for the Poor and Underserved. 1:305–314, 1990.
14. Measuring Cultural Competence in Health Care: Recommendations for National Standards and an Outcome-Focused Research Agenda. Office of Minority Health; Health and Human Services. 1999.
15. "Woman allegedly fired over racial slur complains." Douglas County Sentinel, Douglasville, GA, October 1, 1999.

SECTION V
Lifestyle Approaches:
Translating Research into Practice!

chapter
15

Promoting Lifestyle Modification in the Office Setting

Lawrence J. Appel, M.D., MPH, and Edgar R. Miller, III, M.D., Ph.D.

An impressive body of evidence has documented that lifestyle modifications can lower blood pressure (BP) and potentially control hypertension. With the exception of increased physical activity, most lifestyle recommendations are related to nutrition. Effective nutrition-related lifestyle modifications include reduced salt intake, increased potassium intake, weight loss, moderation of alcohol intake, and the Dietary Approaches to Stop Hypertension (DASH) diet (Table 1).[1] The DASH diet emphasizes fruits, vegetables and low-fat dairy products; includes whole

TABLE 1. Lifestyle Modifications that Effectively Lower Blood Pressure	
Lifestyle Modification	**Recommendation**
Increased physical activity	Half hour of moderate intensity physical activity most days of the week
Reduced salt intake	≤ 100 mmol/day of sodium (2.3 g/day of sodium or 5.8 g/day of sodium chloride [salt])
Weight loss	Lose weight if overweight or obese (Ideally, attainment of a body mass index < 25 kg/m²)
Moderation of alcohol intake	≤ 2 alcohol drinks/day (men)
	≤ 1 alcohol drinks/day (women)
DASH diet*	8–10 servings/day of fruits and vegetables
	2–3 servings/day of low-fat dairy products
	Reduced intake of total fat and cholesterol

* Increased potassium intake (≥ 90 mmol/day [3.5 g/day of potassium]) can also lower blood pressure, but this recommendation is subsumed under the DASH diet, which is rich in potassium.

grains, poultry, fish, and nuts; and is reduced in saturated fat, cholesterol, red meat, sweets, and sugar-containing beverages.[2]

The efficacy of these interventions has been well-documented in controlled clinical trials. To a lessor extent, implementation of lifestyle modifications has also been studied in the office setting.[3] In contrast to rigidly controlled trials, such as feeding studies, implementation of lifestyle modifications in free-living individuals often requires substantial changes in behavior. This chapter highlights strategies that promote lifestyle modification in patients.

Roles of Lifestyle Modification

Lifestyle modification, previously termed nonpharmacologic therapy, has important roles in both hypertensive and nonhypertensive individuals (Table 2). In hypertensive individuals, lifestyle modifications serve as initial treatment before the start of drug therapy and as an adjunct to medication in those already on drug therapy. In hypertensive individuals with BP controlled by pharmacotherapy, lifestyle change can facilitate drug stepdown and potentially medication withdrawal. In nonhypertensive individuals, lifestyle modifications have the potential to prevent hypertension[4] and, more broadly, to reduce BP and thereby lower the risk of BP-related cardiovascular disease in the general population.

Implementing Lifestyle Modifications: General Considerations

Physicians can be important catalysts in promoting lifestyle modification. Physician-directed efforts to promote lifestyle modification should be individualized. In particular, the extent of these efforts should be based on the patient's willingness to make lifestyle changes.[5] Table 3 displays Prochaska's model, which classifies individuals by their readiness

TABLE 2.   Role of Lifestyle Modification in Hypertensive and Nonhypertensive Individuals
Hypertensive Individuals
Serve as initial therapy
Serve as adjunct to drug therapy
Facilitate medication stepdown
Nonhypertensive Individuals
Reduce blood pressure
Prevent hypertension

TABLE 3.   Prochaska's Stages of Change Classification for Motivation to Make Lifestyle Changes

Level	Description
Precontemplation	Not intending to change
Contemplation	Intending to change but no changes made
Preparation	Inconsistently making some lifestyle changes
Action	Making lifestyle changes and meeting goals for < 6 months
Maintenance	Have made lifestyle changes and maintained them for > 6 months

to change. For a patient who is precontemplative, a physician should simply provide brief advice on lifestyle modification. Further efforts would likely be unproductive. For precontemplative patients, the goal is to shift them towards the action stage. In contrast, patients who are in the preparation or action stage of change are typically most ready to modify behaviors; such individuals benefit from more specific direction and guidance.

Traditionally, physicians have focused on provision of advice and information. It is now well recognized that such an approach, which may include brochures and written pamphlets, is typically ineffective by itself. It remains, however, one component of a program designed to accomplish behavior change. To the extent possible, physicians should refer their hypertensive patients to dietitians or skilled health educators.

In addition to assessing diet and providing educational materials, therapists should set goals, provide advice, and arrange regular follow-up visits to monitor progress. Success typically requires multiple visits and contacts, including telephone reminders. For patients unable to afford nutritionists' counseling, referral to community resources such as Weight Watchers can provide a more affordable support system to encourage lifestyle modification, at least for weight loss. Without the assistance of dietitians, physicians should nonetheless encourage lifestyle modification routinely.

General principles used to promote behavior change are listed in Table 4. Specific behavioral strategies, such as goal setting and self-monitoring, can aide patients in adopting and maintaining healthy lifestyle behaviors. Self-monitoring allows patients to initially assess their current behaviors and to subsequently set goals for change. A useful acronym that describes key aspects of setting goals is SMART (specific, measurable, attainable, realistic, and time-related) (Table 5). Written contracts with patients for specific outcomes can then be used to enhance compliance with these goals. Focusing on one lifestyle change is likely to be

TABLE 4.   General Principles for Promoting Lifestyle Modifications

Assess readiness to change and focus efforts on individuals who are willing to make changes.

Set SMART goals for physical activity and diet (see Table 5)

Use contracts, signed by patient, for agreed-upon goals (see Table 6)

To the extent possible, engage paraprofessionals (e.g., dietitians), both for initial evaluation and for follow-up

Encourage self-monitoring of physical activity and diet

Encourage gradual changes

Focus on one lifestyle change at a time

Discourage unproven therapies (e.g., fad diets, vitamin supplements, herbal and botanical remedies)

Use positive messages and provide feedback on a regular basis

SMART = specific, measurable, attainable, realistic, time.

TABLE 5.   SMART Goals

		Examples
S	Specific	SMART weight loss goal: "I will lose 4 pounds in the next 2 months
M	Measurable	by walking 30 minutes per day in the morning, substituting diet soda
A	Attainable	for the usual soda that I drink, and eliminating desserts."
R	Realistic	SMART DASH goal: "I will increase my fruits and vegetable intake by
T	Time-related	drinking orange juice in the morning and eating a banana with my cereal. I will eat a salad for lunch on most days of the week."

more practical and effective than attempting multiple changes simultaneously, especially in the context of brief medical visits.

Encouraging Increased Physical Activity

Moderate intensity physical activity, defined as an intensity that is well within the individual's current capacity and that can be comfortably sustained for a prolonged period of time, can effectively lower BP.[6] An efficient means to promote exercise is to provide a written exercise prescription tailored to the patient's motivational readiness, ability, and interests. This advice should be based on the patient's baseline level of activity and stage of change (see Table 3). The Physician-based Assessment and Counseling for Exercise (PACE) study used written prescriptions that follow the acronym FITT (frequency, intensity, type of exercise, and time spent exercising per week).[7] To reinforce the commitment, the patient is asked to sign the prescription, as one would a

TABLE 6. Example of a FITT Exercise Prescription
Any Hospital

Name of patient: Jane Doe   Date: January 3, 2003
I intend to exercise:

F	Five days per week (Saturday, Sunday, Monday, Wednesday and Friday)
I	Moderate intensity (brisk)
T	Walk during lunch breaks on weekdays and before breakfast on weekends
T	At least 30 minutes each of these days

I agree to try this plan starting on: January 4, 2003
I intend to continue this plan at least through: May 1, 2003

_____   _____
Patient's signature   Physician's signature

contract (Table 6). A simple but effective strategy to set goals and monitor progress is to set weekly goals for minutes of physical activity and then record actual minutes on a calender. Other hints for promoting physical activity are listed in Table 7. Note that before making recommendations on physical activity, physicians should determine if a medical examination and exercise test are indicated (Table 8).[8]

Encouraging Weight Loss

Modest weight loss, such as 10 pounds, can reduce BP even without attainment of desirable body weight.[9] Core principles are to reduce caloric intake and increase caloric expenditure. A multitude of strategies have been proposed. Despite the popularity of fad diets, modification of dietary composition has a subsidiary role as a means to accomplish and sustain weight loss. However, adoption of a healthy dietary pattern, such as the DASH diet, can, by itself, lower BP. Similar to physical activity, a "weight loss prescription" can be a powerful motivational tool. Structured weight loss programs (e.g., healthcare-system–based, employer-based, and certain commercial-based programs) can be very useful; however, because several weight loss programs promote diets, products, and strategies that are ineffective, potentially harmful, and often expensive, physicians should provide some guidance to their patients (see Table 7). Note that after weight loss has been achieved, one of the strongest determinants of maintaining weight loss is sustained physical activity.

TABLE 7. Helpful Hints to Promote Physical Activity, Weight Loss, Sodium Reduction, and the DASH Diet
Physical Activity
Encourage a "buddy system" with spouse, child, friend, or coworker
Make physical activity routine (e.g., part of lunch break or afternoon break)
Include physical activity at all major events (e.g., holiday celebrations, vacations, business trips)
Double-task (e.g., exercising on a treadmill while watching the news on TV)
Set weekly goals for minutes of physical activity (e.g., 180 minutes per week) and record actual minutes on a calender
Weight Loss
Avoid fad diets
Cut down on portion sizes
Choose water and seltzer more often
Check calories per serving (and serving size) on food labels
Avoid calorie-dense foods (e.g. sweets, desserts, heavy sauces)
Increase physical activity (especially important for maintaining weight loss)
Consider structured programs that provide skill building, motivation, and group support
Reduced Sodium (Salt) Intake
Check food labels carefully; similar products can have vastly different sodium levels
Use reduced sodium or no-salt-added products
Buy fresh, plain frozen, or canned with no-added-salt vegetables
Cut back on canned, smoked, and processed meats
Flavor with spices, herbs, vinegar, lemon, lime, and salt-free-seasoning blends
Remove the salt shaker from the table
Cut back on salt in recipes
Carefully select cereals and bread products
DASH Diet
Start each day with breakfast, which ideally should include fruit, juice and low-fat milk.
Choose fruit or nuts for snacks
Choose fruit juices rather than soda
Treat meat as one part of a meal rather than the focus
Double up on vegetables; most are low in calories and rich in nutrients
Read food labels for saturated fat and cholesterol
Use low-fat (1%) or skim milk

Encouraging Reduced Sodium Intake

A reduced sodium intake is well accepted as a means of lowering BP, especially in older-aged persons, hypertensive individuals, and blacks (see Table 7). Approximately 75% of dietary sodium is added during food processing by manufacturers; only 10% is inherent in the food itself before processing. Just 15% is discretionary, or added by individuals as they prepare or eat food. Hence, the most critical aspect of reducing sodium intake is judicious selection of foods. Canned and processed foods are well-recognized sources of sodium. Less well appreciated is the fact that most baked goods and cereals are also high in sodium and in aggregate

TABLE 8.   Recommendations for Medical Examination and Exercise Testing Before Initiation of a Moderate or Vigorous Exercise Program[1]

	Apparently Healthy		Increased Risk*		
	Younger[†]	Older	No Symptoms	Symptoms	Known Disease[‡]
Moderate exercise[§]	No[¶]	No	No	Yes	Yes
Vigorous exercise**	No	Yes	Yes	Yes	Yes

*Individual with two or more cardiovascular risk factors OR one or more symptoms suggestive of cardio-vascular disease.
[†]Men ≤ 40 years, women ≤ 50 years.
[‡]Known cardiac, pulmonary, or metabolic disease (particularly diabetes).
[§]Moderate is an intensity well within the individual's current capacity, one that can be comfortably sustained for a prolonged period of time (60 minutes).
[¶]"No" indicates not necessary, "yes" indicates exercise test recommended.
**"Vigorous" defined as exercise intensive enough to represent a substantial cardiorespiratory challenge OR enough to result in fatigue within 20 minutes.
Adapted from American College of Sports Medicine, 1995

provide a substantial fraction of total dietary sodium intake—roughly one third. Strategies to reduce sodium consumption are listed in Table 7.

Encouraging the DASH Diet

In controlled feeding studies, the DASH diet can substantially lower BP.[10,11] Strategies to promote the DASH diet in free-living individuals have been published.[12,13] The DASH diet is rich in fruits, vegetables, and low-fat dairy products and reduced in saturated fat and cholesterol. Although the goal of eight to 10 servings of fruits and vegetables per day seems daunting, fruit juices along with dried or fresh fruit can contribute to the total. One practical strategy to adopting the DASH diet is to make meal-by-meal changes, starting with breakfast. A breakfast with fruit juice, a banana, cereal, and milk is a great start and may be necessary in order to meet the fruits, vegetables, and dairy goals. For lunch, a chef salad for lunch on workdays is an excellent way to increase vegetable intake while keeping calorie consumption and sodium intake under control. Finally, doubling up on servings of vegetables at dinner is another strategy. To meet the dairy goal, a yogurt at lunch and milk at dinner are required (see Table 7).

Key Points

∞ Key elements of successful nutritional counseling are patient motivation, commitment to change, and plans for movement toward desired goals.   *(continued)*

Key Points (*Continued*)

↪ Irrespective of the behavior to be changed, several important strategies should be used to enhance adherence: set specific, reasonable dietary and physical activity goals within a specified, rather than open-ended period: schedule frequent follow-up visits (or contacts) early in the process to assess progress, solve problems, and identify barriers to adherence: use the services of skilled therapists, such as dietitians, to facilitate sodium reduction, adoption of the DASH diet, and weight loss; and provide information (brochures, handouts, and web site addresses) that might encourage or reinforce lifestyle modification (Table 9).

↪ Ultimately, physician-directed strategies that promote lifestyle modification should lower BP and improve hypertension control.

TABLE 9. Patient Resources for Lifestyle Modification	
Books	**Comments**
The DASH Diet for Hypertension[13]	Extensive guide to the DASH diet with sections on sodium reduction and weight loss
American Heart Association cookbooks	Numerous cookbooks, typically with easy recipes, all of which have been tested; in addition to a general cookbook, some cookbooks focus on low sodium, low saturated fat and low cholesterol meals.
Handouts	
The *DASH* Diet (NIH Publication 01–4082), from the National Heart, Lung and Blood Institute (NHLBI)	Summary of DASH diet with helpful hints; PDF file available on the NHLBI web site below
How do I follow a healthy diet?, from the American Heart Association	Tips on how to eat a health diet; PDF file available on the AHA web site below
Nutrition and your Health: Dietary Guidelines for Americans, prepared by Office of Disease Prevention and Health Promotion	Detailed handout on core principles of a healthy diet; PDF file available on the web site below
Web Sites	
http://www.nhlbi.nih.gov/health/public	Web site with resources prepared by NHLBI for the general public; several deal with implementing lifestyle modifications (general diet, physical activity, and weight loss); patient handouts can be downloaded
http://www.americanheart.org	Web site with information and advice about living a healthy lifestyle; several cookbooks available; some patient handouts can be downloaded
	(*continued*)

TABLE 9.	Patient Resources for Lifestyle Modification (*Continued*)
Web Sites	
http://www.health.gov/dietaryguidelines	Web site on dietary guidelines for Americans
http://www.healthfinder.gov	Web site that searches resource for the best government and nonprofit health and human services information on the Internet
http://www.nutrition.gov	Web site with fact sheets on common nutrition-related issues
http://www.eatright.com/	Web site of the American Dietetic Association with fact sheets and handouts, some of which can be downloaded

References

1. Joint National Committee on Prevention, Detection, Evaluation, and Treatment of High Blood Pressure: The Sixth Report of the Joint National Committee on the Prevention, Detection, Evaluation, and Treatment of High Blood Pressure. Arch Intern Med 1997, 157:2413–2446.
2. Karanja NM, Obarzanek E, Lin PH, et al. for the DASH Collaborative Research Group: Descriptive characteristics of the dietary patterns used in the dietary approaches to stop hypertension trial. J Am Diet Assoc 1999, 99(suppl):19–27.
3. Miller ER, Erlinger TP, Young D, et al: Lifestyle changes that reduce blood pressure: implementation in clinical practice. J Clin Hypertens 1999, 1:191–198.
4. Whelton PK, He J, Appel LJ, et al: Primary prevention of hypertension: clinical and public health advisory from the National High Blood Pressure Education Program. JAMA 2002, 288:1882–1888.
5. Prochaska JO, DiClemente CC: States and processes of self-change in smoking: towards an integrative model of change. J Consult Clin Psychol 1983, 51:390–395.
6. Whelton SP, Chin A, Xin X, He J: Effect of aerobic exercise on blood pressure: a meta-analysis of randomized, controlled trials. Ann Intern Med 2002, 136:493–503.
7. Calfas KJ, Long BJ, Sallis JF, et al: A controlled trial of physician counseling to promote the adoption of physical activity. Prev Med 1996, 25:225–233.
8. Health screening and risk stratification. In Kenney WL (ed): ACSM's Guidelines for Exercise Testing and Prescription. Baltimore, Williams and Wilkins, 1995, p 25.
9. National Institutes of Health: Clinical guidelines on the identification, evaluation, and treatment of overweight and obesity in adults. National Heart, Lung, and Blood Institute, U.S. Department of Health and Human Services, 1998.
10. Appel LJ, Moore TJ, Obarzanek E, et al. for the DASH Collaborative Research Group: A clinical trial of the effects of dietary patterns on blood pressure. N Eng J Med 1997, 336:1117–1124.
11. Sacks FM, Svetkey LP, Vollmer WM, et al. for the DASH-Sodium Collaborative Research Group: A clinical trial of the effects on blood pressure of reduced dietary sodium and the DASH dietary pattern (The DASH-Sodium Trial). N Engl J Med 2001, 344:3–10.
12. Kolasa KM: Dietary approachs to Stop Hypertension (DASH) in clinical practice. Clin Cardiol 1999, 22:16–22.
13. Moore T, Svetkey L, Lin P-H, Karanja N (eds): The DASH Diet for Hypertension. New York, Simon and Schuster, 2001.

Dietary Cations and Hypertension

Paul K. Muntner, Ph.D., MHS,
Paul K. Whelton M.D., M.Sc., and
Jiang He, M.D., Ph.D.

chapter 16

Clinical trials have overwhelmingly demonstrated that dietary modification offers the potential for lowering blood pressure (BP) and the concomitant risk of cardiovascular disease (CVD) with minimal risk.[1–3] Using this evidence, recent national guidelines recommend dietary modification as (1) a means to prevent hypertension, (2) an initial approach for treating high-normal BP (HNBP) and stage 1 hypertension among persons without target organ damage and CVD and (3) a useful concurrent treatment for persons taking pharmacologic therapy.[4,5] This chapter provides an update of the most recently available evidence on the use of dietary cation alteration as a means for preventing and treating hypertension.

The dietary intake of low sodium and high potassium, calcium, and magnesium is highly confluent. However, the most rigorous evidence regarding the efficacy of a reduced sodium or an increased intake of potassium, calcium, and magnesium in modulating levels of BP has been assessed in trials that have independently tested the effect of these cations on BP.[6,7] As such, evidence of a BP-lowering effect for dietary sodium reduction and increased potassium, calcium, and magnesium are discussed individually here. The beneficial effects of an overall dietary approach for reducing BP from two recent clinical trials are reviewed at the end of this chapter.[8,9]

Sodium Reduction

Effects of dietary sodium on CVD risk were noted more than 5000 years ago. However, clear evidence showing that reducing sodium intake lowers BP was not assembled until the 20th century. In the 1940s, Kempner reported that a low-sodium rice diet substantially reduced BP in a majority of patients with severe hypertension.[10] In 1960, Dahl showed that dietary sodium was a major determinant of BP across human populations.[11] Animal experiments;[12–15] observational studies;[16]

and randomized, controlled trials are consistent in demonstrating that reducing dietary sodium lowers BP.

Clinical Trials

During the past 30 years, more than 80 randomized, controlled trials have explored the efficacy and effectiveness of reductions in dietary sodium on BP in hypertensive and normotensive subjects. The findings from these trials have been summarized in four recent meta-analyses.[17–20] Although the meta-analyses differed in their methodologies including inclusion or exclusion criteria and statistical analyses, they all concluded that a reduction in sodium intake lowers BP. Specifically, compared with control subjects, the mean reduction in BP was −3.9 to −5.9 mmHg for systolic BP and −1.9 to −3.8 mmHg for diastolic BP in hypertensive subjects and −1.2 to −1.9 mmHg for systolic BP and −0.3 to −1.1 mmHg for diastolic BP in normotensive subjects (Fig. 1). All of these results were statistically significant ($P < 0.05$). The results of these analyses also indicate that the relationship between sodium reduction and BP is greater for persons of older age, those with higher BP levels, and those with a longer duration of sodium reduction.

Several large clinical trials that included sodium reduction but were not included in the previously mentioned meta-analyses had concordant findings.[9,21] The Trial of Nonpharmacologic Interventions in the Elderly (TONE) was a randomized, controlled trial designed to determine whether counseling in weight loss, a reduction in dietary sodium intake, or both enhance BP control and reduce the need for antihypertensive

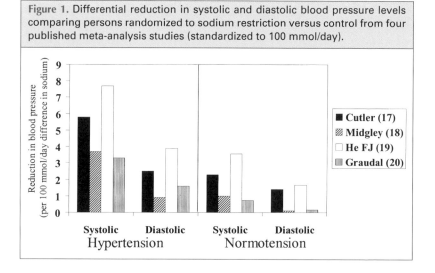

Figure 1. Differential reduction in systolic and diastolic blood pressure levels comparing persons randomized to sodium restriction versus control from four published meta-analysis studies (standardized to 100 mmol/day).

drug therapy in older people with hypertension.[22] The trial was conducted in 975 patients with baseline systolic BP < 145 mmHg and diastolic BP < 85 mmHg who were currently taking one antihypertensive medication. Mean 24-hour urinary sodium excretion was reduced by 40 mmol in those assigned to counseling in sodium reduction alone and by 24 mmol for those assigned to combined counseling in sodium reduction and weight loss. Compared with those randomized to usual care, average systolic BP was reduced by 3.4 mmHg in those assigned to counseling in sodium reduction and by 5.3 mmHg in those assigned to counseling in both sodium reduction and weight loss (Fig. 2). Additionally, participants randomized to usual care were 1.45 times more likely to have BP > 150/90 mmHg, resumption of antihypertensive medication, or a BP-related clinical complication during 2.5 years of follow-up compared with persons assigned to receive counseling for sodium reduction (P < 0.001). Among obese participants, those assigned to usual care were 1.67 and 2.13 times more likely to have these outcomes compared with those randomized to receive counseling for sodium reduction alone and sodium reduction and weight loss counseling, respectively.

The Reduced Sodium Dietary Approaches to Stop Hypertension trial studied the effects of sodium reduction in the context of a diet high in fruits and vegetables and low-fat dairy products.[9] This study reported

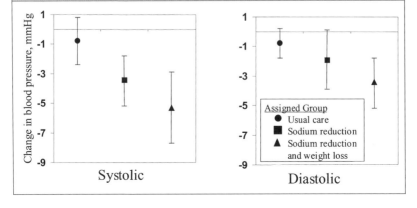

Figure 2. Change in systolic and diastolic blood pressure associated with usual care, sodium reduction counseling alone, and sodium reduction and weight loss counseling together in the Trials of Nonpharmacologic Intervention in the Elderly randomized, controlled trial.(From Whelton PK, Appel LJ, Espeland MA, et al: Sodium reduction and weight loss in the treatment of hypertension in older persons: A randomized controlled trial of nonpharmacologic interventions in the elderly (TONE). TONE Collaborative Research Group. JAMA 279: 839–846, 1998.)

large declines in BP after reductions in sodium intake and are reviewed in the section on overall dietary approaches for lowering BP. No safety concerns were reported in studies of moderate reductions in sodium intake.

Sodium Intake and Cardiovascular Disease Outcomes

No data are available from randomized, controlled trials showing the benefits of sodium reduction on CVD risk. Two cohort studies have been conducted using data from the First National Health and Nutrition Examination Survey (NHANES I) Epidemiological Follow-up study, a representative sample of the U.S. population that has been actively followed for 17 to 21 years.[23,24] Although, they used the same data, these studies reached different conclusions. One study did not find an association between higher sodium intake and an increase in CVD mortality. A subsequent study found a significant increased risk of mortality from stroke, CVD, coronary heart disease (CHD), and all causes among overweight participants. In the latter study, among overweight adults, for each 100-mmol sodium higher intake per 24 hours, the risk of mortality increased by 89% for stroke, 44% for CHD, 61% for CVD, and 39% for death from all causes (each $P \leq 0.02$). Differences in the results between these two studies may have resulted from differences in the hypotheses explored, exclusion criteria, analysis methodology, and the interaction between being overweight and sodium intake on CVD. In a more recent study of 1173 men and 1263 women living in Finland, a 100-mmol higher level of urinary sodium excretion was associated with an increased risk of CVD, CHD, and all-cause mortality of 45%, 51%, and 26%, respectively.[25] The relationship was stronger in overweight participants and was further increased after correction for regression-dilution bias.

Implications

In summary, a large body of scientific evidence shows a clinically important benefit of reducing dietary sodium intake for lowering BP as well as, the development of hypertension and cardiovascular disease. As such, the American Heart Association (AHA) and the National Heart Lung and Blood Institute (NHLBI) advocate limiting dietary sodium to ≤ 100 mmol per day.[5] Analysis of observational experience from a broad range of communities suggests that reducing dietary sodium by 100 mmol per day lowers systolic BP by an average of 3 to 6 mmHg.[26] Furthermore, the results from TONE show that counseling patients regarding sodium reduction is effective in the clinical setting. Although the response may vary by population group, sodium reduction to meet the AHA and NHLBI guidelines is strongly recommended.

Potassium Supplementation

The impact of potassium supplementation on BP reduction has been studied in clinical trials since the early 20th century.[27] The balance of evidence supports the role of potassium supplementation in lowering BP and it is recommended for the prevention and treatment of high BP.[4]

Clinical Trials

Since the first report of a benefit from potassium supplementation in lowering BP in 1928, more than 60 clinical trials have been published.[28,29] Because many of these randomized, controlled trials were small and underpowered, meta-analysis of their results have yielded the best evidence that potassium supplementation lowers BP.[30] In the largest and most recent of these meta-analyses, 33 randomized clinical trials that met prespecified inclusion requirements were analyzed.[28] One of these trials was an outlier; an extreme reduction of 41 and 17 mmHg in systolic and diastolic BP, respectively, was noted in the potassium supplementation group. Even after excluding an outlier trial that observed a 41/17-mmHg BP reduction, potassium supplementation was associated with a significant reduction in mean (95% confidence interval [CI]) systolic and diastolic BP of 3.11 mmHg (1.91, 4.31) and 1.97 mmHg (0.52, 3.42), respectively. Systolic BP reductions were significantly greater for the six trials with > 80% black participants than the 25 trials with > 80% white participants ($P = 0.03$; Table 1). The reduction in systolic and diastolic BP among those receiving potassium supplementation was also larger at higher levels of sodium intake. Although most clinical trials of potassium supplementation used potassium chloride pills, there is little reason to suspect different outcomes depending on whether potassium is administered as a dietary supplement, as a nonchloride salt, or by increasing fruit and vegetable intake.

Potassium Intake and Cardiovascular Disease Events

The presence of an inverse relationship between potassium intake and stroke mortality and a positive relationship between sodium to potassium ratio and stroke mortality have been reported from ecologic studies.[31,32] Several within-population studies that have indicated that high-potassium diets are protective against stroke and kidney disease.[33,34] Khaw et al. reported that dietary potassium intake was protective against stroke mortality in a 12-year prospective study of an elderly population in Southern California.[35] Specifically, among 859 residents of a retirement community, each 10-mmol higher level of dietary potassium intake was associated with a relative risk (95% CI) of stroke of 0.60 (0.44, 0.82) after adjustment for gender, age, systolic BP, serum total choles-

TABLE 1. Reduction in Systolic and Diastolic Blood Pressure in Those Receiving a Higher Versus Lower Level of Potassium*

Subgroup	Systolic, mmHg (95% CI)	Diastolic, mmHg (95% CI)
Overall	−3.1 (−14.3, −1.9)	−2.0 (−3.4, −0.5)
Hypertension	−4.4 (−6.6, −2.2)	−2.5 (−4.9, −0.1)
Normotension	−1.8 (−2.9, −0.6)	−1.0 (−2.1, 0.0)
Black	−5.6 (−18.7, −2.4)	−3.0 (−0.7, −5.3)
White	−2.0 (−3.0, −0.9)	−1.1 (−2.1, −0.1)
Urinary sodium excretion		
< 5 mmol/day	−1.2 (−2.4, 0.0)	0.1 (−1.0, 1.1)
5–12 mmol/day	−2.1 (−4.0, −0.3)	−1.4 (−2.8, 0.0)
≥ 12 mmol/day	−7.3 (−10.1, −4.6)	−4.7 (−8.3, −1.1)

* 32 randomized controlled trials by sub-group
CI = confidence interval
Adapted from Whelton PK, He J, Cutler JA, et al: Effects of oral potassium on blood pressure: Meta-analysis of randomized controlled clinical trials. JAMA 277:1624–1632, 1997.

terol, fasting plasma glucose, body mass index (BMI), and current smoking. In a 19-year prospective analysis of the NHANES I study, Bazzano et al. noted that after adjustment for age and energy intake, persons consuming < 34.6 mmol potassium per day had a 37% (relative hazards = 1.37; 95% CI: 1.20, 1.54; P < 0.001) higher hazard of stroke than their counterparts who were consuming higher levels of potassium.[36] The relative hazards estimate was not substantially altered by additional adjustment for established CVD risk factors and dietary factors. After adjustment for age, race, gender, systolic BP, serum cholesterol, BMI, history of diabetes, physical activity, education level, regular alcohol consumption, current cigarette smoking, vitamin supplement use, and other dietary factors, persons consuming < 34.6 mmol potassium per day experienced a 28% higher hazard of stroke than their counterparts consuming more potassium.

Implications

Evidence from clinical trials of potassium supplementation is consistent and supports a beneficial effect on BP. Also, low dietary potassium intake has been found to increase stroke risk. Current guidelines recommend an intake of potassium ≥ 90 mmol per day, preferably from food sources such as fresh fruits and vegetables.[5]

Calcium Supplementation

The hypothesis of an inverse relationship between dietary calcium and BP stemmed from reports in the 1960s relating hard drinking water to lower mortality from CVD.[37–39] Additional observational evidence in the 1970s and early 1980s found a correlation between higher calcium intake and lower BP levels. Since these early observations, many controlled trials have studied the effects of calcium supplementation on BP and hypertension. The balance of evidence indicates the positive benefit of calcium supplementation is too small to warrant its inclusion for the prevention or treatment of hypertension.[40,41]

Clinical Trials

Many randomized, controlled trials and several meta-analyses of these studies have been conducted to assess whether calcium supplementation lowers BP.[42–44] Trials of the efficacy of calcium supplementation in lowering BP have varied in size, duration, level of calcium supplementation, and level of baseline calcium intake within the study population. Results from meta-analyses of these trials provide the best estimate of efficacy.

In 1989, Cappuccio et al. pooled 15 randomized, controlled clinical trials that included almost 400 participants and reported no decrease in supine BP and a reduction of 0.91 (0.21, 1.61) and 0.56 mmHg (0.01, 1.12) in standing systolic and diastolic BP among those receiving calcium supplementation.[45] In 1996, Bucher et al. published a pooled analysis that showed a reduction (95% CI) in systolic BP of 1.27 mmHg (2.25, 0.29) and in diastolic BP of 0.24 mm Hg (0.92, +0.44). The most recent and largest meta-analysis was an update of the findings by this group.[42] This update was restricted to randomized, controlled trials conducted in nonpregnant patients. Overall, this meta-analysis included 42 studies with 4560 participants. A majority of the trials lasted for 4 to 14 weeks. Compared with their previous meta-analysis, calcium supplementation was associated with a slightly greater reduction in systolic and diastolic BP pressure. Compared with the control group, calcium supplementation was associated with an overall mean decline of 1.44 mmHg (95% CI: 2.20, 0.68) in systolic BP and 0.84 (95% CI: 1.44, 0.24) in diastolic BP. The authors concluded: "The modest response in systolic and diastolic blood pressure reduction we found does not justify the use of calcium supplementation as a sole treatment for patients with mild hypertension."[42]

Calcium Intake and Cardiovascular Disease Outcomes

Data from several large cohort studies have been used to investigate the association between calcium intake and risk of CVD, CHD, and stroke. During 28 years of follow-up, the adjusted relative risk (95% CI) of CVD and CHD mortality comparing the lowest to highest quintiles of calcium intake among 2605 Dutch civil servants was 1.3 (0.8, 1.9) and

0.9 (0.6, 1.6) for men and 1.1 (0.6, 2.0) and 1.1 (0.5, 2.5) for women, respectively.[46] Among Iowa's Women's Health Study Cohort participants who were not taking calcium supplementation, the relative risk (95% CI) of ischemic heart disease mortality was 0.63 (0.40, 0.98) for women in the highest versus lowest quintile of dietary calcium intake.[47] However, no association was noted between total calcium intake and ischemic heart disease mortality. Also, calcium supplementation did not significantly lower the risk of ischemic heart disease for women with an otherwise low level of dietary calcium intake (relative risk: 0.66, 95% CI: 0.36, 1.23).

Data from the initial 8 years of the Health Professionals Follow-up study indicated that a higher calcium intake was not associated with stroke risk. Specifically, men in the highest quintile of calcium intake had a 0.88 (0.63,1.23) risk of stroke compared with their counterparts in the lowest quintile.[34] In contrast, among 85,764 women in the Nurses' Health Study, the risk of ischemic and intraparenchymal stroke was 0.72 (0.53, 0.98) and 0.56 (0.24, 1.30), respectively, for those in the highest compared with the lowest quintile of calcium intake.[33] However, a higher quintile of calcium intake was associated with an increased risk of subarachnoid hemorrhage. In a pooled analysis, a significant association was not present between calcium intake and any stroke outcomes.

Implication

In summary, the overall consensus is that if calcium supplementation reduces blood pressure, its effect is minimal. The current Joint National Committee (JNC) VI guidelines state: "Although it is important to maintain an adequate amount of calcium intake for general health, there is no rationale for recommending calcium supplements for lowering blood pressure."[5]

Magnesium Supplementation

Early animal experiments and ecologic analyses suggested that magnesium intake might be inversely related to BP.[37,39,48] Since then, an inverse association between dietary magnesium intake and BP has been noted in several observational epidemiologic studies.[49,50] A review of evidence from observational studies has highlighted the limitations of inferences from these reports.[51,52] Limitations noted include imprecision of the dietary data and the concordance of dietary intake of magnesium with other micro-and macronutrients.

TABLE 2. Effect of Sodium Reduction on Systolic and Diastolic Blood Pressure in Those On Control and DASH Diet

	Control Diet			DASH Diet		
	High sodium to low sodium	High sodium to medium sodium	Medium sodium to low sodium	High sodium to low sodium	High sodium to medium sodium	Medium sodium to low sodium
Sodium reduction						
Systolic	−6.7 (−8.0, −5.4)	−2.1 (−3.4, −0.8)	−4.6 (−5.9, −3.2)	−3.0 (−4.3, −1.7)	−1.3 (−2.6, 0.0)	−1.7 (−3.0, −0.4)
Diastolic	−3.5 (−4.3, −2.6)	−1.1 (−1.9, −0.2)	−2.4 (−3.3, −1.5)	−1.6 (−2.5, −0.8)	−0.6 (−1.5, 0.2)	−1.0 (−1.9, −0.1)

Adapted from Sacks FM, Svetkey LP, Vollmer WM, et al: Effects on blood pressure of reduced dietary sodium and the Dietary Approaches to Stop Hypertension (DASH) diet. DASH-Sodium Collaborative Research Group. N Engl J Med 344:3–10, 2001.

Clinical Trials

A quantitative review of randomized trials was published in August 2002.[53] This review used a comprehensive search strategy to identify published English language reports on magnesium supplementation and BP in humans published before May 2001. Overall, 20 clinical trials met the authors' inclusion criteria. Magnesium supplementation was associated with a decline in systolic BP in 14 of the 20 (70%) trials, although statistically significant (P < 0.05) reductions were noted in only two of these studies. An overall pooled reduction in systolic BP of 0.6 mmHg (95% CI: 2.2 to +1.0) was seen for those randomized to the magnesium supplementation versus those in the control group. The analogous reduction in diastolic BP was 0.8 (95% CI: 2.1 to +0.5). In meta-regression analysis, high doses of magnesium supplementation were associated with a greater reduction in systolic and diastolic BP. Specifically, for each 10-mmol/day higher intake of magnesium, systolic and diastolic BP were lowered by 4.3 mmHg (6.3 to 2.2; P<0.01) and 2.3 mmHg (4.9 to 0.0; P = 0.09), respectively.

Dietary Magnesium Intake and Cardiovascular Disease

Although in many studies, serum magnesium correlated inversely with the incidence of CVD, evidence from prospective cohort studies relating dietary magnesium intake to CVD incidence is sparse.[54,55] The large population-based Atherosclerosis Risk in Communities (ARIC) study examined the relationship between dietary magnesium intake and CVD incidence among 13,922 participants free of CHD at baseline.[56] Over 6 years of follow-up, 96 women and 233 men had an incident CHD event. Dietary magnesium intake was weakly associated with risk of CHD in men but not in women. Compared with the lowest quartile of dietary magnesium consumption, the relative risk of CHD for the second lowest, third lowest, and highest quartile was 0.85 (0.60, 1.22), 0.79 (0.54, 1.16), and 0.69 (0.45, 1.05) in men and 1.20 (0.61, 2.34), 1.42 (0.74, 2.73), and 1.32 (0.68, 2.55) in women, respectively. Among this same population, serum magnesium showed a strong inverse relationship with CHD incidence. In the ARIC study, dietary magnesium showed only minimal correlation to serum magnesium (Pearson r = 0.04 for women and 0.09 for men).

Implications

Although supplementation with large doses of magnesium may provide a small benefit in lowering BP, the clinical value of such supplementation is uncertain. Given the minimal evidence in favor of the benefits of dietary supplementation, magnesium is not recommended as a means to lower BP or prevent hypertension.[5]

An Overall Dietary Approach

Trials that tested the ability of individual nutrients to lower BP often produced reductions in BP that were small. The presence of a synergistic effect such that consumption of increased amounts of these nutrients in sum results in a more substantial and important reduction in BP has been proposed. Two rigorously conducted controlled trials provide important data on the impact of overall change in diet on BP.[8]

Dietary Approaches to Stop Hypertension (DASH)

The DASH clinical trial compared the BPs of adults randomized to three different diets, which included a control or usual American diet, a diet rich in fruit and vegetables but retaining the same fat intake as the control diet, and a "combined" diet rich in fruits and vegetables with reduced saturated and total fat and low-fat dairy products. Volunteers were given three meals daily as well as between meal snacks throughout the study.

The DASH intervention, which includes multiple beneficial dietary changes (i.e., potassium, magnesium, fiber, antioxidants, and calcium [low-fat dairy products]) lowered BP more effectively than what has been reported for the individual components. A follow-up study, the reduced sodium DASH, clearly documented the benefits of salt restriction for lowering BP, both with the usual diet and with the DASH intervention. The BP-lowering effect of dietary sodium reduction was approximately twice as great in those assigned to the control diet than those assigned the DASH diet (Table 2). Compared with the high-sodium control diet, the DASH diet with a low level of sodium was associated with 11.5-and 7.1-mmHg larger reductions in systolic BP among participants with and without hypertension.

Implications

The DASH "combination" diet provided reductions in BP similar to those seen in clinical trials of drug monotherapy in mild hypertension. Moreover, a low sodium intake resulted in a substantial decrease of BP regardless of overall dietary pattern (i.e., the typical American diet or a healthy diet high in fruits and vegetables). Encouraging a combined approach of a diet rich in fruits, vegetables, and low-fat dairy products with a low saturated fat intake and reduced dietary sodium consumption appears to be a useful tool for treating and preventing hypertension.

Conclusions

In November 20002, a clinical and public health advisory on the primary prevention of hypertension from the National High Blood Pressure

> **TABLE 3.   Dietary Micronutrient Recommendations Contained in the 2002 Clinical and Public Health Advisory from the National High Blood Pressure Education Program**
>
> - Reduce dietary sodium intake to ≤ 100 mmol/day (2.4 g of sodium)
> - Maintain adequate intake of dietary potassium (> 90 mmol [3500 mg]day)
> - Consume a diet that is rich in fruits and vegetables and in low-fat dairy products with a reduced content of saturated and total fat (Dietary Approaches to Stop Hypertension [DASH] eating plan)
>
> Adapted Whelton PK, He J, Appel LJ, et al: Primary prevention of hypertension: Clinical and public health advisory from The National High Blood Pressure Education Program. JAMA 288:1882–1888, 2002.

Education Program was published.[4] The goal of that report was to update previous guidelines using the most recent available evidence. Consistent with evidence from clinical trials and relevant to dietary cations, these guidelines suggest a multifaceted approach for prevention of hypertension, including specific dietary recommendations (Table 3). First, dietary sodium intake should be limited to < 100 mmol/day. Second, these guidelines recommend an adequate intake of dietary potassium (> 90 mmol [3500 mg] per day). Finally, a diet rich in fruits, vegetables, and low-fat dairy products and low in saturated fat (i.e., the DASH diet) was recommended as a means for prevention. Promoting dietary modification, including a reduction in sodium intake, potassium supplementation, and undertaking an overall dietary approach, is challenging but provides a great potential for improving BP levels.

References

1. Stamler J, Stamler R, Neaton J: Blood pressure, systolic and diastolic, and cardiovascular risks. Arch Int Med 153:598–615, 1993.
2. Neaton JD, Grimm RH Jr., Prineas RJ, et al: Treatment of Mild Hypertension Study. Final results. Treatment of Mild Hypertension Study Research Group. JAMA 270:713–724, 1993.
3. Flack JM, Neaton J, Grimm R Jr., et al: Blood pressure and mortality among men with prior myocardial infarction. Multiple Risk Factor Intervention Trial Research Group. Circulation 92:2437–2445, 1995.
4. Whelton PK, He J, Appel LJ, et al: Primary prevention of hypertension: Clinical and public health advisory from The National High Blood Pressure Education Program. JAMA 288:1882–1888, 2002.
5. The sixth report of the Joint National Committee on Prevention, Detection, Evaluation, and Treatment of High Blood Pressure. Arch Intern Med 157: 2413–2446, 1997.
6. Whelton PK, He J, Appel LJ: Treatment and prevention of hypertension. In Manson JE, Ridker PM, Gaziano JM, Hennekens CH (eds): Prevention of Myocardial Infarction. New York: Oxford University Press, 1996, pp 154–171.

7. Whelton PK, He J: Blood pressure reduction treatment trials. In Hennekens CH, Buring J, Furberg C (eds): Clinical Trials in Cardiovascular Disease. Philadelphia: W.B. Saunders, 1998.

8. Appel LJ, Moore TJ, Obarzanek E, et al: A clinical trial of the effects of dietary patterns on blood pressure. DASH Collaborative Research Group. N Engl J Med 336: 1117–1124, 1997.

9. Sacks FM, Svetkey LP, Vollmer WM, et al: Effects on blood pressure of reduced dietary sodium and the Dietary Approaches to Stop Hypertension (DASH) diet. DASH-Sodium Collaborative Research Group. N Engl J Med 344:3–10, 2001.

10. Kempner W: Treatment of kidney disease and hypertensive vascular disease with rice diet. Am J Med 4:545–577, 1948.

11. Dahl LK: Possible role of salt intake in the development of essential hypertension. In Bock KD, Cottier PT (eds): Essential Hypertension. Berlin: Springer-Verlag, 1960, pp 53–65.

12. Swales JD: Dietary salt and hypertension. Lancet 1:1177–1179, 1980.

13. MacGregor GA: Sodium and potassium intake and high blood pressure. Eur Heart J 8(suppl)B:3–8, 1987.

14. Weinberger MH: Sodium chloride and blood pressure. N Engl J Med 317:1084–1086, 1987.

15. Denton D, Weisinger R, Mundy NI, et al: The effect of increased salt intake on blood pressure of chimpanzees. Nat Med 1:1009–1016, 1995.

16. Stamler R, Shipley M, Elliott P, et al: Higher blood pressure in adults with less education. Some explanations from INTERSALT. Hypertension 19:237–241, 1992.

17. Cutler JA, Follmann D, Allender PS: Randomized trials of sodium reduction: An overview. Am J Clin Nutr 65:643S–651S, 1997.

18. Midgley JP, Matthew AG, Greenwood CM, Logan AG: Effect of reduced dietary sodium on blood pressure: A meta-analysis of randomized controlled trials. JAMA 275:1590–1597, 1996.

19. He FJ, MacGregor GA: Effect of modest salt reduction on blood pressure: A meta-analysis of randomized trials. Implications for public health. J Hum Hypertens 16: 761–770, 2002.

20. Graudal NA, Galloe AM, Garred P: Effects of sodium restriction on blood pressure, renin, aldosterone, catecholamines, cholesterols, and triglyceride: A meta-analysis. JAMA 279:1383–1391, 1998.

21. Whelton PK, Appel LJ, Espeland MA, et al: Sodium reduction and weight loss in the treatment of hypertension in older persons: A randomized controlled trial of nonpharmacologic interventions in the elderly (TONE). TONE Collaborative Research Group. JAMA 279:839–846, 1998.

22. Whelton PK, Kumanyika SK, Cook NR, et al: Efficacy of nonpharmacologic interventions in adults with high-normal blood pressure: Results from phase 1 of the Trials of Hypertension Prevention. Trials of Hypertension Prevention Collaborative Research Group. Am J Clin Nutr 65:652S–660S, 1997.

23. He J, Ogden LG, Vupputuri S, et al: Dietary sodium intake and subsequent risk of cardiovascular disease in overweight adults. JAMA 282:2027–2034, 1999.

24. Alderman MH, Madhavan S, Cohen H, et al: Low urinary sodium is associated with greater risk of myocardial infarction among treated hypertensive men. Hypertension 25:1144–1152, 1995.

25. Tuomilehto J, Jousilahti P, Rastenyte D, et al: Urinary sodium excretion and cardiovascular mortality in Finland: A prospective study. Lancet 357:848–851, 2001.

26. Stamler J, Elliott P, Stamler R, et al: Non-pharmacological treatment of hypertension. Lancet 344:884–885, 1994.

27. Addison WL: The use of sodium chloride, potassium chloride, sodium bromide, and potassium bromide in cases of arterial hypertension which are amenable to potassium chloride. Can Med Assoc J 18:281–285, 1928.

28. Whelton PK, He J, Cutler JA, et al: Effects of oral potassium on blood pressure: Meta-analysis of randomized controlled clinical trials. JAMA 277:1624–1632, 1997.

29. Cappuccio FP, MacGregor GA: Does potassium supplementation lower blood pressure? A meta-analysis of published trials. J.Hypertens 9:465–473, 1991.

30. Greenland S: Meta-analysis. In Modern Epidemiology. 1998, 643–675.

31. Xie JX, Sasaki S, Joossens JV: The relationship between urinary cations obtained from the Intersalt study and cerebrovascular mortality. J Hum Hypertens 6:17–21, 1992.

32. Yamori Y, Nara Y, Mizushima S: Nutritional factors for stroke and major cardiovascular diseases: International epidemiological comparison of dietary prevention. Health Reports 6:22–27, 1994.

33. Iso H, Stampfer MJ, Manson JE, et al: Prospective study of calcium, potassium, and magnesium intake and risk of stroke in women. Stroke 30:1772–1779, 1999.

34. Ascherio A, Rimm EB, Hernan MA, et al: Intake of potassium, magnesium, calcium, and fiber and risk of stroke among US men. Circulation 98:1198–1204, 1998.

35. Khaw KT, Barrett-Connor E: Dietary potassium and stroke-associated mortality. A 12-year prospective population study. N Engl J Med 316:235–240, 1987.

36. Bazzano LA, He J, Ogden LG, et al: Dietary potassium intake and risk of stroke in US men and women: NHANES I epidemiologic follow-up study. Stroke 32:1473–1480, 2001.

37. Stitt FW, Clayton DG, Crawford MD, Morris JN: Clinical and biochemical indicators of cardiovascular disease among men living in hard and soft water areas. Lancet 1:122–126, 1973.

38. Neri LC, Johansen HL: Water hardness and cardiovascular mortality. Ann N Y Acad Sci 304:203–221, 1978.

39. Schroeder HA: Relationship between mortality from cardiovascular disease and treated water supplies; variation in states and 163 largest municipalities of the United States. JAMA 172:1902–1908, 1960.

40. Birkett NJ: Comments on a meta-analysis of the relation between dietary calcium intake and blood pressure. Am J Epidemiol 148:223–228, 1998.

41. Bucher HC, Guyatt GH, Cook RJ: Dietary calcium and blood pressure. Ann Intern Med 126:492–493, 1997.

42. Griffith LE, Guyatt GH, Cook RJ, et al: The influence of dietary and nondietary calcium supplementation on blood pressure: an updated metaanalysis of randomized controlled trials. Am J Hypertens 12:84–92, 1999.

43. Cappuccio FP, Elliott P, Allender PS, et al: Epidemiologic association between dietary calcium intake and blood pressure: A meta-analysis of published data. Am J Epidemiol 142:935–945, 1995.

44. Cutler JA, Brittain E: Calcium and blood pressure. An epidemiologic perspective. Am J Hypertens 3:137S–146S, 1990.

45. Cappuccio FP, Siani A, Strazzullo P: Oral calcium supplementation and blood pressure: An overview of randomized controlled trials. J Hypertens 7:941–946, 1989.

46. Van der Vijver LP, van der Waal MA, Weterings KG, et al: Calcium intake and 28-year cardiovascular and coronary heart disease mortality in Dutch civil servants. Int J Epidemiol 21:36–39, 1992.

47. Bostick RM, Kushi LH, Wu Y, et al: Relation of calcium, vitamin D, and dairy food intake to ischemic heart disease mortality among postmenopausal women. Am J Epidemiol 149:151–161, 1999.

48. Berthelot A, Esposito J: Effects of dietary magnesium on the development of hypertension in the spontaneously hypertensive rat. J Am Coll Nutr 2:343–353, 1983.

49. Rubenowitz E, Axelsson G, Rylander R: Magnesium in drinking water and death from acute myocardial infarction. Am J Epidemiol 143:456–462, 1996.

50. Joffres MR, Reed DM, Yano K: Relationship of magnesium intake and other dietary factors to blood pressure: The Honolulu heart study. Am J Clin Nutr 45:469–475, 1987.

51. Whelton PK, Klag MJ: Magnesium and blood pressure: Review of the epidemiologic and clinical trial experience. Am J Cardiol 63:26G–30G, 1989.

52. Mizushima S, Cappuccio FP, Nichols R, Elliott P: Dietary magnesium intake and blood pressure: A qualitative overview of the observational studies. J Hum Hypertens 12:447–453, 1998.

53. Jee SH, Miller ER, III, Guallar E, et al: The effect of magnesium supplementation on blood pressure: A meta- analysis of randomized clinical trials. Am J Hypertens 15:691–696, 2002.

54. Yamori Y, Mizushima S: A review of the link between dietary magnesium and cardiovascular risk. J Cardiovasc Risk 7:31–35, 2000.

55. Cappuccio FP: Sodium, potassium, calcium and magnesium and cardiovascular risk. J Cardiovasc Risk 7:1–3, 2000.

56. Liao F, Folsom AR, Brancati FL: Is low magnesium concentration a risk factor for coronary heart disease? The Atherosclerosis Risk in Communities (ARIC) Study. Am Heart J 136:480–490, 1998.

57. Svetkey LP, Sacks FM, Obarzanek E, et al: The DASH Diet, Sodium Intake and Blood Pressure Trial (DASH-sodium): Rationale and design. DASH-Sodium Collaborative Research Group. J Am Diet Assoc 99:S96–104, 1999.

Nutrition, Dietary Supplements, and Nutraceuticals in Hypertension

chapter 17

Mark C. Houston, M.D., SCH

New and future treatment guidelines for lower target blood pressure (BP) levels in the general hypertensive population as well as in specific populations of hypertensive patients will demand a combination of non-pharmacologic (lifestyle modification) and pharmacologic therapy.[7,27] Hypertensive patients with diabetes mellitus (DM), renal insufficiency (RI), proteinuria, congestive heart failure (CHF), or coronary heart disease (CHD), as well as those with previous myocardial infarction (MI), cerebrovascular accidents (CVA), or transient ischemic attacks (TIA) often require three to four antihypertensive medications to reach a BP of 140/90 mm Hg or less.[7,27] Lower recommended target BP goals of 130/80 mm Hg or perhaps 110/70 mm Hg cannot be attained without aggressive use of *balanced* drug and nondrug treatments. Nutrition, dietary supplements, nutraceuticals, achieving ideal body weight, exercise (i.e., aerobic and resistance training), and restriction of caffeine and alcohol are crucial ingredients of this *combination* approach to reduce BP and subsequent target organ damage (TOD) (Fig. 1).

Hypertension, Nutrition, and Vascular Biology

Hypertension (HTN) is a consequence of the interaction of environment and genetics. *Macronutrients* and *micronutrients* are crucial in the regulation of BP, subsequent TOD, and atherosclerosis (AS). *Nutrient–gene interactions,* oxidative stress, and subsequent gene expression have either positive or negative influences on vascular biology in humans. *Endothelial dysfunction* and vascular smooth muscle cell dysfunction are the initiating and perpetuating factors in essential hypertension. The correct combination of macronutrients and micronutrients significantly influences prevention and treatment of hypertension and subsequent

181

vascular complications. Treatment directed at the blood vessel, as well as the BP, should include identification and optimal management of cardiovascular (CV) risk factors and oxidative stress in order to reduce AS and TOD (Figs. 1 and 2). TOD reduction is dependent on *both hypertensive and nonhypertensive* mechanisms.

Nutritional needs have been imposed on the population during our evolution from a pre-agricultural, hunter–gatherer milieu to a highly technological agricultural industry that is dependent on mechanical processing for our food supply.[18,48] The paleolithic diet consisted of low sodium, high potassium, high fiber, low fat, lean animal protein, low refined carbohydrate, and low cholesterol intake composed of fruits, vegetables, berries, nuts, fish, fowl, wild game, and other nutrient-dense foods. On the other hand, the modern diet of processed, chemically altered, fast, fried, and frozen food has resulted in an epidemic of nutritionally related diseases such as hypertension, hyperlipidemia diabetes and obesity.

Figure 1. The importance of combination therapy, sequence, and variety of treatment options (non-drug and drug) improve vascular biology and blood pressure.

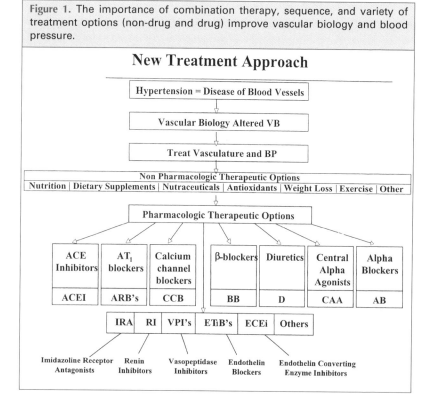

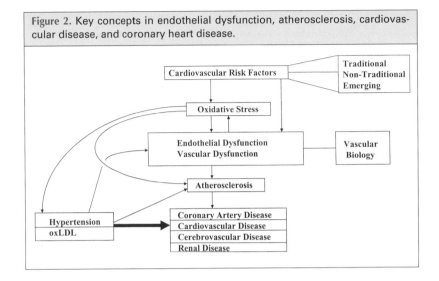

Figure 2. Key concepts in endothelial dysfunction, atherosclerosis, cardiovascular disease, and coronary heart disease.

Nutrition Trials and Hypertension

Reduction in BP as well as reductions in cardiovascular morbidity and mortality have been demonstrated in numerous short- and long-term clinical hypertension nutritional trials.[4,5,12,44,45,47] Up to 50% of hypertensive patients in the appropriate stage and risk category may be initially treated with lifestyle modifications for 6 to 12 months based on Joint National Committee-VI (JNC-VI) guidelines.[27] However, specific patients with existing cardiovascular, cerebrovascular, renal, or other TOD, diabetes or multiple cardiovascular risk factors usually require immediate drug therapy in conjunction with lifestyle modifications.[27] Combined nutrients present in food, especially fruits and vegetables, as well as single and combined nutraceutical and nutrient or dietary supplementation have been demonstrated to reduce BP (Table 1).[43]

The combined low-sodium Dash II diet[45] reduced BP 11.5/6.8 mm Hg within 2 weeks maintained this BP for the duration of the 2-month study and improved quality of life. This level of BP reduction is equivalent to that achieved with pharmacologic monotherapy.

Sodium. A reduction in sodium intake to 2400 mg/day lowers BP an average of 4 to 6 mm Hg systolic and 2 to 3 mm Hg diastolic BP in salt-sensitive hypertensive patients.[3] Reduced sodium intake also reduces renal dysfunction, proteinuria, CHF, CVA, vascular hypertrophy, and left ventricular hypertrophy. Further reductions of BP can be achieved with progressive restriction from 150 mmol to 100 mmol to 50 mmol of dietary sodium per day in the DASH II diet.[45]

TABLE 1. Lifestyle Changes and SBP Meta-analysis of Clinical Diet Trials	
Intervention	Reduction in SBP (mm Hg)
↑ Mg^{++}	0–1
↑ Ca^{++}	2
↑ K^+	4
↓ ETOH	4
Fish Oil	6
↓ Na^+	6
↓ Weight	8
Exercise	10
DASH diet	12

Adapted from Reaven P, Parthasarathy S, Grasse BJ, et al: Effects of oleate-rich and linoleate-rich diets on the susceptibility of low density lipoprotein to oxidative modification in mildly hypercholesterolemic subjects. J Clin Invest 1993, 91:668–676.

Potassium. The magnitude of BP reduction with supplementation of 60 to 120 mEq per day of potassium is 4.4 mm Hg systolic and 2.5 mm Hg diastolic BP in hypertensive patients.[3,49] In addition, potassium may reduce cardiovascular events and CVA independent of BP and reduce the risk of cardiac arrhythmias. The recommended dietary intake is a K^+/Na^+ ratio is 5:1.

Magnesium. Magnesium supplementation in the range of 500 to 1000 mg per day reduces systolic BP 2.7 mm Hg and diastolic BP 3.4 mm Hg.[51] Magnesium lowers systemic vascular resistance (SVR) and reduces arrhythmias. The mechanism is blockade of calcium influx into vascular SMCs and increased levels of the vasodilating prostaglandin E_1 (PGE_1).

Calcium. A recent meta-analysis of the effect of calcium supplementation in hypertensive patients demonstrated a reduction in systolic BP of 4.3 mm Hg and diastolic BP of 1.5 mm Hg.[9] Calcium is particularly effective in patients with a high sodium intake and when given in a natural form with potassium and magnesium.[36,41,50] Blacks, elderly, diabetic, salt sensitive, pregnant, postmenopausal women, and low-renin hypertensives have the best response.

Protein. High intake of non-animal protein (1 mg/kg/day) (Intersalt Study, Intermap Study) is associated with a lower BP.[3,19] Hydrolyzed whey protein[29] and sardine muscle extract[28] significantly lower BP in humans through an angiotensin-converting enzyme (ACE) inhibitor mechanism.

Fats. Consumption of omega-3 fatty acids (polyunsaturated fatty acids [PUFA]) such as EPA (eicosapentaenoic acid) and DHA (docosahexanoic acid) significantly reduce mean BP in humans by 5.8 to 8.1 mm Hg.[8,32,37,42] This combined with omega-9 fatty acids (olive oil) (monounsaturated, oleic acid), low saturated fat, elimination of trans-fatty acids, and increased gamma linolenic acid (GLA) may have dramatic effects on blood pressure, vascular biology, and AS. The omega-3 to omega-6 fatty acid ratio should be 1:1 to 4:1 with consumption of cold water fish (e.g., cod, tuna, mackerel, salmon), flax seed or oil, fish oil (15 g/day), cod liver oil supplements, and EPA/DHA supplements (3 to 4 g/day). The olive oil dose is 40 grams of extra-virgin olive oil per day (4 tablespoons).[20]

Garlic. The prospective placebo-controlled studies utilizing the correct form (wild garlic is best) and dose of garlic demonstrate only minimal decreases in systolic BP of 5 to 8 mm Hg or mean BP of 2% to 3%.[1] However, garlic may have numerous other beneficial vascular effects because it is a natural ACE inhibitor and calcium channel blocker (CCB).[11]

Seaweed. Wakame seaweed in doses of 3.3 g/day significantly lowered BP in hypertensive humans within 4 weeks because of ACE inhibitor activity.[38] The average reduction in BP was 14/5 mm Hg. Long-term use appears to be safe based on the Japanese experience.

Fiber. Clinical trials with various types of fiber to reduce BP have been inconsistent.[3,25] The average BP reduction in prospective studies using 60 g/day of oatmeal fiber (3 g/day of beta glucan, glucomannan or 7 g/day of psyllium) is 7.5 mm Hg/5.5 mm Hg.

Vitamin. Vitamin C at doses of 250 to 500 mg twice a day lowers BP, especially in hypertensive patients with initially low plasma ascorbate levels.[16,21,39] Vitamin C improves endothelial dysfunciton, increases nitric oxide levels, is a potent antioxidant, decreases systemic vascular resistance, and decreases BP by an average of 7/4 mm Hg. The greater the initial BP and the lower the plasma ascorbate level, the greater the response. Combinations with other antioxidants and vitamins may have synergistic antihypertensive effects.

Vitamin B6 Pyridoxine. Supplemental vitamin B6 at 5 mg/kg/day reduced BP 14/10 mm Hg over 4 weeks.[6] Vitamin B6 reduces central sympathetic nervous system activity and acts as a central alpha agonist (i.e., clonidine), a CCB, and a diuretic. Pyridoxine also improves insulin sensitivity and carbohydrate metabolism, which improves BP. Daily doses should probably not exceed 200 mg to avoid neuropathy.

Lycopene. Paran et al[40] evaluated 30 subjects with grade I hypertensive given tomato lycopene extract for 8 weeks. The BP decreased 9/7 mm Hg within 8 weeks. Lycopene is found in high concentrations in tomatoes and tomato products, guava, pink grapefruit, watermelon, papaya, and apricots.

Coenzyme Q10 (Ubiquinone). Enzymatic assays show a deficiency of coenzyme Q-10 (coQ-10) in 39% of essential hypertensive patients versus only a 6% deficiency in control subjects.[34] Human studies demonstrate significant and consistent reductions in BP averaging 15/10 mm Hg in all reported prospective clinical trials.[13,14,15,31,33] Doses of 100 to 225 mg per day (1 to 2 mg/kg/day) to achieve a therapeutic plasma level of over 2 μ/mL are effective within 4 to 8 weeks in reducing BP. The BP remains steady at this level and returns to baseline at 2 weeks after discontinuation of coQ-10. CoQ-10 reduces SVR, catecholamine, and aldosterone levels; improves insulin sensitivity and endothelial function; and increases nitric oxide levels.[13,14,33] No adverse effects have been noted at these doses with chronic use. Patients have been able to stop or reduce the number of antihypertensive drugs by one to three with chronic ingestion of coQ-10. A reputable, certified absorbable form with excellent bioavailability and measurement plasma levels are important clinical considerations.

L-Arginine. L-arginine is the natural predominant precursor for vascular nitric oxide. Administration of 10 g/day orally in food or as a supplement significantly reduces BP in human subjects by 6.2/6.8 mm Hg and improves endothelial dysfunction and blood flow.[30,46]

Taurine. Taurine, a sulfonic beta-amino acid, is significantly reduced in the urine of patients with essential hypertension.[2] Administration of 6 g/day of taurine lowers BP 9/4 mm Hg.[22] Taurine induces sodium-water diuresis and vasodilation, increases atrial natriuretic factor, reduces sympathetic nervous system activity and aldosterone levels, improves insulin sensitivity, and reduces homocysteine levels.

Celery. Celery has antihypertensive properties caused by 3-N-butyl phthalide, apigenin, and other substances that act like ACE inhibitors or CCB blockers. Four stalks per day or the equivalent in celery juice, oil, or celery seed extract reduces BP in animals and humans.[10,17,26,34,35]

Combinations. Combinations of various nutraceutical or dietary supplements, vitamins, and antioxidants may further enhance BP reduction, reduce oxidative stress, and improve vascular function and structure.[24] Optimal doses and combinations are yet to be determined, but future research will provide important data. Finally, the addition of lifestyle modification with low-dose combination antihypertensive drugs provides additive or synergistic BP reduction to achieve these lower BP goals; improves risk factors, metabolic parameters, vascular structure, and function; and allows for lower doses and number of drugs with reduced side effects to reduce TOD.

Natural Antihypertensive Compounds Categorized by Antihypertensive Class

As discussed previously, many of the natural compounds such as food, nutraceutical and dietary supplements, vitamins, antioxidants, or minerals function in a similar fashion to a specific class of antihypertensive drugs. Although the potency of these natural compounds may be less than or equal to the antihypertensive drug and the onset of action slower when used in combination, the antihypertensive effect is magnified. In addition, many of these natural compounds have varied, additive, or synergistic mechanisms of action in lowering BP. Table 2 summarizes these natural compounds into the major antihypertensive drug classes such as diuretics, beta-blockers, central alpha agonists, CCBs, ACE inhibitors, and ARBs.

TABLE 2. Natural Antihypertensive Compounds Categorized by Antihypertensive Class

Diuretics

Hawthorne berry	Mg^{++}
Vitamin B6 (pyridoxine)	Ca^{++}
Taurine	Protein
Celery	Fiber
GLA	Coenzyme Q-10
Vitamin C (ascorbic acid)	L-Carnitine (?)
K^+	

Beta-blockers

Hawthorne berry

Central alpha agonists

Taurine	Vitamin C
K^+	Vitamin B6
Zinc	Coenzyme Q-10
Na^+ restriction	Celery
Protein	GLA/DGLA
Fiber	Garlic

Direct vasodilators

Omega-3 fatty acids	Flavonoids
MUFA (omega-9 fatty acids)	Vitamin C
K^+	Vitamin E
Mg^{++}	Coenzyme Q-10
Ca^{++}	L-Arginine
Soy	Taurine
Fiber	Celery
Garlic	Alpha lipoic acid

Calcium channel blockers

Alpha lipoic acid (ALA)	Hawthorne berry
Vitamin C (ascorbic acid)	Celery
Vitamin B-6 (pyridoxine)	Omega-3 fatty acids (EPA and DHA)
Magnesium (Mg^{++})	Calcium
N-Acetyl cysteine (NAC)	Garlic
Vitamin E	

ACE inhibitors

Garlic	Geletin
Seaweed—various (Wakame, etc.)	Sake
Tuna protein or muscle	Essential fatty acids (omega-3 fatty acids)
Sardine protein or muscle	Chicken egg yolks

(continued)

TABLE 2. Natural Antihypertensive Compounds Categorized by Antihypertensive Class (*Continued*)

Hawthorne berry	Zein
Bonito fish (dried)	Dried salted fish
Pycnogenol	Fish sauce
Casein	Zinc
Hydrolyzed whey protein	Hydrolyzed wheat germ isolate
Sour milk	

Angiostensin receptor blockers
Potassium (K+)
Fiber
Garlic
Vitamin C
Vitamin B6 (pyridoxine)
Coenzyme Q-10
Celery
Gamma linolenic acid (GLA) and DGLA

References

1. Ackermann RT, Mulrow CD, Ramirez G, et al: Garlic shows promise for improving some cardiovascular risk factors. Arch Intern Med 2001, 161:813–824.
2. Ando K, Fujita T: Etiological and physiopathological significance of taurine in hypertension. Nippon Rinsho 1992, 50:374–381.
3. Appel LJ: The role of diet in the prevention and treatment of hypertension. Curr Atheroscler Rep 2000, 2:521–528.
4. Appel LJ, Moore TJ, Obarzanek E, et al: A clinical trial of the effects of dietary patterns on blood pressure. N Engl J Med 1997, 336:1117–1124.
5. Ascherio A, Rimm EB, Hernan MA, et al: Intake of potassium, magnesium, calcium and fiber and risk of stroke among US men. Circulation 1998, 98:1198–1204.
6. Aybak M, Sermet A, Ayyildiz MO, Karakilcik AZ: Effect of oral pyridoxine hydrochloride supplementation on arterial blood pressure in patients with essential hypertension. Arzneimittelforschung 1995, 45:1271–1273.
7. Bakris GL: A practical approach to achieving recommended blood pressure goals in diabetic patients. Arch Intern Med 2001, 161:2661–2667.
8. Bao DQ, Mori TA, Burke V, et al: Effects of dietary fish and weight reduction on ambulatory blood pressure in overweight hypertensives. Hypertension 1998, 32:710–717.
9. Bucher HC, Cook RJ, Guyatt GH, et al: Effects of dietary calcium supplementation on blood pressure: a meta-analysis of randomized controlled trials. JAMA 1996, 275:1016–1022.
10. Castleman M: The Healing Herbs: The Ultimate Guide to the Curative Power of Nature's Medicines. Emmaus, PA: Rodale Press 1991, 105–107.
11. Clouatre D: European Wild Garlic: The Better Garlic. San Francisco: Pax Publishing, 1995.
12. De Lorgeril M, Salen P, Martin JL, et al: Mediterranean diet, traditional risk factors

and the rate of cardiovascular complications after myocardial infarction: final report of the lyon diet heart study. Circulation 1999, 99:779–785.

13. Digiesi V, Cantini F, Bisi G, et al: Mechanism of action of coenzyme Q10 in essential hypertension. Curr Ther Res 1992, 51:668–672.

14. Digiesi V, Cantini F, Brodbeck B : Effect of coenzyme Q10 on essential hypertension. Curr Ther Res 1990, 47:841–845.

15. Digiesi V, Cantini F, Oradei A, et al: Coenzyme Q-10 in essential hypertension. Mol Aspects Med 1994, 15(suppl):257–263.

16. Duffy SJ, Gokce N, Holbrook M, et al : Treatment of hypertension with ascorbic acid. Lancet 1999, 354:2048–2049.

17. Duke JA: The Green Pharmacy Herbal Handbook. Emmaus, PA: Rodale Press; 2000, 68–69.

18. Eaton SB, Eaton SB III, Konner MJ: Paleolithic nutrition revisited: a twelve-year retrospective on its nature and implications. Eur J Clin Nutr 1997, 51:207–216.

19. Elliott P, Dennis B, Dyer AR, et al: Relation of dietary protein (total, vegetable, animal) to blood pressure: INTERMAP epidemiologic study. Presented at the 18th Scientific Meeting of the International Society of Hypertension, Chicago, IL, August 20–24, 2000.

20. Ferrara LA, Raimondi S, d'Episcopa I, et al: Olive oil and reduced need for antihypertensive medications. Arch Intern Med 2000, 160:837–842.

21. Fotherby MD, Williams JC, Forster LA, et al: Effect of vitamin C on ambulatory blood pressure and plasma lipids in older persons. J Hypertens 2000, 18:411–415.

22. Fujita T, Ando K, Noda H, et al: Effects of increased adrenomedullary activity and taurine in young patients with borderline hypertension. Circulation 1987, 75:525–532.

23. Gaby AR: The role of co-enzyme Q-10 in clinical medicine: Part II. Cardiovascular disease, hypertension, diabetes mellitus and infertility. Alt Med Rev 1996, 1:168–175.

24. Galley HF, Thornton J, Howdle PD, et al: Combination oral antioxidant supplementation reduces blood pressure. Clin Sci 1997, 92:361–365.

25. He J, Welton PK: Effect of dietary fiber and protein intake on blood pressure. A review of epidemiologic evidence. Clin Exp Hypertens 1999, 21:785–796.

26. Heinerman J: Heinerman's New Encyclopedia of Fruits and Vegetables. Paramus, NJ: Prentice Hall 1995, 93–95.

27. Joint National Committee on Prevention, Detection, Evaluation, and Treatment of High Blood Pressure: the sixth report of the Joint National Committee on the prevention, detection, evaluation, and treatment of high blood pressure. Arch Intern Med 1997, 157:2413–2446.

28. Kawasaki T, Seki E, Osajima K, et al: Antihypertensive effect of valyl-tyrosine, a short chain peptide derived from sardine muscle hydrolyzate, on mild hypertensive subjects. J Hum Hypertens 2000, 14:519–523.

29. Kawase M, Hashimoto H, Hosoda M, et al: Effect of administration of fermented milk containing whey protein concentrate to rats and healthy men on serum lipids and blood pressure. J Dairy Sci 2000, 83:255–263.

30. Kelly JJ, Williamson P, Martin A, Whitworth JA: Effects of oral L-arginine on plasma nitrate and blood pressure in cortisol-treated humans. J Hypertens 2001, 19:263–268.

31. Kendler BS: Nutritional strategies in cardiovascular disease control: an update on vitamins and conditionally essential nutrients. Prog Cardiovasc Nurs 1999, 14:124–129.

32. Knapp HR, Fitzgerald GA: The antihypertensive effects of fish oil: a controlled study

of polyunsaturated fatty acid supplements in essential hypertension. N Engl J Med 1989, 320:1037–1043.

33. Langsjoen P, Willis R, Folkers K: Treatment of essential hypertension with coenzyme Q10. Mol Aspects Med 1994, 15(suppl):265-272.

34. Le OT, Elliott WJ: Dose response relationship of blood pressure and serum cholesterol to 3-N-butyl phthalide, a component of celery oil [abstract]. Clinical Research 1991, 39:750A.

35. Le OT, Elliott WJ: Mechanisms of the hypotensive effect of 3-N-butyl phthalide (BUPH): a component of celery oil [abstract]. J Am Hypertens 1992, 40(suppl A):326.

36. McCarron DA: Calcium metabolism in hypertension. Keio J Med 1995, 44:105–114.

37. Morris M, Sacks F, Rosner B: Does fish oil lower blood pressure? A meta-analysis of controlled trials. Circulation 1993, 88:523–533.

38. Nakano T, Hidaka H, Uchida J, et al: Hypotensive effects of wakame. J Jpn Soc Clin Nutr 1998, 20:92.

39. Ness AR, Chee D, Elliot P: Vitamin C and blood pressure—an overview. J Hum Hypertens 1997, 11:343–350.

40. Paran E, Engelhard Y: Effect of tomato's lycopene n blood pressure, serum lipoproteins, plasma homocysteine and oxidative stress markers in grade I hypertensive patients [abstract]. Am J Hypertens 2001, 14:141A.

41. Preuss HG: Diet, genetics and hypertension. J Am Coll Nutr 1997, 16:296–305.

42. Prisco D, Paniccia R, Bandinelli B, et al: Effect of medium-term supplementation with a moderate dose of n-3 polyunsaturated fatty acids on blood pressure in mild hypertensive patients. Thromb Res 1998, 91:105–112.

43. Reaven P, Parthasarathy S, Grasse BJ, et al: Effects of oleate-rich and linoleate-rich diets on the susceptibility of low density lipoprotein to oxidative modification in mildly hypercholesterolemic subjects. J Clin Invest 1993, 91:668–676.

44. Resnick LM, Oparil S, Chait A, et al: Factors affecting blood pressure responses to diet: the Vanguard Study. Am J Hypertens 2000, 13:956–965.

45. Sacks FM, Svetkey LP, Vollmer WM, et al: Effects on blood pressure of reduced dietary sodium and the dietary approaches to stop hypertension (DASH) diet. N Engl J Med 2001, 344:3–10.

46. Siani A, Pagano E, Iacone R, et al: Blood pressure and metabolic changes during dietary L-arginine supplementation in humans. Am J Hypertens 2000, 13:547–551.

47. The Treatment of Mild Hypertension Research Group: The Treatment of Mild Hypertension Study: a randomized, placebo-controlled trial of a nutritional-hygienic regimen along with various drug monotherapies. Arch Intern Med 1991, 151:1413–1423.

48. Weder AB: Your mother was right: eat your fruits and vegetables. Curr Hypertens Rep 1999, 1:11–12.

49. Whelton PK, He J. Potassium in preventing and treating high blood pressure. Semin Nephrol 1999, 19:494–499.

50. Whiting SJ, Wood R, Kim K: Calcium supplementation. J Am Acad Nurse Pract 1997, 9:187–192.

51. Witteman JCM, Grobbee DE, Derkx FHM, et al: Reduction of blood pressure with oral magnesium supplementation in women with mild to moderate hypertension. J Clin Nutr 1994, 60:129–135.

Comorbid Depression and Hypertension-related Chronic Medical Conditions

chapter
18

Leonard E. Egede, M.D., M.S.

Cardiovascular diseases (CVDs) are among the leading causes of death in the United States. About 62 million people (30 million men and 32 million women) had some form of CVD in 2002, and CVD accounted for 960,000 deaths or one of every 2.5 deaths in 1999.[1] In addition, CVD accounted for $329.2 billion in direct and indirect medical costs. Hypertension is a major contributor to CVD in the United States. In 1999, nearly 44 million people had hypertension, and almost 61 million people had one or more types of hypertension-related chronic medical conditions (Table 1).[2] Therefore, hypertension is not only a prevalent comorbid condition; but is also a significant contributor to morbidity and mortality in the United States.

Depression

Depression is a brain disorder that affects about 19 million or 9.5% of the adult population of the United States every year.[3] Depressive disorders affect about 12% of women (12.4 million) and 6.6% of men (6.4 million) each year.[4] Depression is a major cause of workplace absenteeism, decreased or lost productivity, and increased use of health care resources.[5] Suicide is the most dreaded complication of major depression, and it occurs in 10% to 15% of patients previously admitted for depression.[5] Women are two to three times more likely to attempt suicide[6]; however, men are four-times more likely to commit suicide.[7]

191

TABLE 1. Prevalence of Hypertension-related Chronic Medical Conditions, United States 1999

Condition	Population (in millions)	Patients with Condition, %	Patients with Comorbid Hypertension, %
Diabetes	10.7	5.4	60.7
Hypertension	44.1	22.6	100.0
CAD	21.8	11.0	51.3
Stroke	4.1	2.1	68.8
ESRD	2.6	1.3	22.1
All hypertension-related chronic conditions	60.5	30.3	74.4

CAD = coronary artery disease, ESRD = end-stage renal disease

Relationship between Comorbid Depression and Hypertension-related Chronic Medical Conditions

Depression co-occurs in a substantial proportion of patients with various general medication conditions including heart disease, stroke, cancer, diabetes, and chronic renal disease (Table 2).[2]

Hypertension

After controlling for age and gender, almost 9% of adults with hypertension had major depression in 1999 (see Table 2).[2] Depression is predictive of later incidence of hypertension in normotensive subjects.[8] There is also an association between baseline depression and increased mortality in older adults with moderate hypertension independent of other known CVD risk factors.[9] Finally, depression has been associated with noncompliance with antihypertensive medication.[10]

Coronary Artery Disease

Comorbid depression is present in about 11% of adults with coronary artery disease (CAD) (see Table 2).[2] Evidence suggests that baseline de-

TABLE 2. Major Depression in Individuals with Hypertension-related Chronic Medical Conditions

Chronic Medical Conditions	Adjusted for Age and Gender, %	95% CI
Diabetes	10.1	8.4, 11.8
Hypertension	8.9	8.0, 9.8
CAD	11.2	9.9, 12.5
Stroke	16.1	12.4, 19.8
ESRD	17.7	13.3, 22.1

pression increases the risk of subsequent cardiac and total mortality independent of disease severity or type of treatment.[11,12] Data also show that among patients with angiography-proven CAD, depressed patients have more physical limitations, more frequent angina, less satisfaction with care, and lower perceived quality of life than nondepressed patients.[13]

Diabetes Mellitus

Approximately 10% of people with diabetes have major depression (see Table 2).[2] Individuals with diabetes have two times the chance of depression compared with individuals without diabetes.[14,15] Depression in people with diabetes is associated with poor adherence to dietary recommendations,[16] hyperglycemia,[17] poor metabolic control,[18] increased diabetes complications,[19] decreased quality of life,[20] and increased health care use and expenditure.[15]

Stroke

Poststroke depression occurs in roughly 30% of stroke survivors[21,22]; in 1999, about 16% of individuals with stroke had major depression (see Table 2).[2] Poststroke depression prolongs rehabilitation, is associated with worse outcomes, and prolongs hospital length of stay.[23] In addition, the impaired recovery of physical and language function that is caused by depression persists for up to 2 years after the stroke and after the remission of depression.[24] Finally, poststroke depression can last from 12 to 39 weeks and is associated with a mortality rate of 23%.[22]

End-stage Renal Disease

The prevalence of major depression in individuals with end-stage renal disease (ESRD) ranges from 6% to 34%.[25,26] After adjusting for age and gender, 18% of adults with ESRD had major depression in 1999 (see Table 2).[2] Depression is associated with increased risk of mortality and hospitalizations in individuals with ESRD.[26] Adjusting for time on dialysis, age, race, socioeconomic status, comorbidity, and nationality, the risks of death and hospitalization were 1.23 and 1.11, respectively, for physician-diagnosed depression.[26] Similarly, higher levels of depressive affect in ESRD patients have been associated with increased mortality.[27]

In summary, major depression is a significant problem in people with hypertension-related diseases. Untreated depression in these patients impairs physical functioning, decreases quality of life, and increases mortality.

Diagnosis of Depression

The diagnosis of depression is based on clinical findings. Several valid and reliable screening instruments are available for use in primary care.[28–32] Depressed mood and anhedonia plus the presence of additional symptoms of depression listed in Table 3 typically characterize major depressive disorders. These disorders differ quantitatively and qualitatively from normal sadness or grief. Normal grief or sadness is usually time limited and is less pervasive than major depressive disorders. In addition, hopelessness and an inability to experience pleasure may occur in rare instances, but suicidal thoughts or psychotic symptoms are always absent in normal sadness.[5]

Major Depression

Patients experience depressed mood and anhedonia during the same 2-week period plus five or more of the symptoms listed in Table 3.[33]

Dysthymia

Dysthymia is characterized by depressed mood for most of the day, for more days than not, as indicated either by subjective account or observation by others, for at least 2 years. In addition, at least two of the symptoms listed in Table 4 should be present while the patient is depressed.[33]

Minor Depression

Minor depression is similar to major depression in that patients' experience depressed mood and anhedonia during the same 2-week period. However, the patients have fewer symptoms than required to make a diagnosis of major depression.[33]

Bipolar Disorder and Cyclothymia

Bipolar disorder is a recurrent mood disorder featuring one or more episodes of mania or mixed episodes of mania and depression.[33] Cy-

TABLE 3. Symptoms of Major Depression*	
Depressed mood	Fatigue or loss of energy
Markedly diminished interest or pleasure in activities	Feelings of worthlessness or excessive or inappropriate guilt
Significant weight loss when not dieting or weight gain	Diminished ability to think or concentrate
Insomnia or hypersomnia	Recurrent thoughts of death, recurrent suicidal ideation, or a suicide attempt
Psychomotor agitation or retardation	

*These symptoms should represent a change from previous functioning and should occur all day or almost all day.

TABLE 4.	Symptoms of Dysthymia
Poor appetite or overeating	Low self-esteem
Insomnia or hypersomnia	Poor concentration or difficulty making decisions
Low energy or fatigue	Feelings of hopelessness

clothymia is characterized by the presence of many periods with hypomanic symptoms and many periods with depressive symptoms that do not meet the criteria for a major depressive episode for at least 2 years.[33] Patients with bipolar disorder and cyclothymia should be referred to a psychiatrist.

Treatment of Depression

The treatment of patients with depression includes several methods. Pharmacotherapy, psychotherapy, and electroconvulsive therapy (ECT) are effective treatment options. All classes of antidepressant medications are equally effective.[34] Pharmacotherapy is the principal treatment in primary care. Newer pharmacotherapies such as the selective serotonin reuptake inhibitors (SSRIs) are easier to dose, better tolerated by patients, and have fewer side effects and drug–drug interactions than the older agents such as the tricyclic antidepressants (TCAs).[34]

The four stages of treatment include response (4 to 6 weeks), remission (6 to 8 weeks), continuation (6 to 9 months), and maintenance (variable duration). The goal of treatment is full remission.

A total of 50% to 70% of patients respond to the initial agent, and 50% of nonresponders respond to an alternative agent.

The choice of initial agent is based on prior response (individual or family) to the same agent and the side effects experienced. Patient education is critical to adherence and treatment success. Tables 5 and 6 show the classification, dosage, and side effects of commonly used antidepressant medications. Figure 1 shows a simple, evidence-based, algorithm to treat depression in primary care.

Barriers to Recognition and Treatment of Depression in Primary Care

Only about 50% of depressed patients are recognized by their primary care physicians as being depressed. The most important reason is that fewer than 2% of primary care patients complain of depression during the physician–patient encounter.[35] Other important barriers[36–38] to recognition and treatment of depression in primary care are listed in Table 7. The diagnosis of depression should be entertained in all pri-

TABLE 5. Classification and Dosage of Commonly Used Antidepressant Medications

Drug Class	Generic Name	Trade Name	Starting Dose, mg	Optimal Dose, mg	Indications	Precautions
SSRIs	Escitalopram	Lexapro	10	10–20	Depression Anxiety	Decrease dose in liver or renal impairment
	Citalopram	Celexa	20	20–40	Depression OCD	Maximum dose 20 mg in liver disease and elderly persons
	Fluoxetine	Prozac	20 90 weekly	40–60	Depression Bulimia OCD Panic disorder PMDS	Lower dose in liver impairment and elderly persons
	Paroxetine	Paxil, Paxil CR	20 25 for CR	20–60 25–62.5	Depression Panic Disorder OCD Social anxiety disorder PTSD	Start 10 or 12.5 mg, Maximum 40 or 50 mg in renal and liver impairment and elderly persons
	Sertraline	Zoloft	50	100–200 mg	Depression PTSD Panic disorder OCD	No dosage adjustment in renal failure 100 mg maximum in liver disease and elderly persons
SNRIs	Mirtazapine	Remeron	15	15–45	Depression	Decrease dose in liver and renal impairment noradrenaline reuptake
	Venlafaxine	Effexor, Effexor XR	75 BID/TID	75–225 mg BID/TID	Depression GAD	Decrease dose in liver and renal impairment

Class	Generic	Brand	Starting dose	Dose range	Indications	Cautions
DRIs	Bupropion	Wellbutrin, Zyban	200 150 SR	200–300 150–300 SR	Depression Smoking cssation	Decrease dose in liver disease
Triazolopyridine	Trazodone	Desyrel	150	150–400	Depression	Decrease dose in liver disease and elderly persons
TCAs	Amitriptyline	Elavil, Endep	75 day	75–150 day	Depression	Decrease dose in liver disease
	Clomipramine	Anafranil	25 TID	100–250 day	Depression OCD	Caution after MI
	Doxepin	Sinequan, Adapin	75	75–300 day	Depression Pruritus	Decrease dose in liver disease and elderly persons
	Imipramine	Tofranil	50–100 mg QD or TID	150–300 mg QD or TID	Depression Urinary incontinence Enuresis	Decrease dose in liver disease and elderly persons
	Desipramine	Norpramin	100	100–300 QD	Depression	Decrease dose in liver disease and elderly persons
	Nortriptyline	Pamelor	60	60–150	Depression Enuresis ADD	Caution after MI

ADD = attention-deficit disorder; BID = twice daily; DRI = dopamine reuptake inhibitor; GAD = generalized anxiety disorder; MI = myocardial infarction; OCD = obsessive compulsive disorder; PTSD = posttraumatic stress disorder; QD = once daily; SSRI = selective serotonin reuptake inhibitors; SNRI = serotonin-norepinephrine reuptake inhibitors; TID = thrice daily; TCAs = tricyclic antidepressants.

TABLE 6. Commonly Occurring Side Effects of Antidepressant Medications

Generic Name	GI Disturbance	Anticholinergic Effects	Weight Gain	Weight Loss	Sedation	Insomnia	Hypotension	Sexual Dysfunction
SSRIs								
Escitalopram	2+	2+	0	0	0	0	0	2+
Citalopram	2+	1+	0	0	2+	2+	2+	2+
Fluoxetine	2+	1+	0	0	1+	2+	1+	2+
Paroxetine	2+	2+	0	0	1+	2+	1+	2+
Sertraline	2+	1+	0	1+	0	1+	1+	2+
SNRIs								
Mirtazapine	2+	3+	2+	0	4+	0	0	1+
Venlafaxine	3+	2+	0	1+	0	2+	0	2+
DRIs								
Bupropion	2+	1+	2+	3+	4+	0	0	2+
Triazolopyridine								
Trazodone	2+	2+	1+	1+	4+	0	2+	0
TCAs								
Amitriptyline	1+	4+	2+	0	4+	0	4+	1+
Clomipramine	1+	4+	1+	0	4+	0	4+	1+
Doxepin	1+	4+	1+	0	4+	0	4+	1+
Imipramine	1+	4+	1+	0	4+	0	4+	1+
Desipramine	1+	3+	1+	0	3+	0	4+	1+
Nortriptyline	1+	3+	1+	0	3+	0	4+	1+

0 = none or absent; 1+ = < 5%; 2+ = 5%–20%; 3+ = 21%–40%; 4+ = >40%.
Sertraline may cause hypoglycemia.
Mirtazapine is associated with hyperglycemia, hypercholesterolemia, and hypertriglyceridemia.
Effexor may increase blood pressure in 5% of patients.
Bupropion stimulates insulin secretion in individuals with low, threshold, and high glucose levels.

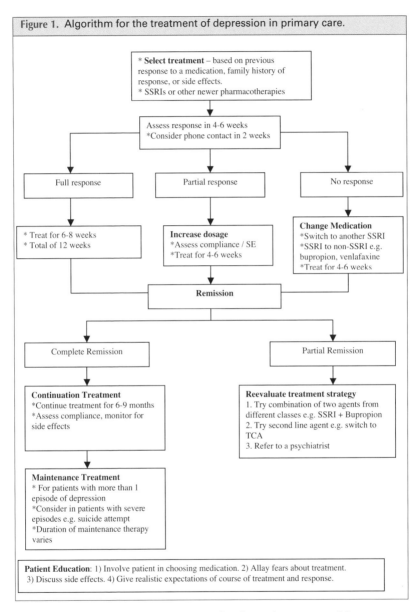

Figure 1. Algorithm for the treatment of depression in primary care.

* **Select treatment** – based on previous response to a medication, family history of response, or side effects.
* SSRIs or other newer pharmacotherapies

Assess response in 4-6 weeks
*Consider phone contact in 2 weeks

Full response

Partial response

No response

* Treat for 6-8 weeks
* Total of 12 weeks

Increase dosage
*Assess compliance / SE
*Treat for 4-6 weeks

Change Medication
*Switch to another SSRI
*SSRI to non-SSRI e.g. bupropion, venlafaxine
*Treat for 4-6 weeks

Remission

Complete Remission

Partial Remission

Continuation Treatment
*Continue treatment for 6-9 months
*Assess compliance, monitor for side effects

Reevaluate treatment strategy
1. Try combination of two agents from different classes e.g. SSRI + Bupropion
2. Try second line agent e.g. switch to TCA
3. Refer to a psychiatrist

Maintenance Treatment
* For patients with more than 1 episode of depression
*Consider in patients with severe episodes e.g. suicide attempt
*Duration of maintenance therapy varies

Patient Education: 1) Involve patient in choosing medication. 2) Allay fears about treatment. 3) Discuss side effects. 4) Give realistic expectations of course of treatment and response.

mary care patients with chronic medical conditions. Health care providers should be aware of their biases, be sensitive to patient concerns, and offer creative solutions when a diagnosis of depression is likely. Finally, the routine inclusion of depression screening questions as part of the history and physical examination in primary care clinics will likely be beneficial.

TABLE 7. Barriers to Recognition and Treatment of Depression in Primary Care

Patient-level Barriers to Recognition and Treatment
Misconceptions about the etiology of depression
Shame and Stigma of depression
Distrust of physicians
Denial
Fear of addiction to anti-depressants
Cost of medications
Religious/Spiritual beliefs

Clinician-level Barriers to Recognition and Treatment
Inadequate knowledge about depression
Provider beliefs and attitudes
Unwillingness to document a diagnosis
Attributing symptoms of depression to the individuals chronic illness
Unwillingness to uncover and discuss psychosocial issues
Time constraints
Disincentives

Health Care System Barriers to Recognition and Treatment
Biomedical vs biopsychosocial model
Limited referral sites
Limitations on third-party coverage
Restriction to particular treatments or medications
Poor ancillary support
Low reimbursement for depression care

Future Directions

At this point, the nature of the relationship between depression and several hypertension-related conditions remains unclear. Further studies are needed to determine whether the relationship is causal and whether any interventions may decrease the adverse effects of depression on morbidity and mortality. Coordinated depression screening and treatment strategies need to be implemented in primary care. Such strategies should draw on the knowledge gained from the concepts of chronic disease management and collaborative care. Finally, effective depression screening and treatment strategies that are easily integrated into the routine care for patients with chronic medical conditions need to be developed.

References

1. American Heart Association: 2002 Heart and Stroke Statistical Update. American Heart Association, Dallas, 2001.
2. Egede LE, Zheng D: Prevalence and correlates of major depression in a national sample of US adults with chronic medical conditions. 1999 National Health Interview Survey. Unpublished.

3. Regier DA, Narrow WE, Rae DS, et al: The de facto mental and addictive disorders service system: Epidemiologic Catchment Area prospective 1-year prevalence rates of disorders and services. Arch Gen Psychiatr 1993, 50:85–94.
4. Narrow WE: One-year prevalence of mental disorders, excluding substance use disorders, in the U.S.: NIMH ECA prospective data. Population estimates based on U.S. Census estimated residential population age 18 and over on July 1, 1998. Unpublished.
5. U.S. Department of Health and Human Services. Mental Health: A Report of the Surgeon General. Rockville, MD: U.S. Department of Health and Human Services, Substance Abuse and Mental Health Services Administration, Center for Mental Health Services, National Institutes of Health, National Institute of Mental Health, 1999.
6. Weissman MM, Bland RC, Canino GJ, et al: Prevalence of suicide ideation and suicide attempts in nine countries. Psychological Med 1999, 29:9–17.
7. Hoyert DL, Kochanek KD, Murphy SL: Deaths: final data for 1997. National Vital Statistics Report, 47(19). DHHS Publication No. 99–1120. Hyattsville, MD: National Center for Health Statistics, 1999. Available at http://www.cdc.gov/nchs/data/nvs47_19.pdf
8. Jonas BS, Franks P, Ingram DD: Are symptoms of anxiety and depression risk factors for hypertension? Longitudinal evidence from the National Health and Nutrition Examination Survey I Epidemiologic Follow-up Study. Arch Fam Med 1997, 6:43–49.
9. Abas M, Hotopf M, Prince M: Depression and mortality in a high-risk population. 11-Year follow-up of the Medical Research Council Elderly Hypertension Trial. Br J Psychiatr 2002, 181:123–128.
10. Wang PS, Bohn RL, Knight E, et al: Noncompliance with antihypertensive medications: the impact of depressive symptoms and psychosocial factors. J Gen Intern Med 2002, 17:504–511.
11. Carney RM, Rich MW, Freedland KE, et al: Major depressive disorder predicts cardiac events in patients with coronary artery disease. Psychosom Med 1988, 50:627–633.
12. Barefoot JC, Helms MJ, Mark DB, et al: Depression and long-term mortality risk in patients with coronary artery disease. Am J Cardiol 1996, 78:613–617.
13. Spertus JA, McDonell M, Woodman CL, Fihn SD: Association between depression and worse disease-specific functional status in outpatients with coronary artery disease. Am Heart J 2000, 140:105–110.
14. Anderson RJ, Freedland KE, Clouse RE, Lustman PJ: The prevalence of comorbid depression in adults with diabetes: a meta-analysis. Diabetes Care 2001, 24:1069–1078.
15. Egede LE, Zheng D, Simpson K: Comorbid depression is associated with increased health care use and expenditures in individuals with diabetes. Diabetes Care 2002, 25:464–470.
16. Ciechanowski PS, Katon WJ, Russo JE: Depression and diabetes: impact of depressive symptoms on adherence, function, and costs. Arch Intern Med 2000, 160:3278–3285.
17. Lustman PJ, Anderson RJ, Freedland KE, et al: Depression and poor glycemic control: a meta-analytic review of the literature. Diabetes Care 2000, 23:934–942.
18. Gary TL, Crum RM, Cooper-Patrick L, et al: Depressive symptoms and metabolic control in African-Americans with type 2 diabetes. Diabetes Care 2000, 23:23–29.
19. de Groot M, Anderson R, Freedland KE, et al: Association of depression and diabetes complications: a meta-analysis. Psychosom Med 2001, 63:619–630.
20. Hanninen JA, Takala JK, Keinanen-Kiukaanniemi SM: Depression in subjects with type 2 diabetes. Predictive factors and relation to quality of life. Diabetes Care 1999, 22:997–998.

21. Andersen G, Vestergaard K, Riis J, Lauritzen L: Incidence of post-stroke depression during the first year in a large unselected stroke population determined using a valid standardized rating scale. Acta Psychiatr Scand 1994, 90:190–195.

22. Morris PL, Robinson RG, Raphael B. Prevalence and course of depressive disorders in hospitalized stroke patients. Int J Psychiatry Med 1990, 20:349–364.

23. Turner-Stokes L, Hassan N: Depression after stroke: a review of the evidence base to inform the development of an integrated care pathway. Part 2: treatment alternatives. Clin Rehabil 2002, 16:248–260.

24. Parikh RM, Robinson RG, Lipsey JR, et al: The impact of poststroke depression on recovery in activities of daily living over a 2-year follow-up. Arch Neurol 1990, 47: 785–789.

25. O'Donnell K, Chung JY: The diagnosis of major depression in end-stage renal disease. Psychother Psychosom 1997, 66:38–43.

26. Lopes AA, Bragg J, Young E, et al: Depression as a predictor of mortality and hospitalization among hemodialysis patients in the United States and Europe. Kidney Int 2002, 62:199–207.

27. Kimmel PL, Peterson RA, Weihs KL, et al: Multiple measurements of depression predict mortality in a longitudinal study of chronic hemodialysis outpatients. Kidney Int 2000, 57:2093–2098.

28. Beck A, Ward C, Mendelson M: An inventory for measuring depression. Arch Gen Psychiatr 1961, 4:53–63.

29. Zung W: A self-rating depression scale. Arch Gen Psychiatr 1965, 12:63–70.

30. Radloff LS: The CES-D scale: a self-report depression scale for research in the general population. Appl Psychol Measurement 1977, 1:385–401.

31. Spitzer RL, Williams JB, Kroenke K, et al: Utility of a new procedure for diagnosing mental disorders in primary care: the PRIME-MD 1000 study. JAMA 1994, 272: 1749–56.

32. Whooley MA, Avins AL, Miranda J, Browner WS: Case-finding instruments for depression: two questions are as good as many. J Gen Intern Med 1997, 12:439–445.

33. American Psychiatric Association: Diagnostic and Statistical Manual for Mental Disorders, fourth edition (DSM-IV). Washington, DC, American Psychiatric Press, 1994.

34. Snow V, Lascher S, Mottur-Pilson C: Pharmacologic treatment of acute major depression and dysthymia: American College of Physicians-American Society of Internal Medicine. Ann Intern Med 2000, 132:738–742.

35. Zung WW, Broadhead WE, Roth ME: Prevalence of depressive symptoms in primary care. J Fam Pract 1993, 37:337–344.

36. Egede LE: Beliefs and attitudes of African Americans with type 2 diabetes toward depression. Diabetes Educ 2002, 28:258–268.

37. Nutting PA, Rost K, Dickinson M, et al: Barriers to initiating depression treatment in primary care practice. J Gen Intern Med 2002, 17:103–111.

38. Goldman LS, Nielsen NH, Champion HC: Awareness, diagnosis, and treatment of depression. J Gen Intern Med 1999, 14:569–580.

Management of Obesity

Patrick Mahlen O'Neil, Ph.D., and
Corby K. Martin, Ph.D.

chapter
19

Obesity is a well-known risk factor for hypertension. Weight loss can improve hypertension for many patients. This chapter describes the definition and measurement of obesity, reasonable weight loss goals as part of hypertension management, and proven elements of successful weight management.

Definition and Measurement of Obesity

Although obesity is defined most precisely as excess body *fat*, accurate assessment of body composition is not available in most outpatient settings, and it is not necessary in the majority of cases. Body mass index (BMI) is a weight-to-height ratio accepted worldwide as an index of weight status as related to health. It is calculated as[2]:

$$BMI = \text{Weight in kg} / (\text{height in m})^2$$
or
$$\text{Weight in lbs} \times 703 / (\text{height in inches})^2$$

BMI calculators are widely available on the Internet for direct use and for downloading into PDAs (see the list of resources at the end of this chapter).

The significance of different BMI levels is shown in Table 1. As can be seen, a BMI between 25.0 and 29.9 is considered overweight, and a BMI ≥ 30 is considered obese. The healthy range of BMI is 18.5 to 25.0. These cutpoints are based on the evidence relating comorbidities and mortality to BMI.[14] These reference ranges are based on epidemiologic data and provide an initial benchmark of a patient's weight status. However, as will be noted below, they should not be used as a table of "ideal" weight. Not every overweight or obese patient needs to lower his or her BMI to the 18.5 to 25.0 range to improve health.

The association of BMI and weight gain with hypertension is well established. Among women in the Nurse's Health Study, every additional BMI unit (1 kg/m²) above 20 increased the risk for hypertension by 12%,

TABLE 1. Weight Classification and Obesity Class by BMI		
	BMI (kg/m²)	Obesity Class
Underweight	< 18.5	N/A
Normal	18.5–24.9	N/A
Overweight	25.0–29.9	N/A
Obesity	30.0–34.9	I
	35.0–39.9	II
Extreme Obesity	≥ 40	III

N/A = not applicable
Adapted from The Practical Guide: Identification, Evaluation, and Treatment of Overweight and Obesity in Adults. (See Appendix: List of Online Resources.)

and women who gained 10.0 to 19.9 kg. from age 18 years were 2.7 times more likely to develop hypertension compared with women who maintained weight within 2.0 kg.[9] The Framingham study found that compared with normal-weight individuals (BMI, 18.5–24.9), overweight (BMI, 25.0–29.9) men and women were 46% and 75% more likely to develop hypertension, respectively, and obese (BMI ≥ 30) men and women had 121% and 175% higher risks, respectively.[22]

Fat distribution also modifies the risk posed by a given level of BMI. Upper-body fat distribution, reflecting excess visceral fat, poses a greater health risk than does lower-body fat distribution. This is especially noteworthy in the case of hypertensive patients, given that hypertension is part of the constellation of symptoms that comprise the metabolic syndrome: abdominal obesity, atherogenic dyslipidemia (elevated triglycerides, small low-density lipoprotein [LDL] particles, low high-density lipoprotein (HDL) cholesterol), elevated blood pressure (BP), insulin resistance, and prothrombotic and proinflammatory states.[13] Waist circumference is a good indicator of the presence of excess upper-body fat. Waist circumference is measured by locating the upper hip bone and right iliac crest, wrapping the tape measure around the abdomen at the level of the iliac crest. A waist circumference > 35 inches for women or > 40 inches for men represents heightened risk and increased justification for weight loss.

Weight Loss Goals for Hypertension Management

Although clear health benefits exist for losing weight, particularly for hypertensive patients, approaching the issue of weight and weight loss requires some sensitivity. In the case of a patient with one or more comorbidities (e.g., hypertension, dyslipidemias, insulin resistance, elevated blood glucose level), the risk to the individual patient is not only theoretical and can clearly be noted. Presenting weight as one of the list of problems may take it out of the "moral" realm and place it in a more constructive context. Asking the patient if he or she is willing to discuss ways to lower weight for health is a necessary first step.

Patients may be relieved to learn that the amount of weight loss needed is less than they may assume. Research has clearly demonstrated that a modest reduction in body weight (e.g., 5% to 10% of original body weight) can have a significant positive impact on health, including reduced BP,[3,7,21] and can reduce the risk of developing hypertension.[19] These benefits can be seen even if the resulting BMI is still in the obese range. Actually, many obese patients desire a much greater loss, and it may be necessary to focus on the above weight loss goal as a first, achievable step.

Many people have unrealistic ideas about the pace of weight loss, in part from long-term exposure to the barrage of exorbitant claims in advertisements for weight loss gimmicks and diets of unproven value. Lost in this din is the reality that calories in (i.e., eating and drinking) should be less than calories out (i.e., resting metabolism plus energy expended in activity). It can be helpful to inform the patient that loss of 1 pound of body fat requires the expenditure of approximately 3500 calories more than is consumed, which means, for example, that a 500-calorie-per-day deficit equates to a 1-pound-per-week loss. This can lead to a weight loss goal of 1 to 2 pounds per week at most.

Elements of Successful Weight Management

A variety of effective methods are available to help patients with their weight loss efforts. The range of options that may be considered increases with increasing degree of obesity (Table 2). The approaches should be tried in the order shown, from top to bottom. For example, for patients at BMI above 40, pharmacotherapy may be tried if lifestyle change has been unsuccessful; if neither is successful, surgery may be considered. However, accumulating evidence suggests that combining treatments (e.g., lifestyle change, meal replacements, medication) may provide significantly more weight loss than single interventions.[20]

Lifestyle Changes

As shown in Table 2, lifestyle change is the basis of all weight loss approaches. Lifestyle change typically consists of changes in dietary and exercise patterns. Because these changes are often difficult, behavior therapy techniques are used to encourage the adoption and maintenance of these changes and to equip patients with self-management skills.

TABLE 2.	Weight Loss Strategies by BMI Classification				
	BMI Classification				
Treatment	**25.0–26.9**	**27.0–29.9**	**30–35**	**35.0–39.9**	**> 40**
Lifestyle change	With comorbidities	With comorbidities	+	+	+
Pharmacotherapy	N/A	With comorbidities	+	+	+
Surgery	N/A	N/A	With comorbidities	+

N/A = not applicable
Adapted from The Practical Guide: Identification, Evaluation, and Treatment of Overweight and Obesity in Adults. (See Appendix: List of Online Resources.)

Diet

Dietary interventions for weight loss can range from simple changes or deletions of single items to highly specific daily menu plans. A useful first step is to obtain a picture of the patient's usual eating and drinking patterns. This can be achieved by simply asking for a recall of the previous day's intake, including snacks and drinks. For more accuracy, the patient can be asked to keep a food record for 3 to 7 days (including at least 1 weekend day), listing everything with calories that is consumed. The records should show what is consumed, the method of preparation, the quantity consumed, and the time of consumption. Such self-monitoring records often increase the patient's awareness of sources of excess calories.

However the intake information is obtained, the physician and patient can review it together briefly to determine fruitful areas of change. Often drinks are an overlooked source of calories, and reduction or elimination of calorically sweetened soft drinks and other beverages (e.g., lattes and other specialty coffee drinks that are high in milk, cream, and sugar) can produce a substantial calorie savings. Substitution of fruits for high-calorie snacks can also reduce caloric intake. Fats that are added at the time of eating (e.g., butter, sour cream, salad dressings) may also add substantially to the day's calorie count and should be reduced or replaced with lower-calorie alternatives. Use of lower-calorie meal replacements such as shakes and pre-portioned meals and entrees can enhance short- and long-term weight loss,[6] although the sodium content of the latter items should be examined.

Most patients can benefit from increasing their intake of fruits and nonstarchy vegetables. The "5-A-Day" goal (five servings of fruits and vegetables each day; see http://www.5aday.gov for information and patient handouts) is infrequently met by most Americans. Selection of higher-volume, less calorically dense fruits and vegetables can allow patients to eat a greater volume of food while reducing calories, as long as the fruits and vegetables displace more calorically dense foods.

Many patients need or request more structured dietary guidance. When a registered dietitian is available, a consultation may be appropriate to help the patient develop an individualized weight loss program. When such services are not available, other sources of meal plans can be recommended or provided to the patient. Several meal plans are provided in *The Practical Guide: Identification, Evaluation, and Treatment of Overweight and Obesity in Adults,* which is available at the sites shown in the Appendix. Numerous diets and diet books are widely available, and some general guidance may help patients select among them. Any books that make claims of rapid, effortless weight loss should be eschewed, as should plans based excessively on food combining. Although most nutrition experts recommend the Food Guide pyramid as a guide to healthful eating for the populace, the numbers of servings generally recommended on most materials may be too high for weight loss. Diets that are suitable for weight loss may not follow the pyramid precisely. For example, protein intake during weight loss may represent a higher proportion of calories, especially at a reduced calorie level, and starches may be somewhat less plentiful. However, many "high-protein" diets (e.g., Atkins-type plans) are high-fat diets, and they are likely not advisable for patients who already have cardiovascular risk factors such as hypertension. Sodium intake should also be addressed when discussing diets. Finally, patients should be advised that a weight-*loss* diet may not be a healthful weight-*maintenance* diet, and that maintenance will require careful attention to energy balance. An excellent review of diets for weight loss is found in Melanson and Dwyer.[12]

The DASH (Dietary Approaches to Stop Hypertension) nutritional program is discussed in Chapter 15 and represents a very appropriate weight maintenance dietary plan for hypertensive patients after weight loss.

Exercise

Exercise is vital to maintenance of weight loss and in itself is an aid to controlling hypertension. Chapter 20 provides additional details of increasing moderate-intensity aerobic activity to 30 minutes per day most days of the week (also see the American College of Sports Medicine website, listed in the resources section). It is important to note that mounting evidence suggests the value of incorporating resistance training as part of an exercise plan for weight management. Such training helps maintain muscle mass, which helps to maintain energy expenditure. Anyone beginning resistance training, particularly hypertensive patients, should be advised to avoid the Valsalva maneuver by continuing to breathe when performing resistance exercises. In addition to increasing activity through intentional exercise by augmenting activity throughout the day, such as climbing stairs rather than taking the elevator, decreases in sedentary activities (e.g., television, video games, reading) may further contribute to increased overall energy expenditure.

Behavior Modification

The important dietary, exercise, and activity changes necessary for weight management often run counter to patients' habits, preferences, and environment. They often require short-term discomfort and the denial of immediate gratification for the promise of future benefit. Behavioral techniques can help patients to offset these factors and can equip patients with self-management skills. Although comprehensive behavioral weight loss programs involve frequent sessions with psychologists or other behavioral specialists, several techniques that are particularly effective for weight loss can efficiently be promoted in a primary care setting. Below is a short list some of these techniques.

- **Self-monitoring:** Recording of daily food and drink *intake* has been convincingly demonstrated to improve weight loss.[15] Patients may also record *exercise time or distance* to track and encourage progress. For long-term success, regular weighing and graphing of *weight* is important; patients should be cautioned against overinterpreting very short-term fluctuations that may reflect shifts in fluid balance. (A weight graph for downloading is included in the list of resources.)

- **Behavioral goal-setting:** Achieving long-term weight loss requires more immediate behavioral changes. Patients should be encouraged to set a small number of specific, attainable behavioral goals to be achieved within a modest time frame. Examples include exercising 30 minutes 4 days in the next week, recording food intake 6 of 7 days, or consuming five servings of fruits and vegetables each day. The patient should designate which behaviors he or she is willing to include in these goals.

- **Rewards:** Behaviors are more often achieved and repeated when they produce immediate rewards. Unfortunately, the immediate consequences of reduced food intake or increased exercise are not always rewarding. Establishing a specific reward that will be earned by achieving a specified behavioral goal can improve these natural contingencies. For example, a patient may agree to watch a favorite nightly television show only when he or she has exercised. Or a patient may state that a desired CD or book will only be bought when the dietary plan has been followed for 1 week.

- **Stimulus control:** Many behaviors occur more frequently in the presence of certain cues or stimuli, such as visible food, place, time, activity, or even mood. For example, unplanned eating may be tied to watching television at certain times, driving, or boredom. Limiting eating to a smaller number of stimuli may make it easier to control, for example, by limiting eating to one location in the home, avoiding the pairing of eating with certain other stimuli, or keeping food items out of sight. Stimuli can also promote desirable behaviors; such as trying to exercise at certain reliable times of day or changing into walking shoes before returning home from work.
- **Recovery from lapses:** Weight management is a long-term process, and setbacks should be expected. Success is enhanced if the patient and provider have nonperfectionistic expectations. Patients should be prepared to recover from inevitable lapses or slips by quantifying how much they have strayed from their goals, analyzing the precipitants of the setback, and revising goals accordingly.

Pharmacotherapy

For patients with BMI > 30, or BMI 27 to 30 with comorbidities, weight loss medications may be considered when lifestyle interventions have not produced adequate weight loss. Currently, two medications are approved by the Food and Drug Administration for long-term use.

Orlistat

Orlistat (Xenical) is a lipase inhibitor that blocks approximately 30% of ingested fat from being absorbed. It is nonsystemic. Orlistat has been found to increase weight loss compared to placebo in trials lasting ≤ 2 years, with reductions in BP commensurate with the greater weight loss.[5] It has also been shown to enhance maintenance of weight previously lost through other means.[8]

The most common side effects of orlistat are related to its pharmacologic effect: oily spotting, flatus with discharge, fecal urgency, and so on. Although these side effects are clearly aversive, they usually are time limited and can be managed by limiting fat intake; use of a psyllium mucilloid fiber also reduces these gastrointestinal events.[4] Patient concern about the negative side effects is also believed to promote a reduction in the amount of dietary fat consumed. Orlistat also impairs the absorption of fat-soluble vitamins, although clinically significant deficiencies are rarely seen. Accordingly, patients taking orlistat should also take a multivitamin daily, separated from orlistat administration by at least 2 hours.

Sibutramine

Sibutramine (Meridia) blocks reuptake of serotonin, norepinephrine, and dopamine. It is thought to enhance satiety and, therefore, should be considered for patients who have trouble controlling food intake. Sibutramine has been found to promote weight loss dose dependently and has been shown to enhance maintenance of weight loss.[10] Dry mouth, insomnia, constipation, and headaches are the most commonly reported side effects. Sibutramine has a dose-dependent tendency to increase BP and heart rate; therefore, monitoring is important, especially with hypertensive patients. In a 12-month trial of sibutramine with medication-controlled hypertensive patients, patients receiving sibutramine lost significantly more weight than did placebo patients (4.7% vs. 0.7%, respectively).[11] Although improvements in HDL cholesterol and uric acid were superior for sibutramine patients, small, generally clinically nonsignificant, increases in systolic and diastolic BP were noted. However, discontinuations because of BP increases were infrequent (5%) among sibutramine patients, indicating that the medication can be appropriate for hypertensive patients with monitoring.

Bupropion

Bupropion is a norepinephrine and dopamine reuptake inhibitor. It is distributed as Wellbutrin for antidepressant therapy and as Zyban for smoking cessation. Although not approved for a weight loss indication, it has been found to produce enhanced weight loss compared with placebo over 6 months, with weight loss maintained through 48 weeks.[1] In this trial, non-significant reductions in BP were observed in all groups.

Weight Loss (Bariatric) Surgery

Weight loss surgery is appropriate for patients with a BMI > 40 for whom other approaches are unsuccessful. It is sometimes also appropriate for patients with a BMI between 35 and 40 who have comorbidities of obesity and who have failed at other approaches. Several surgical methods are currently being used; all involve a drastic reduction in stomach capacity. The most frequently performed are gastric bypass, vertical banded gastroplasty, and laparoscopic placement of an adjustable band. Bariatric surgery is relatively safe, with in-hospital mortality occurring in 0.37% of cases.[16] Bariatric surgery is successful at promoting impressive weight loss, and weight regain is less common compared with other weight loss methods.[18] Not surprisingly, marked weight loss from bariatric surgery has been found to improve hypertension along with a host of other negative health conditions.[18]

Summary

Obesity is a significant contributor to several cardiovascular risk factors, including hypertension. Measurement of BMI should be a standard part of assessment of hypertensive patients. Modest reductions in body weight significantly improve these risk factors, particularly hypertension. An initial weight loss goal of 10% of body weight is appropriate. Lifestyle change is the foundation of all weight management, and it includes changes in dietary, exercise, and activity patterns. Behavioral techniques can be used to encourage success at making these changes. For patients at higher BMI who are unsuccessful with lifestyle change alone, pharmacotherapy and bariatric surgery may be considered. In addition, combining weight loss treatments or using numerous tools to promote weight loss should be associated with more successful treatment. A long-term perspective is as appropriate to the management of obesity as it is to the management of hypertension.

References

1. Anderson JW, Greenway FL, Fujioka K, et al: Bupropion SR enhances weight loss: a 48-week double-blind, placebo- controlled trial. Obes Res 10:633–641, 2002.
2. Appel LJ, Moore TJ, Obarzanek E, et al: A clinical trial of the effects of dietary patterns on blood pressure. DASH Collaborative Research Group. N Engl J Med 336: 1117–1124, 1997.
3. Blumenthal JA, Sherwood A, Gullette EC, et al: Exercise and weight loss reduce blood pressure in men and women with mild hypertension: Effects on cardiovascular, metabolic, and hemodynamic functioning. Arch Intern Med 160:1947–1958, 2000.
4. Cavaliere H, Floriano I, Medeiros-Neto G: Gastrointestinal side effects of orlistat may be prevented by concomitant prescription of natural fibers (psyllium mucilloid). Int J Obes Relat Metab Disord 25:1095–1099, 2001.
5. Davidson MH, Hauptman J, DiGirolamo M, et al: Weight control and risk factor reduction in obese subjects treated for 2 years with orlistat: a randomized controlled trial. JAMA 281:235–242, 1999.
6. Flechtner-Mors M, Ditschuneit HH, Johnson TD, et al: Metabolic and weight loss effects of long-term dietary intervention in obese patients: Four-year results. Obes Res 8:399–402, 2000.
7. Goldstein DJ: Beneficial health effects of modest weight loss. Int J Obes Relat Metab Disord 16:397–415, 1992.
8. Hill JO, Hauptman J, Anderson J, et al: Orlistat, a lipase inhibitor, for weight maintenance after conventional dieting: A 1-y study. Am J Clin Nutr 69:1108–1116, 1999.
9. Huang Z, Willett WC, Manson JE, et al: Body weight, weight change, and risk for hypertension in women. Ann Intern Med 128:81–88, 1998.
10. James WP, Astrup A, Finer N, et al: Effect of sibutramine on weight maintenance after weight loss: A randomised trial. STORM Study Group. Sibutramine Trial of Obesity Reduction and Maintenance. Lancet 356:2119–2125, 2000.

11. McMahon FG, Fujioka K, Singh BN, et al: Efficacy and safety of sibutramine in obese white and African American patients with hypertension: A 1-year, double-blind, placebo-controlled, multicenter trial. Arch Intern Med 160:2185–2191, 2000.

12. Melanson K, Dwyer J: Popular diets for treatment of overweight and obesity. In Wadden TA, Stunkard AJ (eds): Handbook of Obesity Treatment. New York, The Guilford Press, 2002.

13. National Cholesterol Education Program: Third report of the National Cholesterol Education Program (NCEP) on detection, evaluation, and treatment of high blood cholesterol in adults (Adult treatment panel III). NIH Publication No. 01–3670. Washington, DC, U.S. Government Printing Office, 2001.

14. National Heart Lung and Blood Institute: Clinical Guidelines on the Identification, Evaluation, and Treatment of Overweight and Obesity in Adults—The Evidence Report. National Institutes of Health. Obes Res 6 (suppl 2):51S–209S, 1998.

15. O'Neil PM: Assessing dietary intake in the management of obesity. Obes Res 9 (suppl 5):361S–366S; discussion 373S–374S, 2001.

16. Pope GD, Birkmeyer JD, Finlayson SR: National trends in utilization and in-hospital outcomes of bariatric surgery. J Gastrointest Surg 6:855–860; discussion 861, 2002.

17. Sacks FM, Svetkey LP, Vollmer WM, et al: Effects on blood pressure of reduced dietary sodium and the Dietary Approaches to Stop Hypertension (DASH) diet. DASH-Sodium Collaborative Research Group. N Engl J Med 344:3–10, 2001.

18. Sjostrom CD, Lissner L, Wedel H, Sjostrom L: Reduction in incidence of diabetes, hypertension and lipid disturbances after intentional weight loss induced by bariatric surgery: The SOS Intervention Study. Obes Res 7:477–484, 1999.

19. Stevens VJ, Obarzanek E, Cook NR, et al: Long-term weight loss and changes in blood pressure: Results of the Trials of Hypertension Prevention, phase II. Ann Intern Med 134:1–11, 2001.

20. Wadden TA, Berkowitz RI, Sarwer DB et al: Benefits of lifestyle modification in the pharmacologic treatment of obesity: a randomized trial. Arch Intern Med 161:218–227, 2001.

21. Whelton PK, Appel LJ, Espeland MA, et al: Sodium reduction and weight loss in the treatment of hypertension in older persons: a randomized controlled trial of nonpharmacologic interventions in the elderly (TONE). TONE Collaborative Research Group. JAMA 279:839–846, 1998.

22. Wilson PW, D'Agostino RB, Sullivan L, et al: Overweight and obesity as determinants of cardiovascular risk: the Framingham experience. Arch Intern Med 162:1867–1872, 2002.

Appendix: List of Online Resources

The web sites listed here were accessible as of June 2003.

American College of Sports Medicine (health and fitness information, including "Exercise Your Way to Lower Blood Pressure" brochure)
http://www.acsm.org/health+fitness/index.htm

Downloadable BMI calculator for PDAs
http://hin.nhlbi.nih.gov/bmi_palm.htm

Facts About The DASH Diet
http://www.nhlbi.nih.gov/health/public/heart/hbp/dash/index.htm

5-A-Day for Better Health program
http://www.5aday.gov

National Heart, Lung, and Blood Institute (information for professionals and consumers)
http://www.nhlbi.nih.gov/health/public/heart/obesity/lose_wt/index.htm

National Institute of Diabetes & Digestive & Kidney Diseases (documents on obesity and weight loss for consumers)
http://www.niddk.nih.gov/health/nutrit/nutrit.htm

North American Association for the Study of Obesity
http://www.naaso.org

Online BMI calculator
http://www.nhlbisupport.com/bmi

Online CME program: Office Management of Obesity
http://www.obesitycme.org

The Practical Guide: Identification, Evaluation, and Treatment of Overweight and Obesity in Adults
http://www.nhlbi.nih.gov/guidelines/obesity/practgde.htm
Also available from: http://www.naaso.org

Weight graph for downloading
http://www.musc.edu/weight

Physical Activity for Patients with Hypertension

*Nancy S. Diehl, Ph.D., and
Kelly R. Evenson, Ph.D.*

Relatively little exercise is required to achieve major cardiovascular benefits, but many of your patients already know that. Some encouragement from you is often helpful (see definitions in Table 1), but physicians have little time to address patients' medical problems and lifestyle in a 12- to 15-minute visit. This chapter addresses that limitation.

Roughly 60% of American adults are not active enough to obtain substantial health benefits, and 25% of adults are completely sedentary.[9] Blood pressure (BP) can be lowered by regular physical activity; vigorous exercise is not required (Table 2). Physicians should help their patients include regular physical activity in their routines. By quantifying their physical activity in *Minute 1,* you will be able to guide their physical activity goal setting and treatment planning in *Minute 2* and provide feedback to them during *Minute 3.*

Summary of Evidence that Physical Activity is Beneficial for Patients with Hypertension

Participation in regular physical activity can reduce the incidence of hypertension and lower BP in hypertensive patients. Regular physical activity can also improve lipid and carbohydrate metabolism.[2,3,9] Current guidelines for physical activity are provided in Table 3.

Facilitating Change

Compliance is critical to success, and the nature of the barrier is different with medication (e.g., cost, side effects) than with physical activity (e.g., time, safety, motivation, weather). For more sedentary patients, simply relaying the physical activity recommendations listed in Table 3 is unlikely to generate action.

The transtheoretical model, or "stages of change" theory,[8] has been applied to physical activity. Success is more likely if interventions are

TABLE 1.	Key Terms in Exercise
Cardiorespiratory fitness	The ability of the circulatory and respiratory systems to supply oxygen during sustained physical activity
Exercise	Planned, structured, and repetitive bodily movements
Flexibility	The range of motion available at a joint
Health-related fitness	Includes components of physical fitness (e.g., cardio-respiratory endurance, muscular strength and endurance, body composition, flexibility)
Physical activity	Bodily movement produced by the contraction of skeletal muscles that increases energy expenditure above the basal level
Physical fitness	Ability to carry out daily tasks with vigor and alertness, without undue fatigue, and with ample energy to enjoy leisure-time pursuits and meet unforeseen emergencies; the components of fitness include cardiorespiratory endurance, skeletal muscular endurance, skeletal muscular strength, skeletal muscular power, flexibility, agility, balance, speed, reaction time, and body composition
Resistance training	Physical training designed to increase strength, power, and muscular endurance

Adapted from USDHHS.[9]

targeted to patients' stages of change. Five stages are typically described (Fig. 1): precontemplation (not intending to begin physical activity in the next 6 months), contemplation (intending to begin regular physical activity but not yet doing so), preparation (making small changes to begin physical activity), action (regular physical activity for less than 6 consecutive months), and maintenance (regular physical activity for more than 6 months).

TABLE 2.	Examples of Moderate and Vigorous Activities by Type of Activity	
Type	Moderate Activities	Vigorous Activities
Leisure	Golf, brisk walking, ballet dancing, twist, jitterbug, jazz, ballroom	Swimming laps, running, aerobic dancing
Occupational	General carpentry, general custodial work, walking briskly at work	Farming: Baling hay, cleaning barn; forestry: sawing by hand; using heavy tools at work
Transportation	Walking 3 mph on a level surface, biking < 10 mph level surface	Walking 4.5 mph on a level surface; biking ≥ 10 mph on a level surface
Household	Vacuuming sweeping the garage or outside of house mowing lawn with power mower	Moving boxes or items in house, shoveling snow by hand, mowing lawn with hand mower

TABLE 3. Current Guidelines for Physical Activity

Screening: "Exercise stress testing is recommended prior to starting physical conditioning programs for men ≥ 45 years, women ≥ 55 years and those at increased cardiovascular risk (2 or more risk factors or target organ damage) when vigorous exercise is contemplated" (ACSM 2000, page 15).[1]

General activity guideline: All adults should accumulate 30 minutes or more of moderate to vigorous intensity physical activity most days of the week.*

Duration and type of activity: The duration of activity is dependent on the intensity of the activity; therefore, lower-intensity activity should be conducted over a longer period of time. The activity should use large muscle groups, which can be maintained continuously, and should be rhythmic and aerobic in nature (e.g., walking, hiking, jogging, aerobic dance).

Resistance training: Resistance training should be part of an overall exercise program, progressive in nature, individualized, and provide a stimulus to all major muscle groups 2 to 3 days a week. Multiple-set regimens may provide greater benefits. Most persons should complete eight to 12 repetitions of each exercise. BP monitoring in hypertensive patients when starting a resistance training program can help limit excessive pressor responses.

Flexibility: Flexibility exercises sufficient to develop and maintain range of motion in major muscle groups should be performed 2 to 3 days per week.

*Recent guidelines suggest increasing physical activity to 60 minutes daily to increase weight loss and prevent weight regain.[5]

Figure 1. The stages of the transtheoretical model of behavioral change and sample recommendations for patients at each stage.

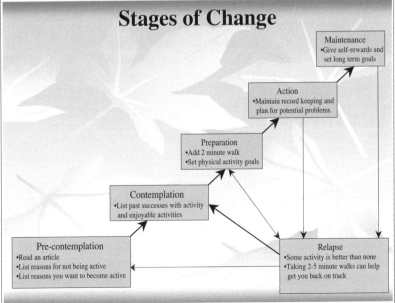

Sedentary patients in the precontemplation stage may need to think or read about the benefits of physical activity before they are ready to try exercise, and they might disregard counseling about increasing physical activity. For patients in the contemplation stage, "prescriptions" of recommended guidelines may be too overwhelming and scare them off. For patients in the action stage, it is appropriate to focus on the guidelines, congratulate them on their success, and encourage them to continue. Patients in the maintenance stage may find relapse prevention solutions, recognition of achievement, and reminders of physical activity benefits helpful.

To get your patients going in 3 minutes or less, *Minute 1* is used to assess the patient's current activity level and readiness to change. *Minute 2* uses this information to prescribe activity and set goals. *Minute 3* involves evaluation of progress and feedback.

Minute 1: Assessment of Current Physical Activity

Assessing current physical activity levels provides crucial information related to the stage of readiness to change. The simplest way to assess current activity is a brief interview. There are four domains to assess: frequency, intensity, type, and time (FITT; Table 4). Ask patients about what they do for regular physical activity. Household activities (e.g., scrubbing, planting, mowing) and walking or biking count as physical activities.

If possible, quantitative data are useful adjuncts. For patients seen frequently, they might keep a physical activity journal or use stepcounters (e.g., Digiwalker stepcounter, www.digiwalker.com) that can be used for goal setting and self-monitoring.

The content of the next 2 minutes depends on the results of minute 1, so it is critical to have an accurate assessment of the patient's activity levels and patterns. People often overreport their exercise. Reminding them that you are asking about their activity to set appropriate goals can reduce bias. Specific and probing questions (e.g., "While doing yard work, how much of the time were you digging or doing something equivalent to a brisk walk?") can also increase accuracy.

An example of someone in the contemplation stage is Bob, age 55 years. He knows the benefits of physical activity for his hypertension,

TABLE 4.   Assessment of Physical Activity Level
Frequency: How often each day does the patient engage in physical activity?
Intensity: Is the activity of moderate (causes some increase in breathing and heart rate) or vigorous (large increases in breathing and heart rate) intensity (see Table 2)?
Type: What kind of activities does the patient engage in? Does he or she enjoy it?
Time: How long does the patient engage in activity during each session? How many sessions per day or week? How long has the patient been doing the current pattern of activity?

excess pounds, and high cholesterol. He is an avid weekend fisherman. He reports that his physical activity is getting the boat ready and cleaning it. He sees people in his neighborhood running and has tried it a couple of times but has not stuck with it. Running is "too hard on my body," and he notes shortness of breath while running and sore knees afterward.

An example of the precontemplation stage is Elizabeth, age 38 years. She is a divorced mother of two and says she has no time to exercise between working full time, talking care of her children and the house, and sleeping. Although high BP runs in her family and she is also overweight, she is not interested in becoming more active. "I am too stressed and don't have time. Taking a pill is faster and easier," she says.

Minute 2: Prescription and Goal Setting

Although doctors and patients set many management goals, physical activity is seldom included. Many patients know about the medical health benefits of exercise, such as reducing risk of cardiovascular disease and helping to control diabetes. But they may need the help of a physician to appreciate exercise's other benefits, such as improved energy, better sleep, and less stress, which may be more relevant in motivating them to change.

The barriers that patients encounter vary. For very obese patients and those with arthritis, exercise may be uncomfortable. Time, money, weather, and family responsibilities are other common barriers. Helping patients to see exercise as a priority can help them increase physical activity. As they begin to appreciate the benefits and start overcoming barriers, they may need help setting activity goals. Setting a long-term goal (4 to 6 months) but focusing on short-term goals (tomorrow or next week) is an effective strategy. PACE (positive, attainable, challenging, and explicit) can facilitate goal setting:

Positive: Goals should be worded in an "I will do . . ." way, keeping a positive attitude.

Attainable: Most resolutions fail because they are too difficult within the time frame.

Challenging: The goal should be moderately challenging but realistic.

Explicit: What exactly do you want to do? "Increasing walking" is not explicit, but "taking a 10-minute walk at lunchtime today" is. Measurement is vital to success.

A potential pitfall is that people often set goals that are too difficult. To maintain motivation, it is critical they meet goals without much difficulty the first time so that they can experience success. Something as simple as an additional 2- to 5-minute walk 4 days of the week is a good starting point. Be specific. Have the patient commit to the time and days he or she will perform the activity (e.g., Tuesday and Thursday mornings between 9 and 10 am).

Minute 3: Evaluation

Providing follow-up and feedback to novice exercisers is very important. When a physician acts as a patient's coach and reviews his or her goals and progress, it validates the effort the patient has made. When patients meet their goals, they deserve heartfelt congratulations. Although it may have been a small step toward a long-term goal, getting started is difficult and critical to the process. You may want to help your patients establish some meaningful rewards in your absence. Ask them to think of simple ideas that they enjoy (e.g., a new pair of running shoes or a new CD) that can be used as small reward that they might feel proud to earn after a week or two.

Patients who did not meet their goals may feel embarrassed. Remind them that goal setting is an iterative process. In some cases, it might make sense to alter the goal to increase their likelihood of success next time. Patients often have black and white thinking about physical activity goals. It is useful to explain the dose–response relationship of physical activity to health. If they do not have time for a 30-minute run, a 10-minute run is acceptable. The physician's feedback as "coach" and health care provider is important. Because patient contact is often limited, it is helpful for them to develop more direct social support for their physical activity (e.g., someone to walk with them). Support is helpful in maintaining a commitment. Other types of support may require less commitment from others yet help patients. Important others (e.g., spouse, coworker, friend) may be enlisted to watch the children for 10 minutes or discuss exercise with the patient.

Something unexpected such as an injury, holiday, work deadline, or vacation can derail a successful routine, and newly active patients is at high risk for "relapse." After they reduce activity, it is easy to default to former patterns. Ask patients to plan for difficult situations and develop strategies for starting back again if something throws them off track. These situations occur, and preparation can prevent the lapse from becoming a relapse.

An example is a patient, Bob, who reports that he ran once but walked three times. He was surprised that he really liked walking, something he has never done before (not real exercise, he had always thought.) He ran 10 minutes the first day "to get the running out of the way" and then walked every other day. He said the walks "cleared my head and gave me more energy." For the next few weeks, he wanted to continue once a week running but increase the walking. At your next appointment with Bob, he reported he got up to 30 minutes of walking 5 days a week during the summer and fall, until it started snowing last week. After congratulating him, you discuss alternatives to walking outside (e.g., treadmill) and ways to make outside more palatable (e.g., comfortable boots, warm hat) to prepare for the upcoming winter months and help Bob maintain his gains.

A second example is Elizabeth, who said she did not have time to read the materials you gave her but she thought about what you told her about having more energy, and that sounded good. Although you might be frustrated at her lack of progress, revisiting the stages-of-change theory helps to reframe her situation. She deserves credit for considering the positive impact of exercise. You might quickly summarize the literature you gave her and encourage her to walk or bike with her children.

Key Points

- ⊙ Physical activity has significant cardiovascular benefits.
- ⊙ Ideally, patients will accumulate 30 minutes of moderate physical activity over the day, most days of the week. Helping patients become more physically active, like any other lifestyle change, is a challenge.
- ⊙ Using the transtheoretical model as a guide, conducting the assessment (Minute 1), goal setting (Minute 2), and providing feedback (Minute 3) helps patients increase their physical activity and improve their health and well-being.

References

1. American College of Sports Medicine: ACSM's Guidelines for Exercise Testing and Prescription. Philadelphia, PA: Lippincott, Williams, and Wilkins, 2000.
2. American College of Sports Medicine (ACSM): Physical activity, physical fitness, and hypertension. Med Sci Sports Exercise 1993, 25:i–x.
3. Fagard RH: Exercise characteristics and the blood pressure response to dynamic physical training. Med Sci Sports Exercise 2001, 33(Suppl 6):484–492.
4. National Heart, Lung, and Blood Institute: The Sixth Report of the Joint National Committee on Prevention, Detection, Evaluation, and Treatment of High Blood Pressure. NIH, 1997.
5. National Academy of Sciences: Dietary Reference Intake for Evergy, Carbohydrates, Fiber, Fat, Protein, and Amino Acids (Macronutrients). National Academy Press; 2002. (http://www4.nationalacademies.org/news.nsf/isbn/0309085373?Open Document)
6. Pate R, Pratt M, Blair S, et al. Physical activity and public health: a recommendation from the CDC and Prevention and American College of Sports Medicine. JAMA 1995, 273:402–427.

7. Pollock M, Gaesser G, Butcher J, et al: The recommended quantity and quality of exercise for developing and maintaining cardiorespiratory and muscular fitness, and flexibility in healthy adults. Med Sci Sports Exercise 1998, 30:975–991.
8. Prochaska JO, DiClemente CC: Transtheoretical therapy: toward a more integrative model of change. Psychother Theory Res Pract 1982, 19:276–288.
9. U.S. Department of Health and Human Services (USDHHS): Physical Activity and Health: a Report of the Surgeon General. Atlanta, GA: U.S. Department of Health and Human Services, Centers for Disease Control and Prevention, National Center for Chronic Disease Prevention and Health Promotion, 1996. (http://www.cdc.gov/nccdphp/sgr/sgr.htm)

Behavioral Approaches in Blood Pressure Reduction

chapter 21

Thomas Pickering M.D., D.Phil.

A fairly consistent body of evidence supports the idea that exposure to chronic stress can accelerate the course of hypertension; therfore, techniques that lead to stress reduction might be expected to lower blood pressure (BP). Although procedures such as autogenic training and progressive muscular relaxation have been around for more than 50 years, the idea really took off in the early 1970s with the popularization of two forms of treatment, one ancient and the other novel—transcendental meditation and biofeedback.[1,2] The early results claimed that these behavioral treatments could provide decreases of BP of the same magnitude as seen with drug treatment.[3] Thirty years later, neither procedure has established a place in the routine treatment of hypertension, although both are used for other purposes. Nevertheless, despite the lack of enthusiasm of the medical profession for this type of treatment, the public is still interested. In a 1993 survey on the use of unconventional medicine in the United States,[4] 11% of hypertensive patients reported using unconventional therapy in the past 12 months, mostly relaxation techniques and homeopathy.

Biofeedback

The original idea of biofeedback was that it would be possible to lower BP by providing the subject with feedback either of the level of BP itself or of some related physiological function such as muscle tone. Typically, the feedback is provided as an auditory or visual signal. During a series of training sessions, subjects focus on changing the signal in the appropriate direction. Although it is well established that transient changes in BP can be produced by these techniques, it has not been well documented that the changes persist during daily life. A meta-analysis reported by Eisenberg et al.[5] included six groups (n = 90) that underwent biofeedback without combination with other behavioral therapies. The BP reduction was minimal (−2.6/0.2 mmHg) in comparison with patients who were wait list control subjects or who underwent sham therapies (−2.9/−1.2 mmHg) and in whom the baseline BP measurements had extended beyond 1 day. Even in the studies that show improvement in BP with direct biofeedback, long-term follow-up data beyond a 6-month period have been inconsistent or lacking. Biofeedback is reportedly effective at lowering elevated clinic BP in patients with "white coat hypertension" without affecting the home BP.[6]

Relaxation Techniques

Relaxation therapy may range from a physician's simple advice to a patient to "relax" to more formal structured techniques. These include meditative techniques such as yoga and Zen based on Eastern philosophy, progressive muscular relaxation,[7] and autogenic training.[8] The common denominator in all these techniques appears to be mental focusing, task awareness, sitting quietly, and relaxing all muscle groups.

Most of the early studies were limited by weaknesses in methodology, including small sample size; absence of control groups; confounding factors such as pharmacologic treatment or placebo response; statistical artifacts, including regression to the mean; and reliance on clinic or laboratory BP measurements.[9] Later studies that used ambulatory BP as the measure of success have provided mixed results. Two have reported positive findings,[10,11] but others have found no effect on ambulatory BP.[12,13] Thus, this issue is still unresolved.

As with biofeedback studies, one of the problems with relaxation studies has been that similar decreases in BP are often seen in both the active treatment and control groups (Fig. 1).[14] One factor that appears to be very important in determining the magnitude of the effects of any of these techniques on BP is the pretreatment level of BP, as reported in an analysis by Jacob et al.[9] Thus, many of the negative studies have included subjects whose initial BPs were essentially normal. The analysis also established that the treatment effect was related to the number of pretreatment baseline readings. Regression to the mean could explain much of the treatment effects in such studies, but then one would expect the same decrease in BP to be seen in both the treatment and control groups (as was observed, for example in the Irvine and Logan study).

An important issue is whether the effects of biofeedback and relaxation can be attributed to placebo effects. One of the issues has to do with the measurements of BP by which the effects of the interventions were judged. The early trials,[1,3,15] used clinic measurements which are

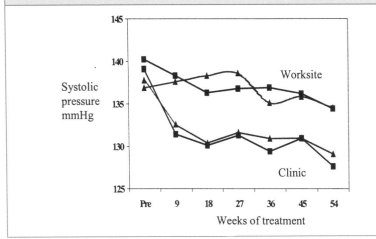

Figure 1. Decline of blood pressure measured both at the worksite and in the clinic during a controlled trial of relaxation therapy. *Solid lines* = changes in the active treatment group; *hatched lines* = the control group. (Data from Chesney MA, Black GW, Swan GE, Ward MM. Relaxation training for essential hypertension at the worksite: I. The untreated mild hypertensive. Psychosom Med 49:250–263, 1987.)

known to be very susceptible to the placebo effect. It is now clearly recognized that BP tends to increase just before a clinic visit, a phenomenon commonly called the "white coat effect" that has been attributed to the anxiety associated with the visit. Thus, any intervention that reduces anxiety may lower the clinic BP without necessarily affecting the BP at other times (Fig. 2). Biofeedback has been found to be of some use in treating patients with white coat hypertension.

One critical aspect of the placebo effect on BP is expectancy of patients, and it has been suggested that an expectancy of positive results is a necessary, if not sufficient, condition for placebo effects.[16] Two lines of evidence support the notion that at least some of the benefits of behavioral forms of treating hypertension derive from placebo effects. First, Agras et al. studied the effects of relaxation training on BP, and divided patients into two groups.[17] One group was informed that the relaxation would not have an immediate effect on BP, but the other was told that it would. The group with the more positive expectations showed the biggest decrease in BP. The second line of evidence comes from the control groups of these studies. In general, it has been found that the more closely the control procedure resembles the "active" treatment, the more likely it is to show a decrease in BP.[18]

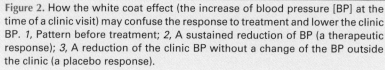

Figure 2. How the white coat effect (the increase of blood pressure [BP] at the time of a clinic visit) may confuse the response to treatment and lower the clinic BP. *1*, Pattern before treatment; *2*, A sustained reduction of BP (a therapeutic response); *3*, A reduction of the clinic BP without a change of the BP outside the clinic (a placebo response).

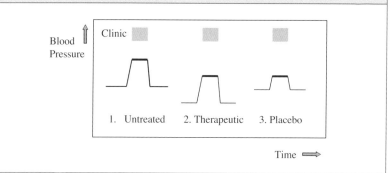

Controlled Breathing Techniques

The most exciting technique in this area is one that combines features of both biofeedback and relaxation training using a novel device that trains patients to lower their breathing rate. The device, which is marketed as the RespeRate, comprises a belt that goes around the chest to record breathing movements, which is linked to a battery-operated monitor that detects the movements. The device emits a series of musical tones that have a different pitch for expiration and inspiration. Patients are instructed to synchronize their breathing to the music. After a few breaths, the device gradually begins to prolong the expiratory phase notes, so that patients gradually slow their breathing rate to a minimum of about 6/min. Patients are encouraged to practice this for about 15 minutes a day. It takes about 4 weeks for the full effects on BP to be realized. Several studies based on the use of the device have been published, and they suggest that the effects are both sustained and substantial Fig. 3.[19]

Current Guidelines on Behavioral Techniques

These changing fortunes of behavioral forms of treatment have been reflected in the Joint National Committee (JNC) recommendations over the years. In 1980, the committee concluded that "these methods are still experimental and cannot yet be recommended for sustained control of hypertension."[20] The 1984 report[21] was more optimistic: "Various relax-

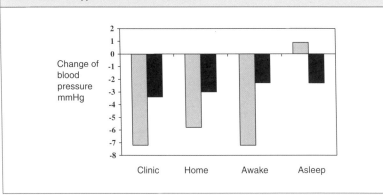

Figure 3. Blood pressure response to treatment with RespeRate, measured in the clinic, at home (self-monitoring), and by ambulatory monitoring (awake and asleep). (Data from Rosenthal T, Alter A, Peleg E, Gavish B: Device-guided breathing exercises reduce blood pressure: Ambulatory and home measurements. Am J Hypertens 14:74–76, 2001.)

ation and biofeedback therapies may consistently produce modest but significant blood pressure reduction," and they "should be considered in the context of a comprehensive treatment program that may include both pharmacologic and nonpharmacologic therapeutic approaches." In 1988, the pendulum had begun to swing the other way: "These promising methods have yet to be subjected to rigorous clinical trial evaluation and should not be considered as definitive treatment for patients with high blood pressure."[22] The latest report[23] (the sixth, published in 1997) stated: "Relaxation therapies and biofeedback have been studied in multiple controlled trials with little effect beyond that seen in control groups. . . . The available literature does not support the use of relaxation therapies for definitive therapy or prevention of hypertension."

Conclusions

Although behavioral forms of treatment are currently out of fashion for the treatment of patients with hypertension, it is facile to dismiss the many positive results of individual studies as merely placebo effects and probably overly simplistic. Encouraging preliminary reports indicate that controlled breathing using a biofeedback device may lower ambulatory BP. Another promising area is the treatment of white coat hypertension, in which the use of antihypertensive drugs is controversial, but in which behavioral techniques appear to be particularly effective. The last word has not yet been said in this area.

References

1. Patel C, Marmot MG, Terry DJ, et al. Trial of relaxation in reducing coronary risk: Four year follow up. Br Med J (Clin Res Ed) 290:1103–1106, 1985.

2. Patel C, Marmot MG, Terry DJ: Controlled trial of biofeedback-aided behavioural methods in reducing mild hypertension. Br Med J (Clin Res Ed) 282:2005–2008, 1981.

3. Benson H, Rosner BA, Marzetta BR, Klemchuk HM: Decreased blood-pressure in pharmacologically treated hypertensive patients who regularly elicited the relaxation response. Lancet 1:289–291, 1974.

4. Eisenberg DM, Kessler RC, Foster C, et al: Unconventional medicine in the United States: Prevalence, costs, and patterns of use. N Engl J Med 328:246–252, 1993.

5. Eisenberg DM, Delbanco TL, Berkey CS, et al: Cognitive behavioral techniques for hypertension: Are they effective [see comments]? Ann Intern Med 118:964–972, 1993.

6. Nakao M, Nomura S, Shimosawa T, et al: Blood pressure biofeedback treatment of white-coat hypertension. J Psychosom Res 48:161–169, 2000.

7. Jacobson E: Progressive Muscular Relaxation. Chicago: University of Chicago Press, 1938.

8. Luthe W: Autogenic Therapy. New York: Grune and Stratton, 1969.

9. Jacob RG, Chesney MA, Williams DM, et al: Relaxation therapy for hypertension: Design effects and treatment effects. Ann Behav Med 13:5–17, 1991.

10. Southam MA, Agras WS, Taylor CB, Kraemer HC: Relaxation training. Blood pressure lowering during the working day. Arch Gen Psychiatry 39:715–717, 1982.

11. Wenneberg SR, Schneider RH, Walton KG, et al: A controlled study of the effects of the Transcendental Meditation program on cardiovascular reactivity and ambulatory blood pressure. Int J Neurosci 89:15–28, 1997.

12. Jacob RG, Shapiro AP, Reeves RA, et al: Relaxation therapy for hypertension. Comparison of effects with concomitant placebo, diuretic, and beta-blocker. Arch Intern Med 146:2335–2340, 1986.

13. van Montfrans GA, Karemaker JM, Wieling W, Dunning AJ: Relaxation therapy and continuous ambulatory blood pressure in mild hypertension: A controlled study. Br Med J 300:1368–1372, 1990.

14. Chesney MA, Black GW, Swan GE, Ward MM: Relaxation training for essential hypertension at the worksite: I. The untreated mild hypertensive. Psychosom Med 49: 250–263, 1987.

15. Patel C, Marmot M: Can general practitioners use training in relaxation and management of stress to reduce mild hypertension? Br Med J (Clin Res Ed) 296:21–24, 1988.

16. Chesney MA, Black GW: Behavioral treatment of borderline hypertension: An overview of results. J Cardiovasc Pharmacol 8(Suppl)5:57–63, 1986.

17. Agras S, Horne M, Taylor CB: Expectation and the blood pressure lowering effects of relaxation. Psychom Med 44:389–395, 1982.

18. Wadden T, Luborski L, Greer S, Crits-Christoph P: The behavioral treatment of essential hypertension: An update and comparison with pharmacological treatment. Clin Psychol Rev 4:403–429, 1984.

19. Rosenthal T, Alter A, Peleg E, Gavish B: Device-guided breathing exercises reduce blood pressure: Ambulatory and home measurements. Am J Hypertens 14:74–76, 2001.

20. The 1980 report of the Joint National Committee on Prevention, Detection, Evaluation, and Treatment of High Blood Pressure. Arch Intern Med 140:1280–1285, 1980.

21. The 1984 report of the Joint National Committee on Prevention, Detection, Evaluation, and Treatment of High Blood Pressure. Arch Intern Med 144:1045–1057, 1984.
22. The 1988 report of the Joint National Committee on Detection, Evaluation, and Treatment of High Blood Pressure. Arch Intern Med 148:1023–1038, 1988.
23. The sixth report of the Joint National Committee on Prevention,Detection, Evaluation, and Treatment of High Blood Pressure. Arch Intern Med 157:2413–2446, 1997.

HOT TOPICS

chapter
22

An Evidence-based Approach to Selecting Initial Antihypertensive Therapy

Jan Basile, M.D.

Clinical Points on Initial Drug Selection

Thiazide-type diuretics should be used as initial drug therapy for most patients with hypertension, either alone or combined with drugs from other classes. Certain high-risk conditions are compelling indications for the initial use of other antihypertensive drug classes such as angiotensin-converting enzyme (ACE) inhibitors, angiotensin receptor blockers (ARBs), beta-blockers, and calcium channel blockers (CCBs). Most hypertensive patients require two or more antihypertensive medications to achieve goal blood pressure (BP). When BP > 20/10 mmHg is necessary to achieve goal BP, consideration should be given to initiating therapy with two agents, one of which should be a thiazide-type diuretic.

The Role of Lifestyle Modification

Although this chapter is devoted to initial drug selection, adoption of a healthy lifestyle (Table 1) can prevent as well as manage hypertension. A healthy lifestyle includes maintaining an ideal body weight, adoption of the Dietary Approaches to Stop Hypertension (DASH) eating plan,[1] limiting alcohol intake, limiting sodium intake, and increasing physical activity. The DASH eating plan established that a diet high in fruits, veg-

TABLE 1.   Key Points in Lifestyle Modification
• Lose weight if needed to maintain ideal body weight
• Adopt the DASH eating plan: Consume a diet rich in fruits, vegetables, and low-fat dairy products with a reduced content of saturated and total fat.
• Limit alcohol intake
→ No more than 2 drinks per day (50% as much in women)
• Get regular exercise
→ Minimum of 30 minutes most days of the week
• Reduce dietary sodium
→ Ideally, < 100 mmol/day (2.4 g sodium or 6 g sodium chloride)
→ Patients with "low renin activity" (e.g., elderly and black individuals) have been shown to have a more significant response to sodium restriction
→ Can enhance BP reduction when the patient is using diuretics as well as minimize the risk of diuretic-induced hypokalemia
• Quit smoking

etables, and low-fat dairy products along with sodium restriction reduced BP more effectively than a typical American diet.[2] Lifestyle modifications can also enhance antihypertensive drug efficacy.

Selecting Initial Antihypertensive Therapy

Clinical trial data has shown that several classes of drugs, including thiazide-type diuretics, beta-blockers, ACE inhibitors, ARBs, and CCBs, all reduce the complications of hypertension (Table 2).

The recently published Antihypertensive and Lipid Lowering Treatment to Prevent Heart Attack Trial (ALLHAT)[3] is the largest hypertension trial ever performed. Conducted in individuals age 55 years and older, ALLHAT was designed to determine whether the newer classes of drugs, a representative dihydropyridine CCB (amlodipine), a representative ACE inhibitor (lisinopril), or a representative alpha-blocker (doxasozin), was superior, equivalent, or inferior to a representative thiazide-type diuretic (chlorthalidone) in lowering the combined incidence of fatal coronary heart disease and nonfatal myocardial infarction (MI). Its

TABLE 2.   Drugs Proven to Reduce Hypertension-related Morbidity and Mortality
• Diuretics
• Beta-blockers
• ACE inhibitors
• CCBs
• ARBs

strength lies in that it included 42,418 subjects, including large numbers of women and blacks as well as a high proportion of smokers, diabetics, and patients with existing cardiovascular disease (groups that have been underrepresented in previous hypertension studies). ALLHAT confirmed that diuretics were unsurpassed in preventing the cardiovascular complications of hypertension (Table 3).

Another recent trial, the Second Australian National Blood Pressure (ANBP2) trial, reported slightly better outcomes in white men with a regimen that began with an ACE inhibitor compared with one that began with a diuretic.[4] It was not as well designed as ALLHAT because it had fewer subjects, a shorter duration of follow-up, and more confounding (based on gender differences) that might have influenced its results.

Accordingly, thiazide-type diuretics should be used as initial therapy for most patients with hypertension unless a compelling indication requires the use of other antihypertensive drugs. Most hypertensive patients require two or more antihypertensive medications to achieve their BP goals. Thiazides can be used in combination with one of the other classes of antihypertensive agents (i.e., ACE inhibitor, ARB, BB, CCB), which have been demonstrated to reduce morbidity and mortality in clinical trials. When used together, thiazides enhance the antihypertensive efficacy of these other antihypertensive classes.

TABLE 3.   General Guidelines for Pharmacologic Treatment

- Clinical trials, viewed collectively, have demonstrated that thiazide-type diuretics, beta-blockers, ACE inhibitors, ARBs, and CCBs are all effective for reducing the complications of hypertension:
  - → Thiazide-type diuretics
    - Thiazides show slightly better results than most drug groups
  - → Beta-blockers
  - → ACE inhibitors
  - → CCBs
  - → ARBs
- Monotherapy is more likely to be effective in controlling BP to goal for patients with:
  - → Stage 1 hypertension in whom a small reduction in BP is required to reach goal
  - → No other comorbidities
  - → No target organ disease
  - → No other major risk factors
- When possible, use long-acting agents, preferably with once-a-day dosing:
  - → Greater consistency of BP control
  - → Better adherence
- Some of the newer low-dose or fixed-dose combinations can be advantageous:
  - → Many have additive BP-lowering effects
  - → Minimize dose-dependent adverse effects
  - → May be used as initial therapy

Compelling Indications for Antihypertensive Treatment

Based on favorable outcome data from clinical trials, certain high-risk conditions represent compelling indications for the use of specific antihypertensive drug classes (Table 4).[5] These agents are often used in combination with other classes of antihypertensive compounds in order to achieve goal BP.

Treatment of Special Groups

Diabetic Hypertension

Combinations of two or more drugs are often required to achieve the targeted BP goal of < 130/80 mmHg. Many classes of antihypertensive agents have been used in diabetics to reduce the rate of cardiovascular disease and stroke. Both ACE inhibitors and ARBs favorably affect the progression of diabetic nephropathy.[5]

Systolic Heart Failure

In patients with an asymptomatic reduction in left ventricular function, typically defined as an ejection fraction < 40%, both ACE inhibitor and beta-blocker therapy are recommended.[5] When patients develop symptoms, aldosterone antagonists have been shown to improve outcomes as well.

Post Myocardial Infarction

ACE inhibitor therapy should be initiated as soon as the patient is hemodynamically stable. Beta-blockers should be used as well. Recently,

TABLE 4. Compelling Indications for Antihypertensive Treatment

• In patients with diabetic hypertension
  → Thiazide diuretics, beta-blockers, ACE inhibitors, ARBs, and CCBs reduce cardiovascular disease and stroke
  → ACE inhibitor– or ARB-based therapy for diabetic nephropathy
• In patients with systolic heart failure
  → For asymptomatic individuals, ACE inhibitors and beta-blockers are recommended
  → For symptomatic individuals, ACE inhibitors, beta-blockers, and aldosterone antagonists are recommended
• For patients who have had an MI
  → Beta-blockers, ACE inhibitors, and aldosterone antagonists have proven beneficial
• In patients with chronic kidney disease
  → ACE inhibitors and ARBs regardless of the cause (both diabetic and nondiabetic)
• In patients with stroke
  → Recurrent stroke reduced with a combination of ACE inhibitors and diuretic

aldosterone antagonists have also improved patient outcomes in clinical trials.[5]

Chronic Kidney Disease

Patients with albuminuiria > 300 mg/day or a reduction in glomerular filtration rate (GFR) < 60 cc/min, which corresponds to a serum creatinine level > 1.5 in men or > 1.3 in women, should attain a goal BP of < 130/80 mmHg. Although ACE inhibitor and ARB therapies have been shown to slow the progression of diabetic and nondiabetic renal disease, three or more drugs are often required to attain the BP goal. ACE inhibitor and ARB therapies should not be used together before the use of a thiazide-type diuretic.

Cerebrovascular Disease

Diuretic, beta-blocker, CCB, ACE inhibitor, and ARB therapies have all been associated with a reduction in stroke risk. In those with a history of stroke, recurrent stroke rates are lowered by using an ACE inhibitor and a thiazide-type diuretic together.

References

1. The Sixth Report of the Joint National Committee on Prevention, Detection, Evaluation, and Treatment of High Blood Pressure. Arch Intern Med 157:2413–2446, 1997.
2. Sacks FM, Svetkey LP, Vollmer WM, et al: Effects on blood pressure of reduced dietary sodium and the Dietary Approaches to Stop Hypertension (DASH) diet. N Engl J Med 344:3–10, 2001.
3. The ALLHAT Officers and Coordinators for the ALLHAT Collaborative Research Group: Major outcomes in high-risk hypertensive patients randomized to angiotensin-converting enzyme inhibitor or calcium channel blocker vs diuretic. The Antihypertensive and Lipid-Lowering Treatment to Prevent Heart Attack Trial (ALLHAT). JAMA 288:2981–2997, 2002.
4. Wing LMH, Reid CM, Ryan P, et al: A comparison of outcomes with angiotensin-converting-enzyme inhibitors and diuretics for hypertension in the elderly. N Engl J Med 348:583–592, 2003.
5. The Seventh Report of the Joint National Committee on Prevention, Detection, Evaluation, and Treatment of High Blood Pressure. JAMA 285:2560–2572, 2003.

Remedies for Single-Dose Therapy Failure

chapter

23

Barry J. Materson, M.D., MBA

When a hypertensive patient has been treated with a single medication and either the desired blood pressure (BP) reduction has not been achieved or the patient has experienced an adverse effect, the clinician still has options. An initial provider checklist is given in Table 1.

TABLE 1.   Initial Provider Checklist When Blood Pressure Is Not Controlled

1. Why did this patient not respond to the initial monotherapy?
   - Does the patient have stage 2 or higher BP?
   - Was his or her baseline systolic BP $\geq$ 15 mm Hg or diastolic BP $\geq$ 10 mm Hg higher than your intended goal BP?
   - Is there evidence for secondary hypertension?
   - Does the patient have unrecognized sleep apnea?
   - Did your patient actually take the drug? Note that 30% of antihypertensive prescriptions are never filled.
   - Is the patient taking something that would counteract the drug?
     a. Nonsteroidal anti-inflammatory drugs, both non-selective and selective cyclo-oxygenase-2 (COX) inhibitors; asking the patient what he or she takes for pain is much more likely to yield a useful answer
     b. Pressor agents such as nasal sprays, older preparations of cold remedies, large amounts of caffeine (e.g., cola beverages), cocaine, excess alcohol
     c. Alternative medications such as Ma Huang or substances containing ephedra
     d. High sodium intake
     e. Immunosupressive drugs such as cyclosporin
   - Is it an age-by-race mismatch? For example, younger white patients are less likely to have a good response to monotherapy with a thiazide diuretic than to an angiotensin-converting enzyme (ACE) inhibitor, angiotensin II receptor blocker (ARB), or beta-blocker, but older patients, including blacks, are more likely to respond to a diuretic.
   - Is the dose high enough?
2. If there has been an adverse effect, is it typical of the drug or is it something unusual? Patients who get physiologically and pharmacologically improbable adverse effects may be giving you a clue to psychological problems such as panic attacks.
3. Is the patient really hypertensive or is "office hypertension" or another measurement artifact (e.g., pseudohypertension or cuff-inflation hypertension) present?
4. Remember that patients with BP elevation induced or aggravated by anxiety almost never respond to antihypertensive drugs. Exceptions may be combined α,β-blockers and clonidine.

Analysis

Let us consider some of the above points. First, you must not reach into the sample drawer and pull out whatever happens to be on top. Informal surveys of referred patients indicate that this is a very common approach to the problem. Do ask yourself *and* your patient: Why was a response lacking?

Single-drug therapy can work in patients with stage 2 hypertension. The problem is that the higher the baseline BP or the greater the gap between baseline and goal, the less likely it is for a single drug to be effective.

Secondary Hypertension

Secondary hypertension is sometimes quite obvious when it presents as documented new-onset severe hypertension or sudden loss of control of established hypertension. Other times, it just sneaks up on you.

Renal artery stenosis, pheochromocytoma, Cushing's syndrome and both hyper-and hypothyroidism are generally easy to diagnose, but they may be quite subtle in elderly individuals. Myxedema and Cushing's disease may not be obvious and require enough thought to request the appropriate diagnostic tests.

On the other hand, primary aldosteronism may not be obvious, even in young patients. If the patient proves to have a primary aldosterone-secreting adenoma, it may be amenable to laparoscopic extirpation. If the patient has bilateral adrenal cortical hyperplasia, treatment must remain medical. If you suspect that this might be the case, some would advise obtaining serum for both aldosterone and renin levels. A ratio of 20:1 or higher should lead to a more detailed investigation, especially if the serum aldosterone level is greater than 14 µg/mL. After the blood is taken, it might be worth prescribing a small dose (25 mg) of spironolactone. A positive result is gratifying and suggests a primary adrenal problem.

Do not forget about sleep apnea, which is often associated with a lack of response to initial therapy. Asking the patient and sleeping partner about the patient's snoring, gasping for air while sleeping, and daytime hypersomnolence might suggest the need for a further evaluation.

Do not overlook obstructive uropathy. A full bladder can elicit sympathetic nervous system discharge and make BP nearly impossible to control. We have cured many cases of severe hypertension with a bladder catheter. Be careful because severe hypotension can occur if the bladder is emptied too fast. Some other considerations include:

- **Nonadherence:** Even well-educated patients sometimes lie about taking their drugs. These are tough cases. You just have to have an index of suspicion and encourage the patient to have greater confidence in you and the therapy. Patients must adhere to the therapeutic plan.

- **Adverse drug effects and interactions:** Many patients fail to achieve control or later lose it because they are taking drugs that interfere with the antihypertensive medication. Both nonselective and Cox-2 selective inhibitors can raise BP. Asking the patient if he or she is taking a nonsteroidal anti-inflammatory drug will not help because few patients will have a clue what you are talking about. You cannot possibly keep up with all of the over-the-counter (OTC) medications (see below). Ask what the patient takes for pain. Keep in mind that some patients borrow and share other people's prescription medications.

- **OTC and alternative therapies:** As noted, ask the patient about all OTC medications he or she is taking. These include nasal sprays, cold remedies, and alternative medications. Ephedrine-containing neutraceuticals, such as Ma Huang, have been associated with stroke. It is essential to obtain a thorough patient medical history.

- **Dietary indiscretion:** Sudden exacerbations of severe hypertension may occur when patients eat a large amount of salt in a short period of time. Large quantities of caffeine may also elevate BP, as will three or more equivalents of alcohol. Remind your patients that a six-pack of beer is equivalent to six shots of whiskey. Patients may also be very reluctant to admit to cocaine abuse.

Improving the Odds in Controlling Patients' Blood Pressure

It is important to use patient profiling when selecting antihypertensive therapy. The chance of initial success with single-drug therapy is improved by use of the age by race paradigm. In brief, this suggests that patients who respond well to an ACE inhibitor, ARB, or beta-blocker (e.g., young white patients) may be less likely to respond to a diuretic or calcium antagonist. The opposite pattern exists for younger and older African American patients who, for example, may require a higher initial dose of an ACE inhibitor, ARB, or beta-blocker to achieve the same BP reduction as in non-blacks.

It is also necessary to give the correct dosage of the drug. If the patient has "office hypertension," you may be chasing a moving target. Similarly, if BP elevation is driven by anxiety, antihypertensive medication will not work. The patient instead needs antianxiety drugs; sometimes he or she needs both antihypertensive and antianxiety medications.

Treatment Recommendations

If you have thought through the above list and still are faced with a patient who has not responded to the initial drug, your choices include adjusting the medications:

- Stop the first drug and prescribe a drug better matched to the patient's age-by-race profile (i.e., sequential therapy).
- Increase the dose of the first drug to its maximum or to toxicity and then add a second drug (i.e., stepped care).
- Stop the first drug and start a combination drug that meets the patient's individual criteria. If a diuretic was not the first drug, it is generally a good idea to make it the second drug.

One rather simplistic method is to consider ACE inhibitors, ARBs, and beta-blockers to be in the same basket and diuretics and calcium antagonists to be in another basket. If a single drug from basket A or B fails, chose one from the other basket. This type of sequential care has a good chance of success, especially if there was an initial age-by-race mismatch.

Stepped care is one of the most successful therapeutic regimens ever designed. However, it drives each drug step to its maximum dose (or toxicity) before adding the next step. Although this works for most patients, it is rather rigid, intellectually unsatisfying, and sometimes makes for unhappy patients.

There may be more than 20 million hypertensive patients in the United States who remain candidates for single-drug therapy. They are the ones with uncomplicated stage 1 hypertension. That means that there are more than 20 million hypertensive patients left who will likely need two or even more drugs to achieve their goal BP. The majority of these patients could benefit from exposure to initial combination therapy. There are abundant fixed-dose combinations on the market today that provide a wide choice. These are combinations of ACE inhibitors or ARBs with a diuretic, both dihydropyridine and nondihydropyridine calcium antagonists with an ACE inhibitor, and beta-blockers with diuretics.

If these recommendations also fail, consider the following:

- Add a diuretic if not already used, or consider a large dose of a loop diuretic, especially if there is edema or renal failure.
- Add a third or even a fourth drug not in the category of one already in use.
- Add a small dose of spironolactone (see previous discussion).
- Consider the combination of a dihydropyridine calcium antagonist with the nondihydropyridine diltiazem. Note that this can be an extremely potent combination. Start low and slowly titrate upward. Edema occurs in about 15% of patients, and some may develop

gingival hyperplasia. Adding an ACE inhibitor will reduce the likelihood of edema.

Thiazide diuretics remain the cornerstone of successful treatment of patients with hypertension. One should use low doses (12.5 mg or hydrochlorothiazide or the equivalent) and titrate to no more than 25 or 50 mg. Watch the serum potassium level carefully. Thiazides do not work if the glomerular filtration rate is reduced to 30 mL/min or lower or if there is severe edema. In that case, use a loop-blocking diuretic. Remember that these tend to be relatively short-acting and they often need to be given at least twice daily. If a low dose does not work, double it.

Many combination regimens fail to counteract alpha-adrenergic vasoconstriction. Clonidine, especially in patch form, can be a valuable adjunct. The problem is that patients taking clonidine tend to get sleepy and have a very dry mouth. Adding reserpine (0.05 to 0.1 mg) can also be useful and is very well tolerated by most patients. If the patient also has obstructive uropathy, addition of an α_1-antagonist may control BP and relieve symptoms as well. Although patients must be warned about orthostatic hypotension with an α_1-antagonist, the problem here is the sensation of dizziness, usually without orthostasis.

In our practice, we no longer use minoxidil because of the potency of diltiazem combined with a dihydropyridine. The cautions are noted above. This combination should not be used lightly, and the patient should understand both the potential benefits and risks.

When all of these recommendations have failed, contact a hypertension specialist. These are physicians certified by the American Society of Hypertension. A list of clinical hypertension specialists is provided on the web (http://www:ash-us.org/ and click on Hypertension Specialists).

Key Point

☞ Knowledge of the particular patient, the pharmacology of the available drugs, a good game plan, and where to go for help are all important tools for controlling BP in the vast majority of patients.

References

1. Materson BJ, Reda DJ, Preston RA, et al: Response to a second single antihypertensive agent used as monotherapy for hypertension after failure of the initial drug. Department of Veterans Affairs Cooperative Study Group on Antihypertensive Agents. Arch Intern Med 1995, 155:1757–1562.
2. Materson BJ, Reda DJ, Cushman WC, Henderson WG: Results of combination anti-

hypertensive therapy after failure of each of the components. Department of Veterans Affairs Cooperative Study Group on Anti-Hypertensive Agents. J Human Hypertens 1995, 9:791–796.

3.   Preston RA, Materson BJ, Reda DJ, et al: Age-race subgroup compared with renin profile as predictors of blood pressure response to antihypertensive therapy. Department of Veterans Affairs Cooperative Study Group on Antihypertensive Agents. JAMA 1998, 280:1168–1172.

4.   Cushman WC, Reda DJ, Perry HM, et al: Regional and racial differences in response to antihypertensive medication use in a randomized controlled trial of men with hypertension in the United States. Department of Veterans Affairs Cooperative Study Group on Antihypertensive Agents. Arch Intern Med 2000, 160:825–831.

The Metabolic Syndrome

William H. Bestermann, Jr., M.D.

chapter

24

The health care needs of the American people have been shifting from care for acute episodic health problems to care for chronic disease conditions.[1] Chronic conditions, including cardiovascular disease, stroke, and end-stage renal disease (ESRD), have become the leading causes of morbidity and mortality and are responsible for billions of dollars annually in avoidable medical care expenditures.[2] Most of these chronic conditions are age related. Given the demographic trends in the United States with a rapidly aging population, projected health care expenditures will require a progressively greater percentage of economic output to meet the costs.[3] A significant proportion of these hospitalizations and expenses are avoidable with aggressive preventive care.[3] The Institute of Medicine (IOM) identified priority conditions of emphasis, including hypertension, high cholesterol, diabetes, stroke, congestive heart failure, and ischemic heart disease.[1] These conditions are components of the risks identified with the metabolic syndrome, which affects nearly 25% of the U.S. adult population, an estimated 47,000,000 individuals.[4] Obesity is the major common factor linked with the metabolic syndrome and the associated cardiovascular and renal risks and complications.[5] Of particular concern are the rapidly increasing rates of obesity. The burden of managing this epidemic will fall heavily on primary care physicians as the number of patients with the cluster of cardiovascular risk factors and related complications increases sharply.[6] Further complicating this situation is the disproportionate burden of the metabolic syndrome among the at-risk low socioeconomic and minority segments of the population, which also are growing more rapidly than the overall population.[7]

Although the prevalence of the metabolic syndrome and subsequent disease outcomes continue to increase, the primary care response has not kept pace. We have powerful medical options at our disposal. Despite the tools at our disposal, our performance in the treatment of the metabolic syndrome has been inadequate. In the HOPE trial,[8] only 28% of patients were on lipid-lowering therapy, and in the RENAAL study[9], the average HbA1c was 8.5. The numbers of patients treated to goal for any given cardiovascular risk factor is on the order of 25% of the total and 50% or fewer of those on treatment. The IOM report considered these treatment accomplishments as evidence of a suboptimal quality of care. The IOM Report stated that:

> *Health care routinely fails to deliver its potential benefits. . . . Americans should be able to count on receiving care that meets their needs and is based on the best scientific knowledge. Yet there is strong evidence that this is frequently not the case. . . . Quality problems are everywhere, affecting many patients. Between the health care that we have and the care that we could have lies not just a gap, but a chasm.*[1]

It seems that the IOM is identifying the poor translation of clinical trials and clinical evidence in the treatment of the metabolic syndrome as a problem in primary medical care practice. As a case in point, although clinical trails and intervention studies have documented the benefit of aggressive treatment of diabetes and hypertension in the risk reduction of ESRD, the incidence rate of dialysis continues to increase.

The IOM has provided recommendations to address the epidemic of metabolic syndrome–related health problems and other common chronic conditions. Thus, improving health outcomes and reversing the health expenditures for avoidable hospitalizations can be achieved with implementation of these strategies in primary care settings. The IOM recommendations include:

1. Organize evidence-based care processes consistent with best practices.
2. Develop the information infrastructure needed to support the provision of care and the ongoing measurement of care processes and patient outcomes.

Elements 1 and 2 have been indispensable components of our efforts to "bust the cluster." A summary of risk factor control results among 289 diabetic hypertensive patients is provided in Table 1. Patients with the metabolic syndrome are especially appropriate for comprehensive management based on evidence and "best practices." These patients have insulin resistance, hypertension, complex hyperlipidemia, impaired glucose tolerance (frank diabetes), hypercoagulation, increased arterial inflammation, and obesity. Although their management is complex, the benefits of successful treatments are enormous.

The medical management of patients with the metabolic syndrome outperforms mechanical revascularization procedures such as angioplasty and bypass surgery. On further reflection, the basis for the superiority of medical management is obvious: vascular disease is often a sys-

TABLE 1. Risk Factor Values and Percent at Goal Among 289 Patients with Diabetes and Hypertension*

Risk Factor	Mean Value	Percent at Goal
Blood pressure	123/77 mmHg	67% < 130/80 mmHg
LDL cholesterol	92 mg/dL	72% < 100 mg/dL
HbA1c	6.5%	74% < 7%

*Patients were drawn from the author's practice.

temic process and is not isolated to the segment of a single or small number of vessels. Whereas surgical management addresses a limited segment of a progressive disease, effective medical management arrests and, in some cases, actually reverses the disease on a systemic basis. Virtually all of the adverse outcomes of type 2 diabetes are vascular, and diabetic patients are at very high risk. They actually have the same risk for a heart attack as patients who have already suffered a first myocardial infarction (MI).[10]

Physicians who treat patients with the metabolic syndrome should focus on one critical fact when they make therapeutic decisions: this collection of diseases is a syndrome. It is most important to realize that these conditions share common genetic and environmental antecedents. Furthermore, this syndrome seems to be a vicious cycle. Impairments of nitric oxide activity may actually be part of the cause of the **metabolic syndrome.** The metabolic syndrome produces severe endothelial dysfunction characterized by diminished nitric oxide activity that worsens as the disease progresses.

The data clearly indicate that treating to goal is very important in achieving certain targets when treating these patients (Table 2).

It is equally important as we work to achieve these goals that we remember the critical fact that the therapeutic target is the metabolic syndrome. For years, the focus of discussion has been which single treatment produced the best outcome for any single risk factor. More recently, there has been a recognition that this argument has limited application in real practice because multiple drugs are required to bring hypertension and other risk factors to goal. However, this very important realization needs to go one step further. Not only are multiple drugs required for treating individual components of the syndrome, but ther-

TABLE 2. Goals for Risk Factor Control in Diabetic Patients

Hypertension	Hyperlipidemia	Type 2 Diabetes
BP < 130/80 mmHg	LDL C < 100 mg/dL	HbA1c < 7%

apies for one component also often have powerful effects on the other risk factors. A comprehensive strategy that takes these factors into account can produce dramatic improvements in the control of multiple risk factors.

The treatment of one component of the syndrome frequently makes management of other components much more difficult. As one example of this complexity, propranolol is an inexpensive and very effective drug for the management of patients with hypertension and those who have had MIs. However, propranolol increases insulin resistance by 33%, causes weight gain, and makes it more likely that patients with impaired glucose tolerance will become diabetic. Propranolol also increases triglycerides and lowers high-density lipoprotein (HDL) level. Thus, primary care doctors must consider the multiple components of the metabolic syndrome when selecting a treatment strategy. The use of a non selective beta-blocker particularly interferes with achieving goal levels for glucose, HDL, and triglycerides. On the other hand, angiotensin-converting enzyme (ACE) inhibitors lower insulin resistance and improve glucose metabolism. Both beta-blockers and ACE inhibitors have positive effects on event reduction in short term-studies, but many beta-blockers actually increase insulin resistance and worsen the findings of the metabolic syndrome. Over the long term, these effects may become a net negative. In the author's practice, beta-blockers in patients with the metabolic syndrome are reserved for those with compelling indications such as previous MI or congestive heart failure.

The same situation exists in the treatment of those with type 2 diabetes. Many patients with type 2 diabetes are treated with two insulin injections daily. In the first year of this treatment, the average patient gains 10 pounds. Because the metabolic syndrome is aggravated by obesity, this is a highly undesirable and counterproductive development. Weight gain adversely impacts the control of glucose, lipids, and hypertension. Metformin treatment is associated with weight loss. Addition of a nighttime insulin injection only replaces a relative insulin deficiency and does not interfere with the weight loss benefit. Metformin plus bedtime insulin offers the best HbA1c, least weight gain, and the fewest episodes of hypoglycemia compared with other combination therapies. Metformin also has another metabolic advantage: when it is combined with a statin, there is a very dramatic effect on all components of the dyslipidemia that accompany the metabolic syndrome.

In fact, metformin is unique among drug therapies for type 2 diabetes in that there is evidence that it reduces the risk of MI by 39%, diabetes-related death by 42%, and all-cause mortality by 36%. This treatment joins statins, ACE inhibitors, and angiotensin receptor blockers (ARBs) in a powerful therapeutic combination to lower events. Similar to these other treatments, metformin has multiple desirable effects on metabolic syndrome patients beyond its effect on the surrogate target, blood glucose. Information from a variety of sources indicates that metformin improves diastolic dysfunction, decreases total cholesterol, decreases very low-density lipoprotein (VLDL) cholesterol, decreases LDL cholesterol, increases HDL cholesterol, decreases oxidative stress, improves vascular relaxation, decreases PAI-1 levels, increases tissue plasminogen activator activity, decreases von Willebrand factor levels, and decreases platelet aggregation and adhesion. It is apparent that metformin has a favorable effect on many parameters in vascular homeostasis that are most desirable in patients at high risk for vascular events.[11]

It is clear that there are clinically important differences in the metabolic effects of drugs that are commonly used to treat components of the metabolic syndrome. Evidence suggests that there are also differential effects on events. Pharmacologic therapies for components of the metabolic syndrome should not be chosen arbitrarily. A coordinated, integrated program that takes all of these factors into consideration in treatment of metabolic syndrome patients has been used in the author's practice (Table 3).

Using this simple protocol, it is possible to achieve excellent control of all risk factors in most patients (see Table 1). For patients with type 2 diabetes, this is a relatively low number of medications compared with usual practice. All of the interventions listed first in each class powerfully reduce events, lower insulin resistance, reduce new cases of diabetes, and improve endothelial function. These interrelationships may explain some of the synergies that seem to be in operation with these treatments.

Joseph Loscalzo at Boston University, an expert on the subject of endothelial function, says: "Since abnormal endothelial physiology is implicated in the genesis and progression of vascular disease, prevention or reversal of endothelial dysfunction represents an attractive goal for therapeutic intervention." Indeed, several interventions have been consistently shown to restore endothelial vasomotor function. These include, among others, lipid-lowering therapy, ACE inhibitor therapy, L-arginine,

TABLE 3. Medications Used to Treat Patients with the Metabolic Syndrome		
Hypertension	**Hyperlipidemia**	**Type 2 Diabetes**
ACE inhibitors/ARBs	Statin	Metformin
Hydrochlorothiazide		HS Insulin
Calcium channel blocker		
β-blocker or reserpine		

antioxidant and estrogen supplementation, smoking cessation, and exercise. Interestingly, these are the very same interventions that attenuate atherosclerosis and improve mortality and morbidity outcomes from cardiovascular disease, suggesting a mechanistic link between endothelial dysfunction and atherosclerosis.

References

1. Chassin MR, Galvin RW: The urgent need to improve health care quality: Institute of Medicine national roundtable on health care quality. JAMA 28:1000–1005, 1998.
2. Institute of Medicine: Crossing the Quality Chasms: A New Health System for the 21st Century. Washington DC, National Academic Press, 2001.
3. US Department of Health and Human Services: Healthy People 2010, Understanding and Improving Health. Washington DC, DHHS.
4. Blackburn GL: I read that nearly a quarter of adult Americans have "metabolic syndrome." What is the malady, and how can I prevent it? Health News 8:12, 2002.
5. Hanson RL, Imperatore G, Bennett PH, Knowler WC: Components of the "metabolic syndrome" and incidence of type 2 diabetes. Diabetes 51:3120–3127, 2002.
6. Wang G, Zheng ZJ, Heath G, et al: Economic burden of cardiovascular disease associated with excess body weight in US adults. Am J Prev Med 23:1–6, 2002.
7. Averett S, Korenmans S: Black-white differences in social and economic consequences of obesity. Int J Obesity Rel Metab Disord 23:166–173, 1999.
8. Heart Outcomes Prevention Evaluation (HOPE) Study Investigators: Effects of an angiotensin-converting-enzyme inhibitor, ramipril, on cardiovascular events in high-risk patients. N Engl J Med 342:145–153, 2000.
9. Brenner BM, Cooper ME, deZeeuw, et al. for the RENAAL Study Investigators: Effects of losartan on renal and cardiovascular outcomes in patients with type 2 diabetes and nephropathy. N Engl J Med 345: 861–869, 2001.
10. Haffner SM, Lehto S, Ronnemau T, et al: Mortality from coronary heart disease in subjects with type 2 diabetes and in nondiabetic subjects with and without prior myocardial infarction. N Engl J Med 339:229–239, 1998.
11. Kirpichnikov D, McFarlane SI, Sowers JR: Metformin: An update. Ann Intern Med 137:25–33, 2002.

Managing Hypertension in Diabetic Patients

chapter

25

Peter D. Hart, M.D., and
George L. Bakris, M.D.

Hypertension in diabetic patients is often associated with cardiovascular disease and progressive renal damage. Seventy-one percent of all diabetic adults in the United States have blood pressure (BP) > 130/85 mmHg.[1] Hypertension and diabetes, together, account for more than 50% of approximately 350,000 patients who begin dialysis in the United States yearly (Fig. 1).[2] Elevated BP in diabetes is analogous to adding gasoline (hypertension) to the fire (diabetes) because high BP potentiates vascular and end-organ injury occurring from diabetes.

The incidence of end-stage renal disease (ESRD) has risen steadily along with the increasing incidence of diabetes in the face of persistent deficiencies in achieving BP goals.[2] Despite recommendations from various public health organizations, physicians have been inadequately aggressive in managing hypertension and other cardiovascular risk factors among diabetic patients in particular. For example, only 11% of diabetic hypertensives are reaching the Joint National Committee (JNC) VI BP goal of < 130/85 mmHg.[3]

This chapter discusses evidence supporting the importance of achieving a BP goal of < 130/80 mmHg and provides guidance on how to get there. To this end, this chapter reviews the derivation and evidence to support a BP goal of less than 130/85 mmHg and, more recently, less than 130/80 mmHg and, outlines an evidence-based approach to achieve the BP goal to maximally reduce morbidity.

Derivation of the Blood Pressure Goal

Most of the evidence comes from post-hoc analyses of clinical trials and large databases that support the need for a lower BP goal in those with diabetes. Available data, completed since the JNC VI report, sup-

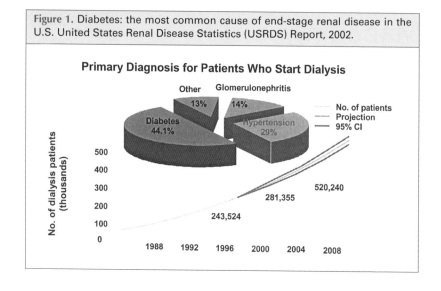

Figure 1. Diabetes: the most common cause of end-stage renal disease in the U.S. United States Renal Disease Statistics (USRDS) Report, 2002.

port the concept of a lower diastolic BP (DBP) goal of less than 130/80 mmHg for those with type 2 diabetes (Table 1).

Post-hoc analyses of clinical trials that support a lower BP goal include the Multiple Risk Factor Intervention Trail (MRFIT). An evaluation of more than 330,000 men supports the concept that BP levels < 120 mmHg have less mortality than any higher level. These data also confirm a much higher mortality rate in those with diabetes regardless of BP level compared with those without diabetes (Fig. 2).[8]

Support for the < 130 mmHg goal also comes from the United Kingdom Prospective Diabetes Study (UKPDS) of 1148 type 2 diabetics randomized to one of two goal BPs: < 150/85 mmHg (the "intensively treated [tight] group") or lower than 180/105 mmHg (the "control [less tight] group"), and followed for an average of 8.4 years. At the end of the trial, the tight BP group had an average BP of 144/82 mmHg, and the "less tight" group was 154/87 mmHg, a BP difference of 10/5 mmHg.[9] Participants in the lower BP group had a risk reduction of 32% in diabetes-related deaths, 24% in diabetes-related endpoints (including amputations), 44% in strokes, and 37% in microvascular complications (i.e., nephropathy and advanced retinopathy). Thus, a lower BP level in this study resulted in a significant risk reduction of diabetes-related cardiovascular and microvascular complications. Although the average achieved systolic BP (SBP) in the aggressively treated group was 144 mmHg, a post-hoc analysis showed that each 10-mmHg reduction in mean systolic BP reduced risk for diabetic-related deaths 15%, myocar-

TABLE 1. Goal BP and Initial Drug Therapy Recommendations in Diabetic Hypertensives

Organization	Year	Goal BP (mmHg)	Initial Therapy
American Diabetes Association	2002	< 130/80	ACEI/ARB
Canadian Hypertension Society	2002	< 130/80	ACEI/ARB
National Kidney Foundation	2000	< 130/80	ACEI
British Hypertension Society	1999	< 140/80	ACEI
WHO & International Society of Hypertension	1999	< 130/85	ACEI
Joint National Committee (JNC VI)	1997	< 130/85	ACEI

dial infarction 11%, diabetic related complications 12%, and microvascular complications by 13%.[10] In this study, no threshold risk for BP level was observed for any endpoint.

The Hypertension Optimal Treatment (HOT) trial randomized patients to different levels of DBP and assessed cardiovascular outcomes.[11] The HOT trial included 18,790 patients of whom 1501 had diabetes. Patients were randomized to one of three diastolic BP goals: < 90 mmHg, < 85 mmHg, or < 80 mmHg. Among the subset of diabetic patients, the lowest relative risk for cardiovascular events was noted in the < 80 mmHg group compared to the < 90 mmHg group (relative risk = 0.49). The risk of major CV events over 10 years was significantly lower in the < 80-

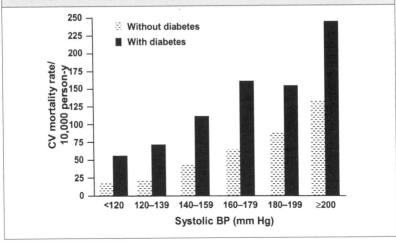

Figure 2. Epidemiological data that show the relationship between CV mortality and level of BP in those with and without diabetes. (From Stamler, et al: Diabetes, other risk factors and 12-yr cardiovascular mortality for men screened in the Multiple Risk Factor Intervention Trial. Diabetes Care 16:434, 1993; with permission.)

mmHg group compared with the < 90-mmHg group (11.9% vs. 24.4%). This benefit of the lower DBP was present for diabetic but not nondiabetic hypertensive patients. The average achieved SBP in this trial was 138 mmHg, although lower trends in CV events were noted < 130 mmHg.

Data for the benefit of a low SBP also come from the post-hoc analyses of the Systolic Hypertension in Elderly People (SHEP) and Systolic Hypertension in Europe (Syst-Eur) trials.[12,13] This is especially important because systolic BP increases with age, and the most rapidly growing segment of the population is elderly. Moreover, SBP becomes more important than DBP in predicting complications in older hypertensive patients. In post-hoc analyses of both SHEP and Syst-Eur, diabetics whose BP was < 140 mmHg had significantly greater CV risk reduction than higher BP levels. Moreover, those who could get levels < 130 mmHg had even greater reduction in CV risk. In the overwhelming majority of diabetics, the diastolic BP is < 80 if the SBP is controlled to < 130 mmHg.

Goals in Kidney Disease

In addition to CV risk reduction, several post-hoc analyses of clinical trials examining outcomes of kidney disease in diabetes provide strong support for lowering SBP to < 140 mmHg. The evidence in nephropathy secondary to type 2 diabetes, however, is scant to support < 130 mmHg unless more than 1000 mg/day of albuminuria is present.[3] However, data in nephropathy from type 1 diabetes do support a BP < 130 mmHg.[14]

One prospective trial in people with type 2 diabetes, the Appropriate Blood Pressure Control in Diabetes (ABCD) trial, randomized participants to two levels of BP control. This study showed no difference in decline of renal function over a 5-year follow-up period.[15] However, it should be noted that a trend toward even slower declines in kidney function were noted among people with a SBP ≤ 130 mmHg.[16] Collectively, these studies in people with nephropathy demonstrate that achieved SBP between 130 and 135 mmHg improves kidney disease outcome compared with levels > 140 mmHg, (Fig. 3).[3,17,18,19] Sub-analyses of these studies indicate that people with > 1 g/day of proteinuria should definitely have a SBP to < 130 mmHg to slow kidney disease progression.[3,20] Given a stable rate of decline in kidney function, a 55-year-old diabetic man with serum creatinine of 2 mg/dL and mean SBP of 144 mmHg would start dialysis 4.5 years earlier than a matched patient whose systolic BP was 134 mmHg (see Fig. 3).

In summary, these trials as well as recent recommendations by the American Diabetes Association, National Kidney Foundation, and

Figure 3. Relationship between achieved level of BP and rate of decline in kidney function. Data from both diabetic and nondiabetic trials are included. (Modified from Bakris GL, et al: Preserving renal function in adults with hypertension and diabetes: A consensus approach. Am J Kidney Dis 2000.)

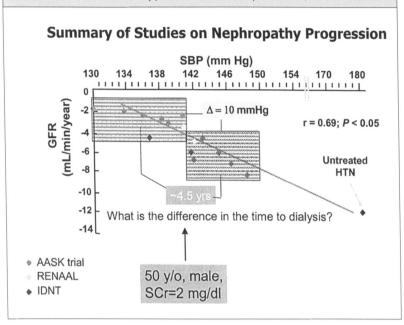

Canadian Hypertension Society strongly suggest that the lower BP goal of 130/80 mmHg is required for reducing cardiovascular morbidity and mortality and to maximally preserve renal function in patients with diabetes and hypertension.

An Approach to Assess and Achieve Goal Blood Pressure

Accurate measurement of BP is mandatory to establish the diagnosis of hypertension.[21,22].

Screening for micro- and macroalbuminuria with a spot urine for albumin:creatinine test is strongly recommended in all diabetic patients during the initial visit and annually thereafter. Microalbuminuria is an independent marker of increased risk for CVD and nephropathy.[23] Several long-term clinical trials in patients with or without diabetes show reducing proteinuria approximately 35% compared with baseline correlates with significant delay in progression to end-stage renal disease (Table 2). This corroborates the National Kidney Foundation's recom-

TABLE 2. Clinical Trials and Renal Outcomes Based on Proteinuria Reduction

Prolonged time to dialysis (~35% proteinuria reduction)
- Captopril trial[50]
- AASK trial[19]
- RENAAL trial[36]
- IDNT[35]

No change in time to dialysis (no proteinuria reduction)
- DHPCCB arm, IDNT[35]
- DHPCCB arm, AASK[19]

mendation that therapy for BP control should also target reduction in proteinuria in these patients.[20]

Nondrug Therapy

Based on all guidelines including the JNC VI, drug therapy to achieve BP goal should be initiated in all people with diabetes; however, lifestyle interventions should also be discussed and reinforced because they can profoundly improve BP control, especially in stage I hypertension.[2,24–27] A summary of lifestyle approaches is summarized in Table 3.

Drug Therapy

All antihypertensive agents reduce BP similarly (10–15/5–10 mmHg) when used at available maximal doses. However, some antihypertensive agents confer more cardiovascular and renal protection than others.

A review of clinical trials that randomized patients with either diabetes or renal impairment to two different levels of BP control demon-

TABLE 3. Nonpharmacologic Intervention

Weight reduction: Weight reduction should be considered an effective tool in the initial management of diabetic patients who have hypertension, especially if they are obese. Weight reduction can reduce BP independent of sodium intake and may improve blood glucose and lipid levels. The loss of 2.2 lbs (1 kg) body weight may result in decreases in mean arterial BP of approximately 1 mmHg.

Sodium restriction or increased potassium intake: In controlled trials in essential hypertension, moderate sodium intake (2.3 g/day) led to a reduction of 5 mmHg in SBP and 2 to 3 mmHg in DPB. Additionally, when drug therapy has been initiated, concomitant sodium restriction often leads to a better BP response. Potassium intake has been shown in the DASH study to be very useful for lowering BP.

Physical activity: Moderate intense physical activity such as 30- to 45-minute brisk walking daily has been shown to lower BP and is recommended by JNC VI.

strate two key results. First, to achieve the desired lower BP goal, an average of 3.2 different antihypertensive medications per day was required (Fig.4).[3,28] Second, initial therapy with an agent that blocks the renin-angiotensin-aldosterone system (RAAS) is preferred over other agents because the risk reduction for both cardiovascular and renal outcomes is greater than with other agents.[2,3,29] Based on the results of clinical trials, a treatment algorithm has been proposed by the National Kidney Foundation to achieve the recommended BP goal for patients with diabetes with or without renal insufficiency (Fig. 5).

If SBP or DBP is 15/10 mmHg above the recommended goal, respectively, at least two different antihypertensive agents are needed.[3] Thus, if the goal BP is 130/80 mmHg and the patient has a clinic BP reading of > 152/96 mmHg and is not receiving treatment, the physician needs to prescribe two different agents to achieve the goal BP. The recently completed Study of Hypertension and the Efficacy of Lotrel in Diabetes (SHIELD) examined > 200 diabetic hypertensives, randomized to either initial fixed-dose combination therapy that included an angiotensin-converting enzyme (ACE) inhibitor or monotherapy with an ACE inhibitor. This study showed that more than twice as many patients achieved the SBP goal of < 130 within the first 2 months on combination therapy than on monotherapy.[30] Even after addition of a diuretic to the monotherapy group, greater control rates persisted in the combination group (Fig. 6).

Initial treatment with an ACE inhibitor, either alone or with a diuretic added, is the initial therapy to achieve a BP of < 130/80 mmHg. Di-

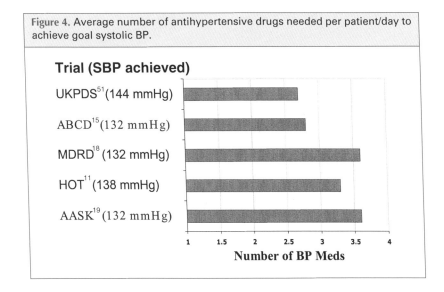

Figure 4. Average number of antihypertensive drugs needed per patient/day to achieve goal systolic BP.

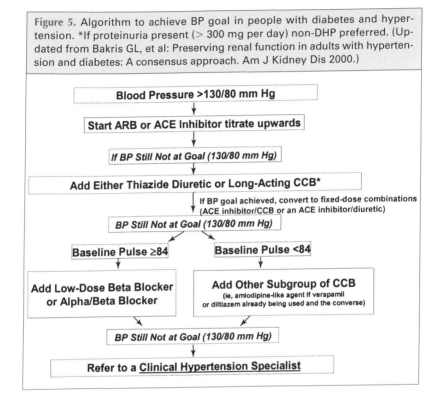

Figure 5. Algorithm to achieve BP goal in people with diabetes and hypertension. *If proteinuria present (> 300 mg per day) non-DHP preferred. (Updated from Bakris GL, et al: Preserving renal function in adults with hypertension and diabetes: A consensus approach. Am J Kidney Dis 2000.)

uretics potentiate the BP-lowering effects of ACE inhibitors, especially in African Americans and elderly individuals. If ACE inhibitors are not tolerated, angiotensin receptor blockers (ARBs) should be substituted.[29,31] ACE inhibitors are the preferred initial therapy in diabetic patients with a SBP > 130 mmHg unless nephropathy and proteinuria are present in type 2 diabetics, in whom ARBs are first-line therapy.[31] ACE inhibitors reduce cardiovascular risks and prevent or delay progression of diabetic nephropathy more than expected from BP lowering alone.

Furthermore, in the MICRO-HOPE (Heart Outcomes Prevention Evaluation[32]) substudy, 3577 diabetic patients with the same eligibility criteria as the HOPE study (age > 55 years, history of cardiovascular disease or diabetes, and one other cardiovascular risk factor) were randomly assigned to ACE inhibitor or placebo, and a primary outcome was development of proteinuria.[33] At the end of the study, there was a 24% relative risk reduction of overt nephropathy (i.e., development of albuminuria) in the ramipril group, (absolute risk reduction [ARR] = 1.9; number needed to treat [NNT] = 52).

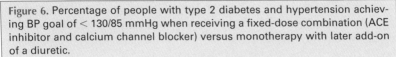

Figure 6. Percentage of people with type 2 diabetes and hypertension achieving BP goal of < 130/85 mmHg when receiving a fixed-dose combination (ACE inhibitor and calcium channel blocker) versus monotherapy with later add-on of a diuretic.

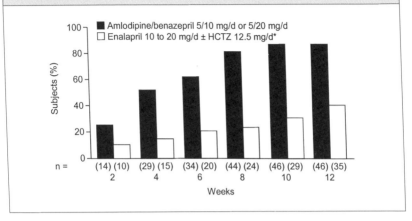

The most common side effects of ACE inhibitors are cough, angioedema and hyperkalemia, and an increase in serum creatinine level. Although intolerant side effects may preclude the use of ACE inhibitors, they should not be withheld from patients with mild renal insufficiency or an initial increase in serum creatinine < 30% above baseline. An analysis of recent renal trials supports the view that acute increases in serum creatinine ≤ 30% above baseline that stabilize within the first 2 months correlate with long-term preservation of renal function.[34]

ARBs have renoprotective effects in type 2 diabetics with nephropathy. Two clinical trials involving > 3000 patients with nephropathy associated with type 2 diabetes provide solid evidence of renoprotection with ARBs. The Irbesartan Diabetic Nephropathy Trial (IDNT) and the Reduction of Endpoints in NIDDM with the AII Antagonist Losartan (RENAAL) study both demonstrate a 16% to 20% risk reduction of nephropathy progression compared with conventional therapy.[35,36]

There are limited data about the effect of ARBs on cardiovascular outcomes. In a prespecified subgroup analysis of the Losartan Intervention For Endpoint reduction in hypertension (LIFE) trial that compared the effect of an ARB based therapy with a beta blocker–based therapy in the high-risk diabetic hypertensive, the ARB was more effective than the beta-blocker with an overall risk reduction of 24% for MI, stroke, or cardiovascular mortality.[37] ARR = 5%; NNT = 20). ARBs are also less likely to cause angioedema or hyperkalemia than ACE inhibitors.[38]

Addition of low-dose thiazide diuretics 12.5 to 25.0 mg/day are recommended as second-line therapy with either an ACE inhibitor or ARB because they are associated with a reduction in cardiovascular events in elderly diabetics with isolated systolic hypertension and potentiate the BP reduction seen with inhibitors of the RAAS.[3]

If the BP is not at goal after these two agents have been used, then calcium channel blockers (CCBs) should be added because they demonstrate an additive BP-lowering capability when used with either ACE inhibitors or ARBs. Moreover, in secondary analyses of clinical trials and when ACE inhibitors are used in concert with CCBs, they have decreased cardiovascular events.[3,39–41]

The role of CCBs in reducing cardiovascular events in diabetic hypertensives is controversial. Although the HOT and Syst-Eur trials showed that long-acting dihydropyridine CCBs reduced cardiovascular events, the Fosinopril Amlodipine Cardiac Events Trial (FACET) and the ABCD Trial demonstrated no reduction in cardiovascular risk.[11–13,15,39] However, 73% of patients in HOT and 43% in Syst-Eur received ACE inhibitors concomitantly. In FACET, the ACE inhibitor group had a markedly reduced CV risk compared with the CCB alone. Two recent meta-analyses suggest that CCBs are safe and can be used alone to lower BP in people without kidney disease and especially when agents that block the RAAS are used in concert to achieve CV risk reduction.[40,41]

Dihydropyridine CCBs, such as amlodipine, should never be used as alternatives to agents that block the RAAS in diabetic renal disease. The IDNT clearly demonstrates that dihydropyridine CCBs are not different from placebo in slowing progressive renal damage in type 2 diabetes and do not offer the protection of an ARB or ACE inhibitor. The nondihydropyridine CCBs such as verapamil and diltiazem reduce proteinuria, a finding that correlates with positive renal outcomes in all trials in patients with diabetic nephropathy; however, no long-term studies exist to demonstrate delay in progressive renal damage.[42,43] Taken together, these data suggest that CCBs are good BP-reducing agents but should not be the initial therapy to lower BP in diabetic patients.

If BP is still not at goal after all these agents are titrated to maximal doses then beta-blockers should be strongly considered because they reduce cardiovascular risk despite their adverse metabolic effects.[44] Carvedilol is currently the only beta-blocker that has demonstrated cardiovascular risk reduction with neutral metabolic effects.[45] Also, beta-blockers have additive BP-lowering effects to most antihypertensive agents in patients with baseline pulse rates > 84 bpm.[3]

If BP is still not at goal, other agents such as α-blockers at bedtime, hydralazine, clonidine or methyldopa, and minoxidil can be used as adjunctive therapy to reach goal BP. Patients whose BP is still not at goal or who remain uncontrolled should be referred to a board certified Hypertension Specialist (see www.ash-us.org for a list in your area).

Ways to Reduce Pill Counts

The use of combination antihypertensive medications, such as an ACE inhibitor combined with either a diuretic or CCB, is useful to reduce pill counts and improve patient adherence. These combinations achieve BP goals in more than 80% of diabetic patients with hypertension, thus resulting in more consistent and cost-effective BP control.[46-48]

Summary

The available evidence indicates the goal BP to protect against cardiovascular disease and nephropathy in diabetic hypertensives should be < 130/80 mmHg. The antihypertensive regimen should include ACE inhibitors or ARBs as initial agents. In most patients with diabetes and hypertension, three different antihypertensive medications, including diuretics, CCBs, or beta-blockers, are needed to achieve the recommended BP of < 130/80 mmHg. Physicians must make every effort to achieve the BP goal by the least intrusive means possible. This minimizes drug-related side effects, improves patient adherence, and reduces cardiovascular and renal morbidity and mortality.

References

1. Geiss LS, Rolka DB, Engelgau MM: Elevated blood pressure among U.S. adults with diabetes, 1988–1994. Am J Prev Med 2002, 22: 42–48.
2. Joint National Committee on Detection, Evaluation, and Treatment of High Blood Pressure: The sixth report of the Joint National Committee on Detection, Evaluation, and Treatment of High Blood Pressure (JNC VI). Arch Intern Med 1997, 154:2413–2446.
3. Bakris GL, Williams M, Dworkin L, et al: Preserving renal function in adults with hypertension and diabetes: a consensus approach. National Kidney Foundation Hypertension and Diabetes executive Committees working group. Am J Kidney Diseases 2000, 36: 646–661.
4. www.usrds.gov
5. Coresh J, Wei GL, McQuillan G, et al: Prevalence of high blood pressure and elevated serum creatinine level in the United States: findings from the third National Health and Nutrition Examination Survey (1988–1994). Arch Intern Med 2001, 161:1207–1216.
6. Perry, HM Jr, Miller JP, Fornoff JR, et al: Early predictors of 15-year end-stage renal disease in hypertensive patients. Hypertension 1995,25(4 Pt 1):587–594.
7. Franklin SS, Gustin W, Wong ND, et al: Hemodynamic patterns of age-related changes in blood pressure: the Framingham Heart Study. Circulation 1997, 96:308–315.
8. Stamler J, Vaccaro O, Neaton JD, Wentworth D: Diabetes, other risk factors, and

12-yr cardiovascular mortality for men screened in the Multiple Risk Factor Intervention Trial. Diabetes Care 1993, 16:434–444.

9. Tight blood pressure control and risk of macrovascular and microvascular complications in type 2 diabetes: UKPDS 38. UK Prospective Diabetes Study Group. Br Med J 1998, 317:703–713.

10. Adler AI, Stratton IM, Neil HA, et al: Association of systolic blood pressure with macrovascular or microvascular complications of type 2 diabetes (UKPDS 36), Br Med J 2000, 312:412–419.

11. Hansson L, Zanchetti A, Carruthers SG, et al: Effects of intensive blood pressure lowering and low-dose aspirin in patients with hypertension: principal results of the Hypertension Optimal Treatment (HOT) randomised trial. The HOT Study Group. Lancet 1998, 351:1755–1762.

12. Curb JD, Pressel SL, Cutler JA, et al: Effect of diuretic-based antihypertensive treatment on cardiovascular disease risk in older diabetic patients with isolated systolic hypertension. Systolic Hypertension in the Elderly Program Cooperative Research Group. JAMA 1996, 276:1886–1892.

13. Tuomilehto J, Rastenyte D, Birkenhager WH, et al: Effects of calcium-channel blockade in older patients with diabetes and systolic hypertension. Systolic Hypertension in Europe Trial Investigators. N Engl J Med 1999, 340:677–684 .

14. Lewis JB, Berl T, Bain RP, et al: Effect of intensive blood pressure control on the course of type 1 diabetic nephropathy. Collaborative Study Group. Am J Kidney Dis 1999,34:809–817.

15. Estacio RO, Jeffers BW, Gifford N, Schrier RW: Effect of blood pressure control on diabetic microvascular complications in patients with hypertension and type 2 diabetes. Diabetes Care 2000, 23(suppl 2):B54-B64.

16. Schrier RW, Estacio RO, Esler A, Mehler P: Effects of aggressive blood pressure control in normotensive type 2 diabetic patients on albuminuria, retinopathy and strokes. Kidney Int 2002, 61:1086–1097.

17. Ravid M, Lang R, Rachmani R, Lishner M: Long-term renoprotective effect of angiotensin-converting enzyme inhibition in non-insulin-dependent diabetes mellitus: a 7-year follow-up study. Arch Intern Med 1996, 156:286–289.

18. Lazarus JM, Bourgoignie JJ, Buckalew VM, et al: Achievement and safety of a low BP goal in chronic renal disease. The Modification of Diet in Renal Disease Study Group. Hypertension 1997, 29:641–650.

19. Wright, JT Jr, Bakris G, Greene, T, et al for the AAKS Study group. Effect of Blood Pressure Lowering and Antihypertensive Drug Class on Progression of Hypertensive Kidney Disease: Results from the AASK Trial. JAMA 2002, 288:2421–2431.

20. Keane WF, Eknoyan G: Proteinuria, Albuminuria, Risk Assessment, Detection, Elimination (PARADE): a position paper of the National Kidney Foundation. Am J Kidney Dis 1999, 33:1004–1010.

21. Hart PD, Bakris GB: Treatment of diabetic hypertension: goals and choices. In Hypertension Therapy Annual 2002. Kaplan NM (ed). London: Dunitz p 41–54.

22. Black HR, Bakris GL, Elliott WJ: Hypertension: epidemiology, pathophysiology, diagnosis and treatment. In: Fuster V, Alexander W, O'Rourke R, et al (eds.) Hurst's The Heart. New York: McGraw-Hill, 2001 pp 1553–1604.

23. Garg J, Bakris GL: Microalbuminuria: marker of vascular dysfunction, risk factor for cardiovascular disease J. Vasc Med 2002, 7:35–43.

24. Midgley JP, Matthew AG, Greenwood CM, Logan AG: Effect of reduced dietary sodium on blood pressure: a metanalysis of randomized controlled trials. JAMA 1996, 275:1590–1597.

25. Geleijnse JM, Witteman JC, et al: Reduction in blood pressure with low sodium, high

potassium, high magnesium salt in older subjects with mild to moderate hypertension. Br Med J 1994, 309:436–440.

26. Moore TJ, McKnight JA: Dietary factors and blood pressure regulation. Endocrinol Metab Clin North Am 1995, 24:543–555.

27. Sacks FM, Svetkey LP, Vollmer WM, et al: Effects on blood pressure of reduced dietary sodium and the Dietary Approaches to Stop Hypertension (DASH) diet. DASH-Sodium Collaborative Research Group. N Engl J Med 2001, 344:3–10.

28. Bakris GL: Maximizing cardio-renal benefits: achieve blood pressure goals. J Clin Hypertens 1999, 1:141–148.

29. Anonymous: Clinical practice guidelines for chronic kidney disease: evaluation, classification and stratification. Am J Kidney Dis 2002, 39(suppl 1):1-231.

30. Bakris GL, Weir MR, Neutel J: Safety and efficacy of an ACE inhibitor/calcium channel blocker combination versus an ACE inhibitor alone in hypertensive patients with type 2 diabetes. Am J Hypertens. 2002, 15(part 2):173A.

31. Anonymous: American Diabetes Association: clinical practice recommendations 2002. Diabetes Care 2002,25(suppl 1):1–147.

32. Effects of an angiotensin-converting-enzyme inhibitor, ramipril, on cardiovascular events in high-risk patients. The Heart Outcomes Prevention Evaluation Study Investigators. N Engl J Med 2000, 342:145–153.

33. Heart Outcomes Prevention Evaluation (HOPE) Study Investigators: Effects of ramipril on cardiovascular and microvascular outcomes in people with diabetes mellitus: results of the HOPE study and MICRO-HOPE substudy. Lancet 2000, 355:253–259.

34. Bakris GL, Weir MR: ACE inhibitor-associated elevations in serum creatinine: is this a cause for concern? Arch Intern Med 2000, 160:685–693.

35. Lewis EJ, Hunsicker LG, Clarke WR, et al: Renoprotective effect of the angiotensin-receptor antagonist irbesartan in patients with nephropathy due to type 2 diabetes. N Engl J Med 2001, 345:851–860.

36. Brenner BM, Cooper ME, de Zeeuw D, et al: Effects of losartan on renal and cardiovascular outcomes in patients with type 2 diabetes and nephropathy. N Engl J Med 2001, 345:861–869.

37. Lindholm LH, Ibsen H, Danloff B, et al: Cardiovascular morbidity and mortality in patients with diabetes in the Losartan intervention for endpoint reduction in hypertension study (LIFE): a randomized trial against atenolol. Lancet 2002, 359:1004–1010.

38. Bakris GL, Siomos M, Richardson D, et al. for the VAL-K study group. ACE inhibition or angiotensin receptor blockade: impact on potassium in renal failure. Kidney Int 2000, 58:2084–2092.

39. Tatti P, Pahor M, Byington RP, et al: Outcome results of the Fosinopril versus Amlodipine Cardiovascular Events randomized Trial (FACET) in patients with hypertension and NIDDM. Diabetes Care 1998, 21:597–610.

40. Neal B, Macmahon S, Chapman N: Effects of ACE inhibitors, calcium antagonists, and other blood pressure lowering drugs: results of prospectively designed overviews of randomized trials. Blood Pressure Lowering Treatment Trialists' Collaboration. Lancet 2000, 356:1955–1964.

41. Staessen, JA, Wang, JG, Thijs, L. Cardiovascular protection and blood pressure reduction: a meta-analysis. Lancet 2001, 358:1305–1315.

42. Bakris GL, Copley JB, Vicknair N, et al. Calcium channel blockers versus other antihypertensive therapies on progression of NIDDM associated nephropathy. Kidney Int 1996, 50:1641–1650.

43. Bakris GL, Mangrum A, Copley JB, et al: Calcium channel or beta blockade on pro-

gression of diabetic renal disease in African-Americans Hypertension 1997, 29:744–750.

44. Gress TW, Nieto FJ, Shahar E, et al. for the Atherosclerosis Risk if Communities Study: Hypertension and antihypertensive therapy and the risk factors for the type 2 diabetes mellitus. N Engl J Med 2000, 342:905–912.

45. Giugliano D, Acampora R, Marfella R, et al: Metabolic and cardiovascular effects of carvedilol and atenolol in non-insulin-dependent diabetes mellitus and hypertension: a randomized, controlled trial. Ann Intern Med 1997, 126:955–959.

46. Epstein M, Bakris GL: Newer approaches to antihypertensive therapy: use of fixed-dose combination therapy. Arch Intern Med 1996, 156:1969–1978.

47. Elliott WJ, Weir DR, Black HR: Cost-effectiveness of the new lower blood pressure goal of JNC VI for diabetic hypertensives. Arch Intern Med 2000, 160:1277–1283.

48. Ifudu O: Benefits of combination antihypertensive therapy in progressive chronic renal failure. Am J Manag Care 1999, 5(suppl II):429-448.

49. Reference deleted.

50. Lewis EJ, et al. The effect of angiotensin-converting-enzyme inhibition on diabetic nephropathy. The Collaborative Study Group. N Engl J Med 1993, 329 (20):1456–1462.

51. Anonymous. Tight blood pressure control and risk of macrovascular and microvascular complications in type 2 diabetes: UKPDS 38. UK Prospective Diabetes Study Group. BMJ 1998, 317 (7160):703–713.

HOT TOPICS

Isolated Systolic Hypertension

Stanley S. Franklin, M.D.

chapter

26

Hypertension has changed considerably over the past half century. Formerly, adults in their forties or fifties presented with severe combined systolic-diastolic hypertension, frequently accelerated or malignant in nature, and associated with the rapid onset of cerebral hemorrhage, heart failure or end-stage renal disease. This form of hypertension still occurs, but with greatly diminished frequency. More recently with the aging of the population and the advent of effective antihypertensive therapy, there has been a shift toward a more slowly progressive form of hypertension that is predominately systolic in nature, affecting middle-aged and older persons. This form of hypertension is frequently complicated by long-standing comorbid atherosclerotic events, such as coronary heart disease (CHD), thrombotic stroke, and slowly progressive heart and renal failure. The dictum of that previous era stated that a person's normal systolic blood pressure (SBP) was 100 plus his or her age. More recently, this slowly increasing SBP with aging has become a major public health problem and is referred to as *isolated systolic hypertension* (ISH). Previously, ISH was defined as a SBP of ≥ 160 mmHg and a diastolic blood pressure (DBP) of < 95 or 90 mmHg. With the recognition of its true risk, ISH was redefined as a SBP of ≥ 140 and DBP < 90 mmHg in the 1990s. The purpose of this chapter is to provide a better understanding of ISH and how best to treat it effectively.

Epidemiology of ISH

Most population studies show that SBP rises from adolescence onward, while DBP initially increases with age, levels off at age 50 to 55 years, and decreases after age 60 to 65 years (Fig. 1).[3] Thus, pulse pressure, the difference between SBP and DBP, begins to increase after age 50 years, and this increase accelerates after age 60 years. The National Health and Nutrition Examination Survey (NHANES III, 1988–1991)[8] showed that three of four adults with hypertension were age 50 or older.

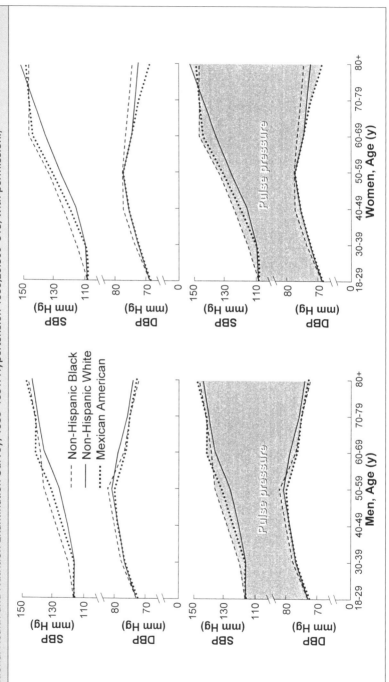

Figure 1. Mean systolic and diastolic blood pressures by age and ethnicity for men and women, U.S. population age 18 years and older, NHANES III. (From Burt VL, Whelton P, Roccella EJ, et al: Prevalence of hypertension in the US adult population: Results from the Third National Health and Nutrition Examination Survey, 1988–1991. Hypertension 1995;25:305–313; with permission.)

TABLE 1. Age-related Hemodynamic Changes in BP Data from the Framingham Heart Study

Age (years)	DBP (mmHg)	SBP (mmHg)	MAP (mmHg)	PP (mmHg)	Hemodynamics
30–49	↑	↑	↑	→↑	R > S
50–59	→	↑	→	↑↑	R = S
≥ 60	↓	↑	→↓	↑↑↑↑	S > R

R = small-vessel resistance; S = large-vessel stiffness.
Adapted from Franklin SS, Gustin W, Wong ND, et al: Hemodynamic patterns of age-related changes in blood pressure. The Framingham Heart Study. Circulation 1997, 96:308–315.

Moreover, about 80% of untreated or inadequately treated individuals with hypertension from age 50 years onward had ISH, which by definition represents wide pulse pressure hypertension.[8] The largest group (75%) of these older hypertensives have stage 1 ISH (140–159 mmHg SBP), but 25% have stage 2 ISH or greater (≥ 160 mmHg SBP). A recent Framingham study showed that persons reaching age 65 years had a 90% lifetime risk of developing hypertension, almost exclusively of the ISH type.[27] The increase in SBP and DBP up to age 50 years can best be explained by the dominance of increased peripheral vascular resistance (Table 1).[9] By contrast, after the fifth decade of life, the decrease in DBP and the widening of pulse pressure become surrogate measurements for increased elastic artery stiffness.[9] Overall, elastic artery stiffness, rather than vascular resistance, becomes the dominant hemodynamic factor in both normotensive and hypertensive subjects after age 50 years. Elevated BP left untreated accelerates stiffening of elastic arteries, which sets up a vicious cycle of further elevation of BP; this leads to the development of either primary ISH (with DBP < 90 mmHg throughout the course) or secondary ISH (starting as combined systolic-diastolic hypertension and becoming ISH as DBP decreases to < 90 mmHg).

Role of Arterial Stiffness

By middle age, long-standing cyclic stress in the media of elastic-bearing arteries produces fatigue and eventual fracturing of elastin along with structural changes of the extracellular matrix that include proliferation of collagen and deposition of calcium.[17] This degenerative process, termed *arteriosclerosis,* is the pathologic process that results in increased central elastic arterial stiffness with widening of pulse pressure. Other disease processes such as diabetes, chronic renal failure, and generalized atherosclerosis can accelerate aging of central elastic arteries with earlier development of arterial stiffness. Although arteriosclerosis is often confused with atherosclerosis, these two disease states are independent but frequently overlapping conditions (Table 2). Atherosclerosis is primarily focal, starts in the intima, and tends to be occlusive. By contrast, arteriosclerosis tends to be defuse, starts in the media, and frequently results in a dilated and tortuous aorta. Moreover, the pathophysiology of atherosclerosis is that of inflammatory disease with lipid-containing plaques and predominantly downstream ischemic disease. In contrast, arteriosclerosis represents degenerative arterial disease, which results in predominantly upstream increased thoracic aortic stiffness and elevated left ventricular load.

The pathologic correlates of increase elastic artery stiffness are many.[17] Increased aortic pulsatile load elevates left ventricular systolic wall stress, decreases coronary flow reserve, impairs left ventricular relaxation, and may lead to diastolic dysfunction. Increased aortic pulsatile load is the major factor in the development of left ventricular hypertrophy with increased coronary blood flow requirements. Simultaneously, the decrease in DBP further compromises the oxygen supply–demand ratio by reducing coronary flow. Furthermore, increased pulsatile stress leads to endothelial dysfunction with a greater likelihood of developing atherosclerosis and for rupturing unstable plaques.

Value of Pulse Pressure as a Marker of Increased Cardiovascular Risk

SBP rather than DBP is associated with a greater increased risk for all cardiovascular disease morbid events in middle-aged and older persons.[16] More recently, however, ISH in general and increased pulse pressure in particular have been identified as independent cardiovascular disease risk factors.[2,10,18] Indeed, numerous studies over the past decade have shown that pulse pressure may be a more sensitive indicator of cardiovascular risk than SBP. In the presence of concordant elevations of SBP and DBP, such as systolic-diastolic hypertension, there is no advantage of SBP over pulse pressure in predicting risk.[12] How-

TABLE 2. Atherosclerosis versus Arteriosclerosis		
Features	Atherosclerosis	Arteriosclerosis
Distribution	Focal	Diffuse
Location	Intima	Media
Geometry	Occlusive	Dilatory
Pathology	Plaque	Elastin, collagen, Ca^{++}
Physiology	Inflammation	Large artery stiffness
Hemodynamics	Ischemia	LV workload

Figure 2. Joint influence of systolic and diastolic blood pressure on CHD risk. CHD hazard ratios were determined from level of DBP within SBP groups from the Framingham Heart Study. (From Franklin SS, Khan SA, Wong ND, et al: Is pulse pressure useful in predicting risk for coronary heart disease? The Framingham Heart Study. Circulation 1999, 100:354–360; with permission.)

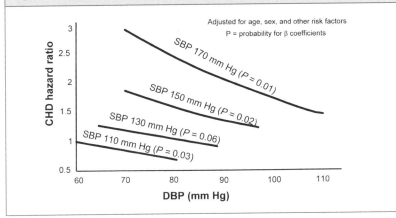

ever, when there is discordantly low DBP along with elevated SBP leading to the development of ISH, pulse pressure becomes dominant in predicting risk. This was shown in the original Framingham cohort (Fig. 2).[10] In normotensive and untreated subjects age 50 to 79 years, using a model adjusted for age, gender, and other risk factors, CHD risk was inversely related to DBP at any given SBP level, suggesting that pulse pressure predicted CHD risk better than either SBP or DBP alone. There was a far greater increase in CHD risk with increments in pulse pressure without a change in SBP than with increments in SBP without a change in pulse pressure. Thus, using increases in pulse pressure as a surrogate for arterial stiffness and parallel increases in SBP and DBP as surrogates for resistance, CHD events relate more to the pulsatile stress of central elastic arterial stiffness than the static stress of peripheral arteriolar resistance. This leads to the conclusion that at any given elevation in SBP, the person with ISH will be at greater risk than the one with systolic-diastolic hypertension.

Benefits of Treatment

Strong evidence in favor of treating ISH came from a recent meta-analysis of 8 random controlled trials,[21] including the two largest studies, Systolic Hypertension in the Elderly Program (SHEP),[19] published in 1991, and systolic Hypertension in Europe Trial (Syst-Eur),[22] published in 1997. Most of these trials, including SHEP and Syst-Eur, were placebo controlled, included both men and women who were age 60 and older, and resulted in an average 10-mmHg SBP reduction with treatment over control arms. The overall results were a 30% reduction in stroke; a 23% decrease in fatal and non-fatal CHD events; an overall 16% reduction in cardiovascular death; and, most striking, a 10% decrease in all-cause mortality.[21] In the Syst-Eur trial, there was a greater benefit in treating diabetic patients with ISH than those without, proving again that in the presence of a greater absolute risk, there is a greater absolute benefit achieved with effective treatment.[26] Furthermore, a second meta-analysis of 1670 individuals, age 80 years and older with ISH selected from these controlled trials, showed a significant reduction in stroke and heart failure but no significant decrease in CHD events or improved all-caused mortality.[13] One can conclude from this study that lowering SBP in octogenarians may not prolong life but can improve quality of life, and therefore, is well worth pursuing.

Targeting Treatment

Within most populations, hypertension carries only a small portion of the total burden of cardiovascular disease risk. The Sixth Report of the Joint National Committee on Prevention, Detection, Evaluation, and Treatment of High Blood Pressure (JNC-VI)[25] has outlined the components of cardiovascular risk (Table 3) and strategies for risk stratification and therapeutic decision making (Tables 4 & 5). For all individuals with high-normal SBP or greater (i.e., 130 mmHg), lifestyle intervention should be started with or without the addition of antihypertensive therapy.

Further refinement of the risk stratification has been outlined in Table 6.

TABLE 3. Components of CVD Risk Stratification in Hypertensive Patients	
Major Risk Factors	**Target Organ Damage or Clinical CVD**
Smoking Dyslipidemia Diabetes Age > 60 years Gender (men and postmenopausal women) Family history of early CVD (women < 65 years; men < 55 years)	Heart diseases • LVH • Angina or prior MI • Prior coronary revascularization • CHF Stroke or TIA Proteinuria, nephropathy: ↑ S_{CR} Peripheral arterial disease Retinopathy

Adapted from The Sixth Joint National Committee on Prevention, Detection, Evaluation, and Treatment of High Blood Pressure. Arch Intern Med 1997,157:2413–2446.

TABLE 4. JNC VI BP Risk Stratification

Risk Group A
- No CV risk factors
- No diabetes, target organ damage, or clinical CVD

Risk Group B
- At least one other risk factor: age > 60 years, male gender or postmenopausal status, dyslipidemia, smoking, +FH
- No diabetes, target organ damage, or clinical CVD

Risk Group C
- Diabetes, target organ damage, or clinical CVD with or without other risk factors

Adapted from The Sixth Joint National Committee on Prevention, Detection, Evaluation, and Treatment of High Blood Pressure: Arch Intern Med 1997,157:2413–2446.

For persons with persistent systolic hypertension of ≥ 160 mmHg, there is evidence from numerous intervention studies favoring the initiation of active drug therapy.[25] In addition, the SHEP placebo control group, although starting with a mean SBP of 170 mmHg, decreased to values of SBP of 150 to 159 mmHg after regression to the mean.[19] Therefore, older persons with persistent SBP values of 150 to 159 mmHg (late stage 1 ISH) also warrant immediate initiation of drug therapy. In contrast, persons with persistent systolic hypertension of 140 to 149 mmHg (early stage 1 ISH) have less clear indications for beginning drug therapy because of the lack of intervention data. In the presence of dyslipidemia[7] (defined by an LDL cholesterol of 160 mg/dL, HDL < 40 mg/dL in men and < 50 mg/dL in women, and serum triglycerides 150 mg/dL), smoking, impaired glucose intolerance (fasting blood sugar of 110 to 125 mg/dL), obesity body mass index [BMI] of ≥ 30), or a wide pulse

TABLE 5. JNC VI Treatment Strategies

BP state (mmHg)	Risk Groups		
	A	B	C
High-normal (130–139/ 85–89)	Lifestyle modification	Lifestyle modification	Drug therapy*†
Stage 1 (140–159/90–99)	Lifestyle modification (≤ 12 mo)	Lifestyle modification (≤ 6 mo)‡	Drug therapy*
Stages 2+ (≥ 160/≥ 100)	Drug therapy*	Drug therapy*	Drug therapy*

*Lifestyle modification should be adjunctive for all patients starting pharmacologic therapy.
†For patients with heart failure, renal insufficiency, or diabetes.
‡For patients with multiple risk factors, drug therapy should be considered in addition to lifestyle modification.
Adapted from The Sixth Joint National Committee on Prevention, Detection, Evaluation, and Treatment of High Blood Pressure: Arch Intern Med 1997,157:2413–2446.

SBP (mmHg)	JNC VI BP Class	Qualifying risks
≥ 160	≥ Stage 2	None necessary (definite)
150–159	Late stage 1	None necessary (probable)
140–149	Early stage 1	Dyslipidemia, IGT, BMI ≥ 30, smoker, pulse pressure ≥ 70
130–139	High normal	LVH, retinopathy, CHD, stroke, PVD, renal disease, diabetes

TABLE 6.   Qualification for Drug Therapy of ISH

pressure of ≥ 70 mmHg, there is justification for initiating immediate drug therapy in older persons with SBP of 140 to 149 mmHg.[11] In the absence of these additional risks, however, one can follow existing recommendations by starting with lifestyle intervention for a prescribed period of time and then initiating drug therapy when lifestyle intervention fails to lower BP significantly.[25] Lastly, one could justify initiating drug therapy for individuals with SBP of 130 to 139 mmHg (high-normal BP) and associated high-risk problems such as (1) hypertensive target organ involvement (left ventricular enlargement, micro- or macro-albuminuria), (2) vascular events (CHD, heart failure, stroke, renal disease, or peripheral vascular disease), or (3) diabetes with or without vascular events.[25]

Therapeutic Target Goals

JNC-VI[25] and World Health Organization (WHO)[29] guidelines exist for the optimal reduction of BP to achieve maximum benefit from antihypertensive therapy. These guidelines, based on observational as well as on outcome data, suggest that low-risk patients (class A or B JNC-VI)[25] should be treated to a target goal of less than 140 mmHg SBP and < 90 mmHg DBP. For class C or high-risk subjects, the therapeutic target goal is < 130 mmHg SBP and < 85 to 80 mmHg DBP mm Hg for secondary prevention of MI, stroke, renal impairment, peripheral vascular disease, or diabetes.

The Value of Lifestyle Intervention

A variety of lifestyle interventions lower BP (Table 7)[5], and the most effective is successful weight reduction in obese hypertensives. Reducing weight is of special importance if the elderly hypertensive has diabetes. Even a reduction of 10 to 15 pounds can have a significant effect in lowering BP.[28] Unfortunately, most patients are refractory to successful weight reduction and even when partially successful tend to have a high percentage of recidivism by 6 to 12 months.[28] Older hypertensive patients are usually more salt sensitive than young ones, but

TABLE 7. Lifestyle Interventions for Prevention or Treatment of Hypertension	
Intervention	Blood Pressure Effect
Exercise	5–10 mmHg ($\geq$ 30 min $\geq$ 3$\times$/wk)
Weight reduction	1–2 mmHg/Kg $\downarrow$
Alcohol intake reduction	1 mmHg/drink/d $\downarrow$
Sodium intake reduction	1–3 mmHg/40 mmol/d $\downarrow$
DASH diet	3–10 mmHg $\downarrow$

Adapted from Cushman W, Dubbert P: Nonpharmacologic approaches to therapy of hypertension Endocrine Practice 1997, 3:106–111.

successful salt restriction depends to a large degree on limiting milk, bread, and a variety of high salt-containing processed foods and substituting fruits, vegetables, and nuts. The DASH diet,[1] which is rich in fruits, vegetables, and high-calcium foods but is low in animal fat foods, has been successful in reducing BP in older hypertensive patients even when consuming average salt intakes. Heavy alcoholic intake can precipitate or worsen hypertension in older patients and is frequently refractory to usual drug therapy. Although lifestyle intervention is generally unsuccessful in fully correcting ISH, it may reduce the need for antihypertensive therapy and minimize associated cardiovascular risk factors. Finally, the greatest chance of success with lifestyle intervention is primary prevention, or preventing high-normal BP from progressing to stage 1 ISH.[25]

Selection of Antihypertensive Drug Therapy

The majority of older persons with ISH ultimately require antihypertensive therapy. Indeed, two or more drugs are needed to achieve BP reductions to levels < 140 mmHg in as many as 70% of nondiabetic patients and to levels of < 130 mmHg in as many as 90% of diabetics and renal disease patients. Although diuretics were recommended as first-line antihypertensive therapy for ISH patients by JNC-VI guidelines on the basis of many previous intervention studies, it was not until the recent publication of the Antihypertensive and Lipid-Lowering Treatment to Prevent Heart Attack Trial (ALLHAT)[23] that there was direct comparisons between the diuretic chlorthalidone, the angiotensin-converting enzyme (ACE) inhibitor lisinopril, and the calcium channel blocker (CCB) amlodipine. The results of ALLHAT showed equivalent benefit from all three antihypertensive drugs in reducing all cause mortality, CHD deaths, myocardial infarctions, and combined CHD endpoints.[23] In addition, chlorthalidone was superior to amlodipine in preventing hospitalized heart failure and superior to lisonipril in reducing both stroke and combined cardiovascular endpoints in African Americans.[23] Therefore, given these findings and the comparative cost savings, diuretics are the first-line therapy for treating middle-aged and older patients with ISH. The results of Syst-Eur[22] favor dihydopyridine CCBs as a second choice if patients are unable to tolerate diuretics.

The Heart Outcomes Prevention Evaluation (HOPE) study[24] results favor the ACE inhibitor ramipril for secondary prevention of CHD, stroke, or diabetes. The Losartan Intervention For Endpoint (LIFE) study[6] and the LIFE substudy in ISH patients[15] showed the advantage of the angiotensin II inhibitor losartan over the beta-blocker atenolol in preventing stroke events in high-risk elderly patients with hypertensive heart disease and severe left ventricular hypertrophy. A large percentage of both the atenolol and losartan arms were receiving diuretics in addition to their study drug. The result of these two landmark studies, together with ALL-HAT, strongly support the combined use of a diuretic with either an ACE inhibitor or an angiotensin II antagonist in treating high-risk JNC-VI class C patients with CHD, stroke, diabetes, or renal disease. CCBs could be used when necessary as a third drug to reach target BP goal. Additional antihypertensives may be used as add-on drugs for further BP control and for specific indications, such as beta-blockers for angina or post-MI and peripheral alpha-blockers for prostatism.[25] Fixed-dose drug combinations can be useful in optimizing treatment. The starting dose in elderly patients with ISH is often one half of that used in younger individuals. Finally, BP should be monitored in the upright as well as sitting position to prevent overtreatment and the development of orthostatic hypotension.

How Effective are Physicians in Controlling ISH?

The JNC-VI[25] and the NHANES III[4] reported on the poor levels of awareness, treatment, and control of hypertension in the United States. Indeed, only one in five elderly patients and one in 10 patients with hypertension and diabetes or renal disease are being treated to goal therapy.[4] As shown in a recent NHANES III study,[8] there were more than four times as many individuals age 50 years or older who had inadequately treated SBP (82%) versus DBP (17%). In general, the older the person, the more difficult it becomes to reach SBP goal. Moreover, untreated or inadequately treated patients required more than a twofold greater reduction in SBP to obtain treatment goals than did their younger counterparts.[8]

Many factors may contribute to the inadequate treatment of patients with hypertension. Physicians' bias toward focusing primarily on DBP rather than on SBP goal and physicians fear of excessive lowering of DBP have contributed to poor SBP control. This fear of excessive therapeutic lowering of DBP—the so-called J curve phenomenon—has been

TABLE 8. Guidelines for Successful Management of ISH

Initial Evaluation

- Evaluate patients for risk factors, target organ damage, and CV complications.
- Note compelling and special indications for CHD, diabetes, and renal disease.
- Classify patient's risk by the JNC-VI risk stratification table.
- Recognize that many patients will have BP goals of < 130/80.
- Set a goal BP for each patient and communicate this to the patient.
- Prepare the patient beforehand that polypharmacy may be required to control BP.
- Promote lifestyle management designed specifically for individual patients.
- Encourage the patient and family to promote healthy lifestyles and BP control.

Follow-up Office Visits

- Tell patients their BP readings in numbers and whether the readings are at goal level.
- Patients with well-controlled hypertension should be told the BP is well controlled because they have been taking their medication and they should continue the same therapy.
- Consider increasing the dosage of a current medication or adding an additional drug to the current regimen of patients with poorly controlled BP.
- Review medications with the patient and provide written list with any medication changes using bold, easily read lettering.
- Consider patient noncompliance when the BP is poorly controlled despite what appears to be adequate therapy.
- Consider secondary causes of hypertension when BP is resistant to multidrug therapy.
- Check medication prescriptions for adequate number of refills.
- Review recent laboratory results with the patient, reassess cardiovascular risk factors (e.g., lipids, blood sugars, smoking) and make appropriate recommendations.
- Determine if the patient can read well. If not, prepare a morning sun and evening moon chart with sample pills attached at the proper times.
- For patients with poor eyesight, solicit a friend or neighbor to assist with medications.
- Tell the patient when to return and make a specific return appointment before he or she leaves the clinic. Asking patients to call back in 3 to 6 months promotes infrequent return visits.

Adapted from Jones D, Basile J, Cushman W, et al: Managing hypertension in the Southeastern United States. Am J of Med Sci 1999, 318:357–364.

exaggerated. If there is any significant risk of precipitating an ischemic cardiac event with therapy-induced low BP, it would occur only with DBP reduction below 60 mmHg, as indicated in a post-hoc analysis of the SHEP study.[20] Other reasons that ISH patients are frequently poorly controlled are failure to use proper doses of medication, failure to use polypharmacy, failure to use a diuretic as a part of polypharmacy, and failure to detect patient nonadherence with therapy. Guidelines for managing patients with ISH are provided in Table 8.

References

1. Appel LJ, Moore TJ, Obarzanek E, et al: The effect of dietary patterns on blood pressure: results from the Dietary Approaches to Stop Hypertension (DASH) randomized clinical trial. N Engl J Med 1997, 336:1117–1124.

2. Benetos A, Safar M, Rudnichji A, et al: Pulse pressure: a predictor of long-term cardiovascular mortality in a French male population. Hypertension 1997, 30:1410–1415.
3. Burt VL, Whelton P, Roccella EJ, et al: Prevalence of hypertension in the US adult population: results from the Third National Health and Nutrition Examination Survey, 1988–1991. Hypertension 1995, 25:305–313.
4. Burt VL, Cutler JA, Higgins M, et al: Trends in the prevalence, awareness, treatment and control of hypertension in the adult US population. Hypertension 1995, 26:60–69.
5. Cushman W, Dubbert P: Nonpharmacologic approaches to therapy of hypertension Endocrine Practice 1997, 3:106–111.
6. Dahlof B, Devereux RB, Kjeldsen SE, et al: Cardiovascular morbidity and mortality in the Losartan Intervention For Endpoint reduction in hypertension study (LIFE): a randomized trial against atenolol. Lancet 2002, 359:995–1003.
7. Executive summary of the third Report of the National Cholesterol Education Program (NCEP) Expert Panel on Detection, Evaluation, and Treatment of High Blood Cholesterol in adult (Adult Treatment Panel III). JAMA 2001, 285:2486–2497.
8. Franklin SS, Jacobs MJ, Wong ND, et al: Predominance of isolated systolic hypertension among middle-aged and elderly US hypertensives. Hypertension 2001, 37:869–874.
9. Franklin SS, Gustin W, Wong ND, et al: Hemodynamic patterns of age-related changes in blood pressure. The Framingham Heart Study. Circulation 1997, 96:308–315.
10. Franklin SS, Khan SA, Wong ND, et al: Is pulse pressure useful in predicting risk for coronary heart disease? The Framingham Heart Study. Circulation 1999, 100:354–360.
11. Franklin SS, Wong ND: Cardiovascular risk evaluation: an inexact science. J Hypertension 2002, 20:1–4.
12. Glynn RJ, L'Italien GJ, Sesso HD, et al: Development of predictive models for long-term cardiovascular risk associated with systolic and diastolic blood pressure. Hypertension 2002, 39:105–110.
13. Gueyffier F, Bulpitt C, Boissel JP, et al: Antihypertensive drugs in very old people: a subgroup meta-analysis of randomized controlled trials. Lancet 1999, 353:793–796.
14. Jones D, Basile J, Cushman W, et al: Managing hypertension in the Southeastern United States. Am J of Med Sci 1999, 318:357–364.
15. Kjeldsen SE, Dahlof B, Devereux RB, et al: Effects of losartan on cardiovascular morbidity and mortality in patients with isolated systolic hypertension and left ventricular hypertrophy. JAMA 2002, 288:1491–1498.
16. Levy D: The role of systolic blood pressure in determining risk for cardiovascular disease. J Hypertens 1999, 17(supp 1):15-18.
17. Nichols WW, O'Rourke MF: McDonald's Blood Flow in Arteries. Philadelphia: Lea & Febiger, 1998.
18. Sagie A, Larson MG, Levy D: The natural history of borderline isolated systolic hypertension. N Engl J Med 1993, 329:1912–1917.
19. SHEP cooperative Research Group: Prevention of stroke by antihypertensive drug in older persons with isolated systolic hypertension. JAMA 1991, 265:3255–3264.
20. Somes GW, Pahor M, Shorr RI, et al: The role of diastolic blood pressure when treating isolated systolic hypertension. Arch Intern Med 1999, 159:2004–2009.
21. Staessen JA, Gasowski J, Wang JG, et al: Risks of untreated and treated isolated systolic hypertension in the elderly: meta-analysis of outcome trials. Lancet 2000, 355:865–872.

22. Staessen JA, Fagard R, Thijs L, et al: Randomized double-blind comparison of placebo and the active treatment for older patients with isolated systolic hypertension. Lancet 1997, 350:757–764.

23. The Antihypertensive and Lipid-Lowering Treatment to Prevent Heart Attack Trial (ALLHAT): Major outcomes in high-risk hypertensive patients randomized to angiotensin-converting enzyme inhibitor or calcium channel blocker VS diuretic. JAMA 2002, 288:2981–2997.

24. The Heart Outcomes Prevention Evaluation Study Investigators: Effects of an angiotensin-converting-enzyme inhibitor, ramipril on cardiovascular events in high-risk patients. N Engl J Med 2000, 342:145–153.

25. The Sixth Joint National Committee on Prevention, Detection, Evaluation, and Treatment of High Blood Pressure: Arch Intern Med 1997, 157:2413–2446.

26. Tuomilehto J, Rastenyte D, Birkenhager WH, et al: Effects of calcium-channel blockade in older patients with diabetes and systolic hypertension. N Engl J Med 1999, 340:677–684.

27. Vasan RS, Beiser A, Seshadri S, et al: Residual lifetime risk for developing hypertension in middle-aged women and men. JAMA 2002, 287:1003–1010.

28. Whelton PK, Appel LJ, Espeland MA, et al: Sodium restriction and weight loss in the treatment of hypertension on older persons: a randomized controlled Trial of Non-Pharmacologic Interventions in the Elderly (TONE). Tone Collaborative Research Group. JAMA 1998, 279:839–846.

29. World Health Organization-International Society of Hypertension Guidelines for the management of hypertension, 1999. Guidelines subcommittee. J Hypertens 1999, 17:151–183.

Management of Refractory Hypertension

chapter

27

Lawrence R. Krakoff, M.D.

The goal for treatment of patients with hypertension is to reduce arterial blood pressure (BP) and, thereby, diminish the likelihood of future cardiovascular mortality and morbidity. Available therapy for hypertension includes nonpharmacologic interventions, often called lifestyle changes, such a weight reduction, reduced salt intake, and increased regular exercise. However, most patients with hypertension, especially those with higher BPs and older than age 50 years, are given antihypertensive medication, together with helpful lifestyle advice. The terms "refractory" and "resistant," when applied to hypertension, mean that BP remains above the desired goal of treatment despite various and multiple measures to decrease it. In practice, refractory hypertension implies that the BP is above recommended goals for treatment systolic and diastolic BP of 140 mm Hg systolic pressure and 90 mm Hg, respectively, as advised in several recent guidelines despite, treatment with lifestyle advice and two to three antihypertensive drugs.[1,2]

Many articles and reviews stress the lack of control for hypertension in patients who are identified and treated. For North American populations, two studies indicate that fewer than 30% of those on medication have BP at or below goal level.[3,4] The lack of more effective control implies a large public health gap between the potential benefits of improved control of blood pressure and the ability of those who detect and treat hypertension to lower BP for those in their practices. This chapter focuses on the assessment of refractory hypertension in adults who receive medical care from internists and family practitioners. Strategies that can lead to better BP control are emphasized. However, after dealing with those issues, a brief perspective, based on evidence from clinical trials, is given concerning the levels of BP control that are achievable.

Refractory Hypertension in Practice

Let us consider a typical patient considered refractory and go through the evaluation. A 58-year-old man had an initial BP of 160/95 mm Hg.

277

TABLE 1. Frequent Causes of Refractory Hypertension
Lack of adherence to prescribed medication
Being overweight
Excessive salt intake
Pseudorefractory hypertension caused by "white-coat effect," inaccurate cuff BP
Inadequate dosing of appropriate medications
Lack of appropriate drug selection
Medical conditions that may reduce responsiveness to treatment: Obesity, sleep apnea, renal disease, LVH
Other medications: Use of NSAIDs or steroids, oral contraceptives, licorice, sympathomimetic substances, immunosuppressive agents, erythropoietin
Unrecognized secondary hypertension: Atherosclerotic renal artery stenosis, primary aldosteronism, excessive salt sensitivity, epithelial sodium channel abnormalities

Despite prescriptions for a thiazide diuretic and beta-blocker, his BP remains 150/90 mm Hg after 6 months of treatment. Table 1 lists many of the conditions that are to be considered.

Lack of adherence to medication is the most often considered cause of inadequate control of BP. Evaluation of this problem is difficult in usual practice, but a few steps may help identify such patients. The patient needs education regarding the necessity of regular medication. Attention should be given to convenience, once-a-day dosing, cost of medication, and consideration of symptoms that may be real adverse reactions or presumed so by the patient. Reviewing prescriptions with the patient may include direct examination of pill bottles and patterns of refilling with the pharmacy. Strategies to monitor use of medication can improve adherence and control of BP.[5]

Failure to achieve goal BP might be caused by the patient's being overweight or having a very high salt intake. Counseling and education by a dietitian or nutritionist who is familiar with cardiovascular risk factors should be considered. Dietary interventions that cause weight reduction can be effective for reducing BP in obese patients. The role of weight-reducing medications is unclear because medications that suppress appetite seem to have little effect on BP. Use of the lipase inhibitor, orlistat, together with a low-calorie diet can be effective for sustained weight reduction and may be beneficial in lowering BP and other risk factors as well.

White coat hypertension has become recognized as the condition when office BPs are elevated, but out-of-office BP taken by ambulatory monitors or accurate home pressure recording are normal. The "white-coat effect" may be present in treated hypertensive patients as well, so that office recordings are misrepresentative of usual daily BP level.[6,7] We recommend use of ambulatory BP monitoring or home BP measurements, taken with recording devices to assess this issue.[8] Recent studies suggest that the byproduct of this intervention is to increase compliance and control with less need for office visits.[9]

Are drug doses adequate? Being overweight or large sized may require higher doses of usual medication. For example, a 250-pound man may need a higher dose of a given drug than one who is 150 pounds. When low doses are used initially, escalation to higher doses is needed before giving up on a specific drug.

Drugs should be chosen that have an additive effect and do not overlap each other's action. A thiazide-type diuretic together with either a beta- blocker or an angiotensin-converting enzyme (ACE) inhibitor or an angiotensin receptor blocker (ARB) can be expected to provide control of many patients with uncomplicated hypertension. In fact, one can almost define true refractory hypertension as failing to respond to such two-drug combinations. On the other hand, clinical evidence suggests that adding a beta-blocker or an ARB to those already on a diuretic ACE inhibitor combination is infrequently effective. For those who remain hypertensive on the two-drug combination, addition of a once-a-day calcium channel blocker (CCB) may achieve control. My advice is to consider a dihydropyridine (DHP) for those not fully controlled on a diuretic and beta-blocker. For those taking a diuretic and ACE inhibitor or ARB, a non-DHP CCB (verapamil or diltiazem) may be as effective as a DHP. Some patients may remain hypertensive despite triple-drug combinations. α-Receptor blockade with doxazosin added may be effective in selected patients.[10] Similarly, the addition of clonidine, as the transdermal patch (TTS system) applied weekly may be helpful. Some still recommend older vasodilator drugs such as hydralazine or minoxidil. Our experience indicates that higher doses of DHPs are highly effective and can be given once daily.[11]

Several medical conditions are associated with drug-resistant hypertension. Obesity may not yield to medical treatment alone so that bariatric surgery may be considered in selected patients. Patients with an obesity-related form of secondary hypertension, sleep apnea syndrome, may yield to treatment with nocturnal nasal positive-pressure ventilation.[12] Chronic renal diseases are often difficult to control with usual medications. These patients may benefit from conversion from thiazide-type diuretics to the loop active drugs, such as furosemide, often at high doses of 80 to 160 mg twice daily. Target organ damage, as defined by the presence of left ventricular hypertrophy (LVH), revealed by either electrocardiography or echocardiography and carotid arterial thickening, has been associated with true refractory hypertension as defined by 24-hour ambulatory BP recording.[13] Although target organ is ordinarily considered to be the consequence of higher BP, there is some evidence that the presence of LVH itself makes hypertension more resistant to treatment, even with multidrug combinations.

A careful history is needed, both during initial visits and later on, for patients with regard to *all* the drugs they take, including over-the-counter (OTC) preparations and unapproved agents. Most patients know to tell about prescription nonsteroidal anti-inflammatory drugs (NSAIDs), steroids, or immunosuppressives (cyclosporine or tacrolimus), if asked. However, if not asked, they might not reveal they are taking them. Some might not consider OTC diet suppressants, NSAIDs (e.g., OTC ibuprofen), or oral contraceptive agents as drugs unless questioned specifically about them. The growing prevalence of ephedra and other "energy" agents suggests that hypertension may, on occasion, be related to their use with the devastating consequences of stroke or sudden death.[14] Cocaine use should be considered as well and requires a frank discussion of illegal substances. Daily licorice ingestion as a flavoring for candy or chewing tobacco can cause a form of salt sensitive hypertension caused by inhibition of renal 11-OH dehydrogenase with potentiation of cortisol as a mineralocorticoid; hypokalemia is usually found.[15] This is a rare but highly reversible form of secondary hypertension. However, the right question must be asked to detect it.

Secondary hypertension remains a possibility when hypertension is resistant to treatment. Renal artery stenosis, especially when it is bilateral, has been well recognized as a cause of refractory hypertension. This condition is usually found in older patients together with multiple risk factors for atherosclerosis and evidence of carotid artery disease, peripheral artery disease, and coronary heart disease (the so-called "vasculopath"). Acute pulmonary congestion (flash pulmonary edema) may add to the picture. Thus, the clinical clues are usually obvious. More recently, case series suggest that primary aldosteronism is increasingly recognized in association with drug-resistant hypertension.[16] Hypokalemia may not be consistently found in patients with this disorder. Workup of the refractory hypertensive patient should then include the screening assessment for primary aldosteronism, measurement of plasma renin activity and serum aldosterone concentration as related to 24-hour urine sodium and potassium excretion. If hormone assays are consistent with primary aldosteronism, the search for an adrenal adenoma (Conn's syndrome) should be undertaken. However, only 30% to 50% of those with suppressed renin and high aldosterone production have an adenoma; most have bilateral adrenal hypersecretion of aldosterone (idiopathic aldosteronism or adrenal hyperplasia). For the latter, addition of spironolactone (an aldosterone antagonist) may be highly effective in reducing BP.[17] Recently, another and more specific aldosterone antagonist, eplerenone, has become available and may be highly effective, with fewer adverse effects (i.e., gynecomastia) for such patients.[18]

A recent study[19] suggests an alternate mechanism for hidden salt sensitive hypertension, namely, a gain of function in the epithelial sodium channel (ENa) of the renal collecting duct. In a small series of patients with refractory hypertension drawn from a hypertension clinic, increased activity of this channel was found in lymphocytes. Adminstration of amiloride, the potassium-sparing agent that specifically blocks ENa, controlled BP in four of nine patients with increased lymphocyte ENa activity.[19] Such research implies that there will be additional detection of mechanisms accounting for apparent drug-resistant hypertension that could lead to more specific and rational therapy. The vascular nitric oxide system is being studied intensively in this regard.[20]

Control or Elimination of Refractory Hypertension

Few clinical trials of drug treatment for hypertension have used the goals of treatment, now recommended, less than 140/90 mm Hg. In all these trials, initial drug treatment was followed by add-on medications with varying combinations. The ALLHAT trial enrolled hypertensive patients who were 55 years old or older, hypertensive ($\geq$ 140/90 mm Hg or on treatment) and had other risk factors or target organ damage. Control rates of 61% to 68% were achieved. The best control occurred in the group given the diuretic chlorthalidone as initial treatment.[21] The INSIGHT trial, compared once-a-day nifedipine with a diuretic combination (amiloride and thiazide) as initial treatment in those with baseline BPs of 150/95 mm Hg or more. Control rates were 58% and 57% in the two groups.[22] The LIFE trial compared losartan and atenolol as initial treatment in patients with baseline BPs of 160/95 mm Hg or more, all of whom had electrocardiographic LVH at entry. Control rates were 48% and 45%.[23] These studies provide benchmarks for control BP within the conditions of clinical trials, which include selected participants, free medication, intensive follow-up, and goal-directed treatment. Whether comparable levels of control can be achieved in usual clinic care is a challenge to health care systems and providers.

Older patients, especially those older than age 75 years, often have isolated systolic hypertension. When these patients stand, BP may drop, and aggressive treatment of hypertension may cause orthostatic hypotension with dizziness or even syncope. This sets a limit to control, as defined by sitting pressures, and indicates the need for measuring BP supine, sitting, and standing in elderly hypertensives, before and during treatment.

When to Seek a Hypertension Consultation

Referral to a hypertension specialist for refractory hypertension has become more accepted and feasible now that such specialists can be identified.[24] Through the efforts of the American Society of Hypertension (ASH) working in conjunction with the National Board of Medical Examiners, a certifying process and examination is available for designating physicians as Clinical Hypertension Specialists. A list of more than 700 hypertension specialists is currently available on the ASH's website (www.ash-us.org). The number of specialists is expected to grow after the next examination in May 2003, which will help ensure convenient and ready access to expertise. After the patient's primary physician has considered the issues given in Table 1, an assessment by a designated clinical hypertension specialist may be helpful, especially when there is need to reevaluate overall drug treatment or consider secondary hypertension. The specialist can offer in-depth experience and a fresh look at the patient's overall status, which may lead to helpful suggestions.

Key Points

- ☞ Refractory or resistant hypertension is a clinical disorder that limits the potential benefit of antihypertensive therapy.
- ☞ Patients whose BPs remain above goals for treatment should be reassessed for many conditions that might account for their condition.
- ☞ Basic clinical skills in taking an accurate and relevant history, knowing the pathophysiology of hypertension and its pharmacology, and persistence in working with each patient for effective continuing care form the basis for achieving optimal control of hypertension and approaching the control rates gained in clinical trials.

References

1. The Sixth Report of the Joint National Committee on Prevention, Detection, Evaluation, and Treatment of High Blood Pressure. Arch Intern Med 1997, 157:2413–2445.
2. Guidelines Subcommittee: 1999 World Health Organization-International Society of Hypertension Guidelines for the Management of Hypertension. J Hypertens 1999, 17:151–183.
3. Meissner I, Whisnant JP, Sheps SG, et al: Detection and control of high blood pressure in the community: do we need a wake-call? Hypertension 1999, 34:466–471.
4. Joffres MR, Ghadirian P, Fodor JG, et al: Awareness, treatment, and control of hypertension in Canada. Am J Hypertens 1997, 10:1097–102.
5. Burnier M, Schneider MP, Chiolero A, et al: Electronic compliance monitoring in resistant hypertension: the basis for rational therapeutic decisions. J Hypertens 2001, 19:335–341.
6. Mezzetti A, Pierdomenico SD, Costantini F, et al: White-coat resistant hypertension. Am J Hypertens 1997, 10:1307.

7. Redon J, Campos C, Rodicio JL, et al: Prognostic value of ambulatory blood pressure monitoring in refractory hypertension: a prospective study. Hypertension 2001, 31:712–718.

8. Jain A, Krakoff LR: Effect of recorded home blood pressure measurements on staging of hypertensive patients. Blood Pressure Monitoring 2002, 7:157–161.

9. Rogers MAM, Small D, Buchan DA, et al: Home monitoring service improves mean arterial pressure in patients with essential hypertension. Ann Intern Med 2001, 134:1024–1032.

10. Black HR, Sollins JS, Garofalo JL: The addition of doxazosin to the therapeutic regimen of hypertensive patients inadequately controlled with other antihypertensive medications: a randomized, placebo-controlled study. Am J Hypertens 2000, 13:468–474.

11. Phillips RA, Ardeljan M, Shimabukuro S, et al: Normalization of left ventricular mass and associated changes in neurohormones and atrial natriuretic peptide afte 1 year of sustained nifedipine therapy for severe hypertension. J Am Coll Cardiol 1991, 17:1595–1602.

12. Suzuki M, Otsuka K, Guilleminault C: Long-term nasal continuous positive airway pressure administration can normalize blood pressure in obstructive sleep apnea patients. Sleep 1993; 16:545–549.

13. Cuspidi C, Macca G, Sampieri L, et al: High prevalence of cardiac and extracardiac target organ damage in refractory hypertension. J Hypertens 2001, 19:2063–2070.

14. Haller CA, Benowitz NL: Adverse cardiovascular and central nervous system events associated with dietary supplements containing ephedra. N Engl J Med 2001, 343:1833–1838.

15. Farese RV, Biglieri EG, Shackleton CHL et al: Licorice-induced hypermineralocorticoidism. N Engl J Med 1991, 325:1223–1227.

16. Lim PO, Jung RT, MacDonald TM: Is aldosterone the missing link in refractory hypertension? Aldosterone-to-renin ratio as a marker of inappropriate aldosterone activity. J Hum Hypertens 2002, 16:153–158.

17. Ouzan J, Perault C, Lincoff AM, et al: The role of spironolactone in the treatment of patients with refractory hypertension. Am J Hypertens 2002, 15(4 pt 1):333–339.

18. Delyani JA, Rocha R, Cook CS, et al: Eplerenone: a selective aldosterone receptor antagonist (SARA). Cardiovasc Drug Rev 2001, 19:185–200.

19. Carter AR, Zhou ZH, Calhoun DA, Bubien JK: Hyperactive ENaC identifies hypertensive individuals amenable to amiloride therapy. Am J Physiol Cell Physiol 2001, 281(suppl C):1413–1421.

20. Thomas GD, Zhang W, Victor RG: Nitric oxide deficiency as a cause of clinical hypertension: promising new drug targets for refractory hypertension. JAMA 2001, 285:2055–2057.

21. The ALLHAT Officers and Coordinators for the ALLHAT Collaborative Research Group: Major outcomes in high-risk hypertensive patients randomized to angiotensin-converting enzyme inhibitor or calcium channel blocker vs diuretic: the Antihypertensive and Lipid-Lowering Treatment to Prevent Heart Attack Trial (ALLHAT). JAMA 2002, 288:2981–2997.

22. Brown MJ, Palmer CR, Castaigne A, et al: Morbidity and mortality in patients randomised to double-blind treatment with a long-acting calcium-channel blocker or diuretic in the International Nifedipine GITS study: Intervention as a Goal in Hypertension Treatment (INSIGHT). Lancet 2000, 356:366–372.

23. Dahlof B, Devereux RB, Kjeldsen SE, et al: Cardiovascular morbidity and mortality in the Losartan Intervention For Endpoint reduction in hypertension (LIFE): a randomised trial against atenolol. Lancet 2002, 359:995–1003.

24. Krakoff LR: The ASH Specialists Program: a progress report. Am J Hypertens 2002, 15:577–579.

SECTION VII
Medical Therapy: Meeting Most
Management Challenges

chapter
28

Hypertension and Congestive Heart Failure

Alan H. Gradman, M.D., and A. Tareq Khawaja, M.D.

Over the past 40 years, epidemiologic studies have shown a progressive reduction in morbidity and mortality in the United States from cardiovascular diseases, including stroke and coronary heart disease.[1] During that time, the incidence and prevalence of congestive heart failure (CHF) rose dramatically (Fig. 1). Heart failure is the most common reason for hospital admission in patients older than age 65 years, and approximately 400,000 new cases are diagnosed annually.

Heart failure represents the final common result of several conditions, including hypertension, coronary artery disease (CAD), idiopathic cardiomyopathy, and valvular heart disease. Two thirds of heart failure patients have a history of coronary disease often complicated by myocardial infarction (MI). Hypertension is the most common precursor of heart failure, and more than 75% of patients have antecedent hypertension. Framingham Study data indicate that hypertension accounts for 39% of attributable risk for heart failure in men and 59% in women (Fig. 2) [2].

Hypertension and heart failure are intimately related at all stages in the natural history of the disease. Elevation in blood pressure (BP) initiates structural changes in the myocardium that alone may lead to heart failure. Hypertension is also a potent risk factor for CAD, which contributes to the pathogenesis of heart failure. In patients who have heart failure caused by systolic dysfunction (as occurs after MI), the presence of hypertension further degrades ventricular performance. Long-term follow-up of more than 1000 patients after MI confirms that hypertensives compared with normotensives had increased inpatient and postdischarge mortality, more inpatient heart failure, and increased re-admission rates for heart failure. Plasma neurohormones were significantly higher in hypertensives, and radionuclide ventriculography demonstrated increased

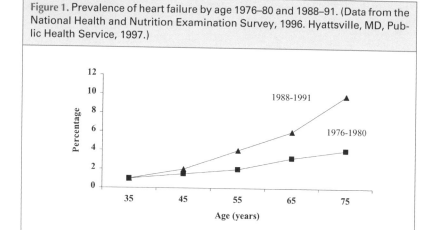

Figure 1. Prevalence of heart failure by age 1976–80 and 1988–91. (Data from the National Health and Nutrition Examination Survey, 1996. Hyattsville, MD, Public Health Service, 1997.)

left ventricular volumes, a major determinant of survival. It is clear that antecedent hypertension interacts with age, neurohumoral activation, and ventricular remodeling to confer greater risk of heart failure after MI.[3]

In the pre–hypertensive drug era, CHF resulted from untreated hypertension and its associated increased left ventricular afterload (the tension developed in the myocardium during systole to pump blood into the aorta), leading first to left ventricular hypertrophy (LVH) and eventually to ventricular systolic dysfunction. Currently, heart failure in hypertensives without CAD occurs most commonly in older patients with hypertension and LVH who demonstrate extramyocytic ventricular fibrosis associated with impaired myocardial relaxation and diastolic ventricular dysfunction. Ejection fraction is usually normal, and symptoms result when a stiff, hypertrophied ventricle impairs diastolic filling, leading to elevation in left ventricular (LV) end-diastolic pressure (Fig. 3), which is transmitted to the pulmonary capillaries, producing dyspnea and pulmonary edema.

Left Ventricular Hypertrophy

LVH is a key pathologic precursor for the development of heart failure in hypertensives. The risk of developing LVH is proportional to BP elevation, and it is estimated that between 40% to 60% of hypertensives have LVH. A 20-mm Hg increase in BP increases the relative risk of LVH by 43% in men and 25% in women.[4]

LVH is not only a hemodynamic adaptation to elevated BP, but also results from a complex array of neurohumoral processes involving the renin-angiotensin-aldosterone system (RAAS) and sympathetic nervous system.[5] Age is also an important risk factor. African Americans are twice as likely

Figure 2. Population-attributable risks for development of CHF. Population-attributable risk is defined as (100 × prevalence × [hazard ratio − 1])/(prevalence × [hazard ratio − 1] + 1). CHF = chronic heart failure; AP = angina pectoris; DM = diabetes mellitus; LVH = left ventricular hypertrophy; VHD = valvular heart disease; HTN = hypertension; MI = myocardial infarction. (From Levy D, Larson MG, Vasan RS: The progression of hypertension to congestive heart failure. JAMA 1996, 275:1557; with permission.)

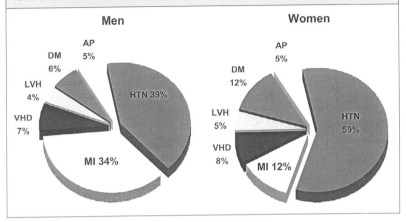

Key Points: LVH and Hypertension

- Hypertension is the single largest risk factor for CHF and is still poorly treated.
- LVH is a hemodynamic adaptation and neurohumoral process involving the RAAS.

to have LVH and to develop cardiac failure compared with whites with similar BP, emphasizing the importance of genetic factors and race.

Pathophysiology

Increased wall tension causes mechanical disruption of the focal adhesion complex that connects the extracellular matrix to the cell cytoplasm. This disruption appears sufficient to modulate cell growth and apoptosis. At the same time, local humoral mechanisms (RAAS) are activated by stretch and likely represent the obligatory link in initiating LVH.[6] Increased synthesis of angiotensin II and aldosterone plays a crucial role and is followed by increased production of fibrous tissue that supports myocyte hypertrophy and surrounds blood vessels. These local events are accompanied by increases in locally and centrally mediated SNS activity.

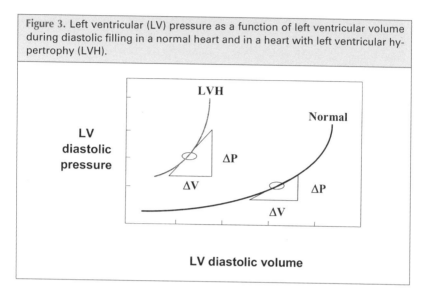

Figure 3. Left ventricular (LV) pressure as a function of left ventricular volume during diastolic filling in a normal heart and in a heart with left ventricular hypertrophy (LVH).

Initial myocyte growth and collagen deposition result in myocardial stiffening and diastolic dysfunction. These patients have an increased mortality rate compared with matched control subjects and develop symptoms of heart failure and poor exercise tolerance, particularly with tachycardia (which impairs LV filling by shortening diastole) and atrial fibrillation.

Diastolic Dysfunction Heart Failure

Heart failure caused primarily by diastolic dysfunction accounts for 25% to 40% to of heart failure admissions to major medical centers.[7] However, the optimal treatment strategy remains unclear. Diuretics and drug treatment to reduce systolic BP are the mainstays of therapy. ACE inhibitors, angiotenin receptor blockers (ARBs), and calcium channel blockers (CCBs) can reduce ventricular collagen content. The diphenylalkylamine CCB verapamil may improve diastolic dysfunction by modifying myocyte Ca^{++} concentrations during cardiac relaxation. Beta-blockers and heart rate–lowering CCBs may be beneficial by prolonging diastole. Unfortunately, well-controlled trials have not been completed. A major clinical trial (CHARM) is underway to assess the value of the ARB candesartan cilexetil in the treatment of patients with heart failure with preserved LV systolic function.

Apoptosis of myocytes, neurohumoral mechanisms and development of fibrosis are collectively termed *ventricular remodeling,* which is the basis for the progression of LVH. Eventually, the LV begins to dilate as a result of the dissolution of collagen fibers from activation of

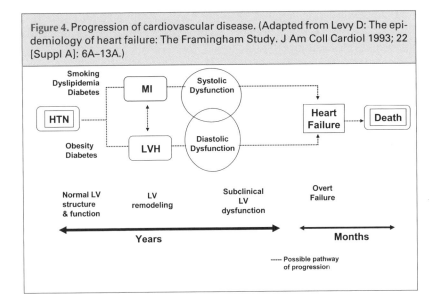

Figure 4. Progression of cardiovascular disease. (Adapted from Levy D: The epidemiology of heart failure: The Framingham Study. J Am Coll Cardiol 1993; 22 [Suppl A]: 6A–13A.)

matrix metalloproteinases and downregulation of their inhibitors, resulting in LV systolic dysfunction and heart failure. In summary, the progression of cardiovascular disease is a complex interplay between hypertension, LVH, and other cardiovascular risk factors that over a period of years, result in the development of LV remodeling, subclinical LV dysfunction, and eventual overt LV systolic dysfunction (Fig. 4).

Key Points: Pathophysiology

- ☞ Myocyte growth and collagen deposition lead to stiffening and diastolic dysfunction.
- ☞ The optimal treatment strategy for patients with diastolic dysfunction is unclear.
- ☞ LV dilatation precedes LV systolic dysfunction.

LVH Regression

The presence of LVH increases the risk of overall mortality by sixfold and the risk of heart failure by fivefold in addition to increasing risk of sudden death, MI, and stroke.[8] Recent evidence suggests a significant benefit of reducing LVH.[9] In retrospective studies, hypertensive patients who achieved similar levels of BP reduction accompanied by a decrease in LV mass had fewer adverse cardiovascular events compared with those with no reduction or with an increase in LV mass. Lifestyle changes such as weight reduction and exercise in obese patients can reduce LV mass independently of BP reduction. Reducing salt and alcohol intake are also effective measures that should be encouraged.[1] Several trials indicate that partial or total LVH regression accompanies antihypertensive therapy.[14] Effective agents include angiotensin converting enzyme (ACE) inhibitors, hydrochlorothiazide, CCBs, ARBs, and (to a lesser extent) beta-blockers. ACE inhibitors and ARBs seem to be the most effective in this regard.[11]

Key Points: LVH Regression

- ⇒ Weight reduction, exercise, and reduced salt and alcohol intake are important
- ⇒ Beneficial agents include ACE inhibitors, ARBs, CCBs, diuretics, and beta-blockers.

Antihypertensive Therapy and Prevention of Heart Failure

The most effective strategy for decreasing the risk of CHF involves the implementation of aggressive antihypertensive therapy. The effects of BP reduction on the risk of developing heart failure are profound. Placebo controlled studies with conventional antihypertensive agents (diuretics and beta-blockers) document reduction in CHF incidence of approximately 50% in patients selected based on elevated diastolic BP.[13] In a meta-analysis of ACE inhibitors or CCBs compared with conventional agents as initial therapy, no statistical difference was noted in heart failure, indicating that these agents produce approximately equal effects, although the trend favored ACE inhibitors.[14] *These data point to the paramount importance of BP reduction in the prevention of heart failure.*

The recently completed LIFE study (Losartan Intervention for Endpoint Reduction in Hypertension) compared atenolol and losartan in their ability to reduce cardiovascular morbidity and mortality in patients with hypertension and electrocardiographic evidence of LVH. More than 9000 patients were randomized, and LVH was significantly reduced in the losartan arm compared with the atenolol arm. Although the overall results of the study favored losartan, there was no difference in the incidence of heart failure.[12] These data suggest that losartan is approximately equivalent to other antihypertensive agents in preventing heart failure.

One agent that appears to be less effective than other drugs in the prevention of heart failure is the alpha-blocker doxazosin. ALLHAT enrolled more than 42,000 patients with BP between 140/90 mmHg untreated and 160/100 mmHg on treatment. The doxazosin arm of the study was discontinued because patients receiving this agent had 25% more cardiovascular events and were twice as likely to be hospitalized for CHF as users of the diuretic chlorthalidone.[15]

Preventing Heart Failure in Elderly Patients with Hypertension

BP increases progressively with age, and a majority of individuals older than age 60 years are hypertensive. Because of reduced compliance in the arterial circulation, systolic BP increases progressively, and diastolic pressure declines. It is now clear that systolic BP elevation is as potent or more potent a determinant of cardiovascular morbidity and mortality as diastolic BP. In the elderly hypertensive population, systolic BP is disproportionately elevated, and two thirds exhibit isolated systolic hypertension (ISH).

Compelling data from clinical trials confirm the benefit of treating hypertension in the elderly, including ISH. Among these benefits is a marked reduction in the development of heart failure. In the placebo-controlled Swedish Trial in Old People with Hypertension (STOP), treatment with beta-blockers and diuretcs reduced the risk of heart failure by 51% in patients with a baseline BP greater than 180/105 mm Hg.[21] In patients with ISH studied in the Systolic Hypertension in the Elderly Program (SHEP), diuretic-based therapy in patients older than 60 years produced a 55% reduction in CHF compared with placebo (Fig. 5).[23] The Systolic Hypertension–Europe trial evaluated the dihydropyridine CCB nitrendipine in a similar patient population and demonstrated comparable reductions in systolic BP and overall cardiovascular risk.[22] The reduction in heart failure endpoint was 29%. STOP-2 randomized 6614 patients between the ages of 70 and 84 years with severe, stage 3 hypertension. In this study, ACE inhibitor treatment proved superior to the CCB in preventing the development of CHF ($P = 0.025$). In patients older than age 80 years, drug treatment remains justified and may give absolute benefit for reduction in CHF (34%), stroke (34%), and major cardiovascular events (22%).[16]

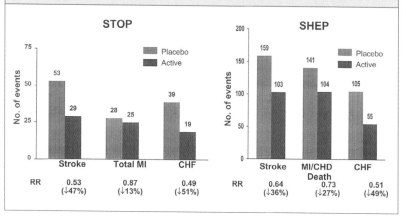

Figure 5. STOP and SHEP Trials: treatment of systolic and diastolic hypertension decreases CHF risk. (STOP = Swedish Trial in Old People with Hypertension; SHEP = Systolic Hypertension in the Elderly Program; CHD = coronary heart disease; RR = relative risk.) (Data from Dahlöf et al. Lancet 1991; 338:1281. Kostis et al. JAMA 1997; 278:212. SHEP Cooperative Research Group. JAMA 1991; 265:3255.)

Diabetes Mellitus, Hypertension, and Heart Failure

Diabetes is associated with a cardiomyopathy affecting primarily diastolic function and is independently associated with the development of CHF. Hypertension occurs in 60% to 70% of diabetics and further augments risk. In the Framingham cohort, the risk of CHF was increased sixfold in male and 10-fold in female diabetics. The UKPDS group reported that "tight" control of hyperglycemia (decreasing the hemoglobin (Hgb) A1c from 7.9% to 7.0%) reduced the risk of heart failure by 9%. Aggressive BP control using an ACE inhibitor or beta-blocker (resulting in a mean BP of 144/82 mmHg compared with 154/87 mmHg) was considerably more effective, decreasing the frequency of CHF development by 56%.[17] The target BP recommended by the American Diabetes Association and National Kidney Foundation is less than 130/80 mm Hg. Most diabetics require multiple antihypertensive agents to reach this goal. Drugs that interrupt the RAAS (ACE inhibitors and ARBs) are preferred. Retrospective analysis of completed trials indicate that beta-blockers are also useful adjuncts to therapy in diabetic patients with heart failure.[18]

Key Points: Special Groups

- Treating hypertension with diuretics with or without beta-blockers, ACE inhibitors, or CCBs but not α_1-blockers reduces CHF.
- Isolated systolic hypertension should be aggressively treated, particularly in elderly patients.
- ACE inhibitors have unique benefits in diabetes.
- African Americans have higher prevalence and more target organ damage at presentation.

Hypertensive Emergency

The profound increase in afterload produced by severe BP elevation may lead to ventricular dysfunction and cardiac failure, even in patients without structural heart disease. Severe hypertension presenting with acute LV failure and pulmonary edema is a hypertensive emergency that requires prompt BP reduction. The initial goal is to reduce mean BP by no more than 25% (within minutes to 2 hours), then toward 160/100 mm Hg within 2 to 6 hours, avoiding excessive decreases in BP. The agent of choice is sodium nitroprusside (0.25 to 10.00 μg/kg/min) intravenously, which produces a rapid BP reduction. The maximum dose should not be used for more than 10 minutes. Concomitant therapy with loop diuretics and intravenous nitroglycerin is usually necessary. After the initial BP goal has been achieved, ACE inhibitors are initiated and maintained, and nitroprusside is tapered to minimize the risks of adverse effects. An alternative is fenoldopam, a peripheral dopamine-1 agonist, which has the added benefit of maintaining or increasing renal perfusion while lowering BP. Enalaprilat, available intravenously, is the active congener of enalapril that may be especially useful for treating patients with severe hypertension complicated by acute heart failure.

Key Points: Emergencies

- Sodium nitroprusside for acute LVF with severe hypertension: Reduce BP by 25% (minutes to 2 hours), then to a target of 160/100 mmHg (2 to 6 hours).
- Avoid sublingual nifedipine.
- An ACE inhibitor (enalaprilat) may be useful for patients with severe hypertension with LV failure.

Treatment of Hypertension and Systolic Heart Failure

Prevention of CHF is the preferred pathway for hypertensive patients. However, after systolic heart failure is present (ejection fraction of less than 40%), the BP should be reduced to the JNC VI goal of less than 130/85 mmHg.[1] We advocate lowering systolic BP even more aggressively to 120 mmHg, if tolerated, to further decrease LV wall stress. A diuretic combined with either an ACE inhibitor or an ARB constitutes usual initial therapy. Beta-blockers (e.g., metoprolol XL, bisoprolol, or carvediolol) are evidence-based additions to the diuretic–ACE inhibitor or diuretic–ARB therapy.[19–21] Beta-blockers can improve ejection fraction and reduce sudden death in patients with heart failure. Beta-blockers should be titrated at intervals of 2 weeks or more as tolerated to recommended maximum doses (Toprol XL 200 mg daily, bisoprolol 10 mg daily, carvedilol 25 mg twice daily). Spironolactone, 25 mg daily, is a useful adjunct for reducing morbidity and mortality.[22] The combination of an ACE inhibitor, ARB, and beta-blocker together in the same patient in the Valsartan Heart Failure Trial did not improve outcomes and raises the possibility of diminishing returns with three or more neurohumoral blockers.

Key Points

- ⧽ Hypertension is a primary etiologic factor in the development of heart failure in the U.S. population.
- ⧽ Its effects are mediated through the development of LV hypertrophy and coronary heart disease.
- ⧽ Treating hypertension aggressively with diuretics, beta-blockers, ACE inhibitors, CCBs, and ARBs is extremely effective in preventing the development of heart failure, and, in many studies, reduced its occurrence by 50%. This is particularly true in the elderly and in patients with isolated systolic hypertension.
- ⧽ Hypertension exacerbates preexisting systolic ventricular dysfunction.
- ⧽ Severe BP elevation may precipitate pulmonary edema, even in patients without structural heart disease, and requires emergent treatment.
- ⧽ Because the morbidity and mortality associated with clinical heart failure are high, prevention is the best option, and physicians should focus on detecting and controlling high BP before structural changes that result in heart failure develop.

References

1. The sixth report of the Joint National Committee on prevention, detection, evaluation and treatment of high blood pressure (JNC VI): Arch Intern Med 1997, 157:2413–2446.
2. Kannel WB: LVH as a risk factor: the Framingham experience. J Hyperten 1991, 9(suppl): 3.
3. Richards AM, Nicholls G, Troughton RW et al: Antecedent hypertension and heart failure after myocardial infarction. J Am Coll Cardiol 2002, 39:1182–1188.
4. Levy D, Larson MG, Vasan RS: The progression of hypertension to congestive heart failure. JAMA 1996, 275:1557.
5. Devereux RB, Roman MJ: LVH in Hypertension: stimuli, patterns and consequences. Hyperten Research 1999, 22:1.
6. Dahlöf B: LVH and angiotensin II antagonists. Am J Hypertens 2001, 14:174.
7. Phillips RA, Diamond JA: Diastolic function in hypertension Curr Card Rep 2001, 3:485-497.
8. Levy D, Garrison RJ, et al: Prognostic implications of echocardiographically determined left ventricular mass in the Framingham Heart Study. N Engl J Med 1990, 322:1561–1566.
9. Dahlöf B, Pennert K, Hansson L: Reversal of LVH in hypertensive patients: a meta analysis of 109 treatment studies. Am J Hypertens 1992, 5:95.
10. Vasan RS, Larson MG, Benjamin EJ: Congestive heart failure in subjects with normal versus reduced LV ejection fractions: prevalence and mortality in a population based cohort. J Am Coll Cardiol 1999, 33:1948.
11. Carson P, Giles T, et al: Angiotensin receptor blockers: evidence for preserving target organs Clin Cardiol 2001, 24:183–190.
12. Dahlöf B, Devereux R, et al: Cardiovascular morbidity and mortality in the losartan intervention for endpoint reduction in hypertension study (LIFE): a randomized trial against atenolol. Lancet 2002, 359:995.
13. Psaty BM, Smith NL: Health outcomes associated with antihypertensive therapy used as first line agents: a systematic review and meta-analysis. JAMA 1997, 277:739–745.
14. Blood Pressure Lowering Treatment Trialists Collaboration: Effects of ACE inhibitors, calcium antagonists and other blood pressure lowering drugs: results of prospectively designed overviews of randomized trials. Lancet 2000, 355:1955–1964.
15. ALLHAT officers and coordinators for the ALLHAT Research Group: Major cardiovascular events in hypertensive patients randomized to doxazosin vs chlorthalidone: The Antihypertensive and Lipid-lowering Treatment to Prevent Heart Attack Trial. JAMA 2000, 283:1967–1975.
16. Gueffner F, Bulpitt C, Boissel J, et al: Anti-hypertensive drugs in very old people: a subgroup meta analysis of randomised controlled trials. Lancet 1999, 353:793–796.
17. UKPDS: Efficacy of atenolol and captopril in reducing risk for macro and microvascular complications in type II diabetes: UKPDS 39. Brit Med J 1998, 317:713–720.
18. Giles TD: Use of β-blockers for heart failure in patients with diabetes mellitus. In A special report: unanswered questions about β-blockers in heart failure. Postgrad Med 2002, pp. 32–37, November, 2002.
19. Hjalmarsan A, Goldstein S, Fagerberg G, et al: Effects of controlled-release metoprolol on total mortality, hospitalizations, and well-being in patients with heart failure: the Metoprolol CR/XL Randomized Intervention Trial in Congestive Heart Failure (MERIT-HF) Study Group. JAMA 2000, 283:1295–1302.
19a. Packer M, Coats AJ, Fowler MB, et al: Effects of carvedilol on survival in servere chronic heart failure. N Engl J Med 2001, 344:1651–1658.

20. The Cardiac Insufficiency Bisoprolol Study II (CIBIS-II): A randomized trial. Lancet 1999, 353:9–13.
21. Dahlöj B, Lindholm LH, Hansson L, et al: Morbidity and mortality in the Swedish Trial in Old People with Hypertension (STOP-Hypertension) Lancet 1991, 338:1281–1285.
22. Staessen JA, Fagard R, Thijs L, et al: Randomized double blind comparison of placebo and active treatment for older patients with isolated systolic hypertension (SYST-EUR). Lancet 1997, 350:757–764.
23. Kostis JB, Davis BR, Cutler J, et al: Prevention of heart failure by antihypertensive drug treatment in older persons with isolated systolic hypertension (SHEP). JAMA 1997, 278:212–216.

Managing Hypertension in Patients with Chronic Renal Insufficiency

chapter
29

Crystal A. Gadegbeku, M.D.

More than 6 million Americans are estimated to have abnormally high serum creatinine levels[1] and are at risk for progressive nephropathy. The population of patients with end-stage renal disease (ESRD) continues to rise and is predicted to reach 600,000 in the United States by 2010.[2] The annual mortality rate for patients on dialysis remains 20% despite advances in ESRD management and technology. Medical therapy must focus on preserving kidney function in susceptible patients.

Approximately 85% of patients with kidney disease have hypertension, and hypertension contributes to the decline in renal function. This chapter provides evidence-based guidelines for optimal antihypertensive therapy and reviews recommendations for timely referral to a nephrologist.

Blood Pressure Control and Progression of Renal Disease

Blood pressure (BP) impacts the rate of progression of kidney disease. Longitudinal clinical trials in diabetic and nondiabetic kidney disease reveal a nearly linear relationship between BP and the rate of decline in renal function (Fig. 1).[3] In 1997, the Joint National Committee (JNC) VI guidelines recommended BP less than 130/85 mm Hg[4] for patients with kidney disease and an even lower target of less than 125/75 mm Hg for patients with more than 1 gram of proteinuria daily based on the Modified Diet and Renal Disease Trial (MDRD). Clinical studies also support the notion of cardiovascular benefit from more strict BP control.[3] The collective evidence for cardiorenal benefit with strict BP control has emerged at a time when hypertension control rates in the general population have stagnated.[5] Therefore, greater emphasis on BP control is necessary to ameliorate the increasing burden of renal disease in the United States. Strict BP

297

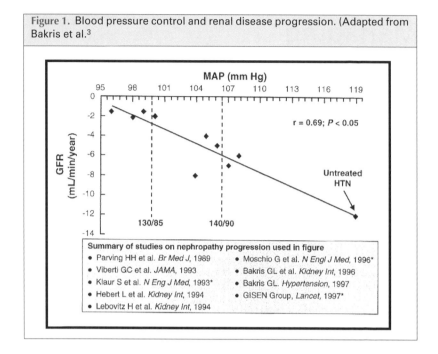

Figure 1. Blood pressure control and renal disease progression. (Adapted from Bakris et al.[3]

control often requires a multidrug regimen (Fig. 2), which highlights the complexity of therapy in patients with kidney disease and illustrates the challenge clinicians face in reaching recommended BP goals.

Proteinuria and Progression of Renal Disease

Even minimal levels of proteinuria and microalbuminuria are important early clinical markers of renal disease. *In vitro* studies suggest that excess renal protein traffic is directly toxic to renal tubules and induces proliferative and inflammatory mediators, which are implicated in nephrosclerosis.[6] In support of the experimental data, clinical studies demonstrate that proteinuria is an independent predictor of renal disease progression. In the MDRD[7] and Ramipril Efficacy in Nephropathy (REIN)[8] studies, urine protein excretion correlated with the rate of progression of kidney failure and risk of ESRD. Not only is proteinuria predictive of renal decline, but treatment that reduces protein excretion by 30% or more slows the progression of renal disease.[3] In addition, microalbuminuria and overt proteinuria are associated with increased cardiovascular risk.[3,9] Therefore, antihypertensive therapy should aim to reduce proteinuria for renal and cardiovascular benefit.

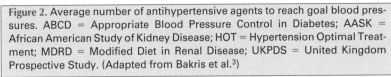

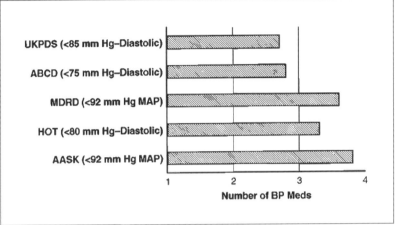

Figure 2. Average number of antihypertensive agents to reach goal blood pressures. ABCD = Appropriate Blood Pressure Control in Diabetes; AASK = African American Study of Kidney Disease; HOT = Hypertension Optimal Treatment; MDRD = Modified Diet in Renal Disease; UKPDS = United Kingdom Prospective Study. (Adapted from Bakris et al.[3])

Quantifying Urine Protein

Microalbuminuria is excessive albuminuria that is undetectable by urine dipstick. Microalbuminuria is defined as albumin excretion of greater than 30 mg in a 24-hour urine sample or greater than 30 mg per gram of creatinine in a spot urine sample. Overt proteinuria, normally detected on routine urinalysis, is albumin excretion greater than 300 mg per 24 hours or greater than 300 mg per gram of creatinine in a spot urine sample. In a 24-hour urine sample, creatinine level should also be measured, along with albumin, to assess the adequacy of the collection. A spot urine sample should be a clean, mid-urine sample in which the ratio of albumin (in milligrams) and creatinine (in grams) is determined. The spot urine sample is more convenient for the patient and results are obtained quickly, while an appropriately collected 24-hour urine sample provides a more accurate assessment of protein and electrolyte excretion as well as creatinine clearance.[9]

False-positive tests for microalbuminuria can occur with either method in patients with urinary tract infections, glycosuria, post-exercise, alkaline urine (pH > 8.0), and highly concentrated urine samples.[9] If microalbuminuria is detected, a repeat test should be performed within 3 months to confirm results.[9]

Effects of Antihypertensive Renin-Angiotensin System Agents on Renal Disease

In experimental models of kidney disease, angiotensin II is a central mediator in glomerular hypertension, a maladaptive hemodynamic response to chronic renal injury. Angiotensin II also increases glomerular basement membrane permeability, which augments proteinuria, stimulates proliferation, inflammation, matrix accumulation, and fibrosis.[7] Evidence from clinical trials support recommendations to use angiotensin converting enzyme (ACE) inhibitors and angiotensin II type 1 receptor blockers (ARBs) in patients with kidney disease.

Angiotensin-Converting Enzyme Inhibitors

ACE inhibitors are effective in decreasing BP, reducing proteinuria, and slowing the rate of decline in kidney function in patients with diabetic and nondiabetic renal disease.[8,10–12] Some authors suggest caution in interpreting the renal benefits of ACE inhibitors because BP was lower in clinical trials of patients receiving these agents.[13,14] However, additional analyses suggest a BP-independent component in the ACE inhibitor renoprotective effect.[10,15–17]

In hypertensive type 1 diabetics with renal disease, captopril reduced the combined endpoints of death, dialysis, or transplantation by 50% compared with placebo during a 4-year period.[10] A meta-analysis of data from 10 small, placebo-controlled, long-term studies of type 1 diabetic patients without hypertension revealed that the use of various ACE inhibitors reduced the risk of developing overt proteinuria 70% and increased regression to normoalbuminuria three-fold.[11] These findings suggest that type 1 diabetics with microalbuminuria benefit from ACE inhibitors irrespective of BP.

Long-term studies support ACE inhibitor use in nondiabetic hypertensive patients with chronic renal disease. In the largest double-blind, prospective trial in renal disease, benezapril decreased progression of renal disease by 70% in patients with glomerular filtration rates (GFR) 45 or greater and by almost 50% in patients with GFR 45 or less mL/min.[18] The REIN trial demonstrated both that ramipril significantly reduced proteinuria and that reduction in proteinuria correlated with renal preservation.[8] Ramipril significantly slowed progression of renal disease in patients with 3 grams or more baseline proteinuria compared with standard therapy, which led to premature termination of this portion of the study. Patients receiving conventional therapy were switched to ramipril, and these patients experienced a similar slowing in the rate of decline in renal function.[19] Patients with less than 3 grams of proteinuria on ramipril also had a significant reduction in risk of ESRD.[20]

Similar to the benazepril study, renal protection was seen in patients with GFR less than 45 mL/min.[21] Thus, ACE inhibitors are beneficial in a variety of kidney diseases including patients with moderate to severe renal dysfunction.

ACE inhibitors are benefical in patients with even lower degrees of proteinuria. The African American Study of Kidney Disease (AASK) is the largest trial in African Americans with hypertensive nephrosclerosis. In AASK, patients with proteinuria greater than 300 mg/day treated with ramipril compared with amlodipine had a 36% slower rate of progression and 48% reduction in the composite endpoint of rapid decline in renal function, ESRD, or death despite similar BP.[22] Previous studies of ACE inhibitors in renal disease included relatively few nonwhite patients. AASK suggests that nonwhite populations with renal disease also benefit from ACE inhibitors.

Because it is established that patients with microalbuminuria and overt proteinuria are at increased cardiovascular risk,[3,9] evidence for cardiovascular protection with ACE inhibitors further supports their use as first-line therapy in this population. In the diabetic component of the Heart Outcomes Prevention Evaluation (MICRO-HOPE), ramipril reduced cardiovascular events 20% to 30% in those with microalbuminuria.[23] Collectively, data from several studies provide compelling evidence for using ACE inhibitors as initial therapy in patients with renal disease.

Angiotensin II Type 1 Receptor Blockers (ARBs)

ARBs differ from ACE inhibitors in the site of blockade of the renin-angiotensin system. However, clinical studies indicate that ARBs and ACE inhibitors have similar systemic and renal hemodynamic effects.[7] ARBs have the added benefit of blocking angiotensin II produced by alternate (non-ACE) pathways. ARBs also cause less hyperkalemia than ACE inhibitors.[24] However, these drugs do not appear to increase the vasodilatory kinins as much as ACE inhibitors. Furthermore, there is less supression of profibrotic substances such as aldosterone and plasminogen activator inhibitor-1 with ARBs compared with ACE inhibitors.[7] The long-term effects of these differences in renal disease are unknown.

The large clinical trials with ARBs to date demonstrate renoprotection in patients with type II diabetes and hypertension. Losartan compared with placebo and irbesartan compared with amlodipine both demonstrated more than 20% risk reduction in ESRD over a 2- to 3-year period in diabetic patients with overt proteinuria.[25,26] In patients with microalbuminuria, hypertension, and type II diabetes, irbesartan also showed a dose-dependent reduction in risk of overt proteinuria with daily doses of 150 and 300 mg compared with placebo despite equivalent BP in all groups.[27] Unfortunately, clinical trials comparing this newer class of medications to ACE inhibitors have not been done. Therefore, the question of which class of drugs is more effective in preserving renal function has not and probably will not be answered.

In theory, the combination of an ACE inhibitor and ARB may provide synergistic renoprotection. Two short-term studies[28,29] suggest that ACE inhibitors and ARBs can be safely used together in patients with renal disease and that the combination therapy can have additive benefits on BP and proteinuria. However, the long-term benefits of the ACE inhibitor ARB combination on proteinuria and progression of renal disease are unknown.

Diuretics

As renal function declines, there is an increased tendency toward salt and water retention. Therefore, diuretics are often necessary to restore euvolemia and treat hypertension. The addition of a low-dose thiazide diuretic, 12.5 to 25.0 mg/day, to the ACE inhibitor leads to additive BP effect[3] in hypertensive patients with normal renal function. Diuretics are particularly effective at enhancing the BP response to ACE inhibitors in African Americans and elderly patients. However, if the serum creatinine level is 1.8 mg/dL or more, thiazides are less effective, and loop diuretics may be required to control volume status and BP. In the setting of significant edema associated with heavy proteinuria, the distal tubule diuretic metolazone (in addition to the loop diuretic) may be necessary for adequate diuresis.

Calcium Channel Blockers

The dihydropyridine (DHP) and nondihydropyridine (non-DHPs) calcium channel blockers (CCBs) (Table 1), have different effects on proteinuria despite similar effects on BP. Whereas the non-DHPs have antiproteinuric effects similar to ACE inhibitors, DHPs, particularly as monotherapy, have less favorable effects on protein excretion[15] and may increase proteinuria.[22,30] However, in combination with ACE in-

TABLE 1. Dihydropyridine and Nondihydropyridine Calcium Channel Blockers	
Dihydropyridines	**Non-dihydropyridines**
Amlodipine	Diltiazem
Felodipine	Verapamil
Isradipine	
Miodipine	
Nicardipine	
Nifedipene	
Nisoldipine	

hibitors, (e.g., the REIN trial), ramipril with a DHP was effective in reducing BP and controlling proteinuria.[30] CCBs have antiproliferative and anti-inflammatory properties that may retard renal injury.[31]

The non-DHP CCBs, either verapamil or diltiazem, in combination with an ACE inhibitor,[32] result in a two-fold greater reduction in proteinuria than either agent alone. If the goal is to minimize proteinuria, then a non-DHP CCB should be the second or third agent (after an ACE inhibitor and a diuretic). If protein excretion is normal and the goal is to reduce BP, either CCB class would be effective.

Beta-Blockers

Beta-blockers are effective in reducing BP and urinary protein excretion, and they have established cardiovascular benefit. The United Kingdom Prospective Diabetes Study (UKPDS)[33] found that atenolol was equivalent to captopril in slowing the progression of proteinuria and renal disease in type 2 diabetic patients. However, this study was performed in predominantly white subjects. In the AASK trial, a study recently completed in African Americans with hypertensive nephrosclerosis, metoprolol, compared with ramipril as first-line therapy, tended to be less effective in reducing the risk of the composite outcome of death, dialysis, and rapid renal decline.[34] These results are consistent with smaller studies including African Americans which suggest that beta-blockers were not as effective at slowing the rate of renal progression as ACE inhibitors and non-DHP CCBs.[35,36] However, in the AASK trial, metoprolol did demonstrate more renal benefit than amlodipine, a DHP CCB.[34]

In patients with congestive heart failure or myocardial infarction, which are often present in patients with chronic kidney disease, beta-blockers are indicated. The combination of beta-blockers and non-DHP CCBs may produce excessive negative inotropic and chronotropic effects and is rarely indicated. Alpha- and beta-blockers can also reduce BP and proteinuria (Table 2).

Other Agents

If BP is still uncontrolled to 130/80 mm Hg or less on a three-drug regimen together with dietary sodium restriction, then referral to a nephrologist or hypertension specialist is recommended. Alpha$_1$-antagonists, central α_2-agonists, and minoxidil are effective antihypertensive agents for patients with renal disease but must be used cautiously in combination with other antihypertensive drugs previously described and may require close monitoring.[3,37] These medications have little, if any, direct antiproteinuric effect but may, nevertheless, be beneficial to the kidney by improving BP control.

TABLE 2. Cardiorenal Effects of Antihypertensive Agents			
Drug Class	**Albuminuria**	**Time to Dialysis**	**Cardiovascular Mortality**
Alpha-blockers	⇔	?	?
ACE Inhibitors	⇓⇓	⇓⇓⇓	⇓⇓
ARBs	⇓⇓	⇓⇓	⇓
Beta-blockers	⇓	⇓	⇓
CCBs-DHP	⇔	⇔	⇔
CCB-NonDHP	⇓	⇓	⇓
Diuretics	⇓	?	⇓

Adapted from table II in MacLeod and McLay[36] with additional data provided by Taal and Brenner[6] and Bakris et al.[3] Most of these data are from experimental and clinical studies in diabetic nephropathy. ⇓ = reduced, ⇔ = little or variable effects. ARB = angiotensin II receptor blockers; CCB = calcium channel blockers; DHP = dihydropyridine

BP control is often achievable in patients with renal disease but likely requires combination therapy and more frequent patient visits. Lifestyle modifications are of greater particular importance in renal patients given their tendency toward sodium retention, resistant hypertension, and progression of kidney disease. Figure 3 illustrates an evidence-based treatment paradigm which can be followed to achieve adequate blood pressure control in patients with renal disease. When BP cannot be controlled to the target of 130/80–85 mm Hg or less, referral to a nephrologist or hypertension specialist is recommended because BP control is critical in preserving renal function.

When and Why to Refer to a Nephrologist

The prevalence of Americans with ESRD continues to increase,[1] and the cost of this therapy will reach $30 billion by the year 2010. Despite improvements in renal replacement therapy and this overwhelming cost, the annual mortality rate of patients on dialysis remains high at 20%.[1] Based on these alarming statistics, it is clear that medical management must focus on preventing or at least delaying the progression of kidney disease.

Delayed nephrology referral is associated with increased morbidity and mortality, hospitalizations, procedures, complications, and cost.[38] In a prospective analysis of 1041 patients, the risk of death was strongly and inversely related to the length of time between referral and initiation of dialysis.[39] Given the evidence of poor prognosis related to late referral, the National Institutes of Health published guidelines in 1993 that recommend referral to a nephrologist of patients with serum creatinine 1.5 mg/dL or more in women and 2.0 mg/dL or more in men.[40]

The recommendations for referral to a nephrologist are not routinely

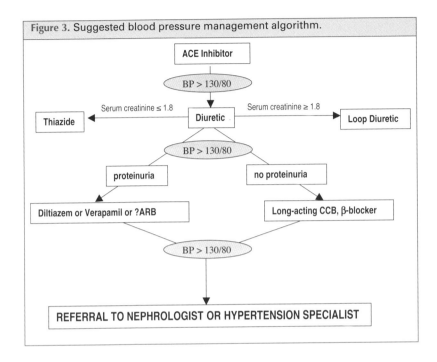

Figure 3. Suggested blood pressure management algorithm.

implemented. The majority of patients are not referred until serum creatinine is 3.0 mg/dL or more,[41] and 70% of patients are referred within 3 months of initiating dialysis.[42] Earlier intervention by a nephrologist can favorably impact patients' quality of life, minimize cost, and improve survival by providing timely therapies to arrest or slow the progressive decline in renal function (Table 3).

Patients with an increase in creatinine of 30% or more after initiation of an ACE inhibitor (or ARB) should be referred to a nephrologist. This may indicate underlying undiagnosed renal disease that requires intervention. In some of these cases, the nephrologist may recommend continuing the ACE inhibitor or ARB with careful follow-up given the evidence for long-term cardiorenal benefit.[3] Patients with persistent proteinuria or nephrotic

TABLE 3.   Reasons for Timely Nephrology Referral
• Initiate therapy to slow the progression of chronic kidney disease.
• Identify and manage comorbidities associated with chronic kidney disease (e.g., diabetes mellitus and heart disease).
• Manage complications of chronic kidney disease (e.g., anemia and renal osteodystrophy).
• Facilitate transition to renal replacement therapy when necessary.

syndrome are at high risk for chronic renal disease and should be referred to a nephrologist. Adherence to the guidelines for nephrology referral has the potential to improve the management of risk factors and other co-morbidities associated with renal disease and could reduce the prevalence, morbidity, and mortality of ESRD.

References

1. Jones CA, McQUillan GM, Kusek JW, et al: Serum creatinine levels in the US Population: Third National Health and Nutrition Examination Survey. Am J Kidney 1998, 32:992–999.
2. US Renal Data System: USRDS, 2001 annual data report: National Institutes of Health, National Institute of Diabetes and Digestive and Kidney Diseases, 2001.
3. Bakris GL, Williams M, Dworkin L, Elliott WJ, et al: Preserving renal function in adults with hypertension and diabetes: a consensus approach. Am J Kidney 2000, 36:646–661.
4. Joint National Committee on Prevention, Detection, Evaluation, and Treatment of High Blood Pressure. Arch Intern Med 1997, 157:2413–2446.
5. Burt VL, Culter JA, Higgins M, et al: Trends in the prevalence and awareness treatments and control of hypertension in the adult US population: data from the health examination surveys, 1960 to 1991. Hypertension 1995, 26:60–69.
6. Taal MW, Brenner BM: Renoprotective benefits of RAS inhibition: from ACEI to angiotensin II antagonists. Kid Intern 2000, 57:1803–1817.
7. Hunsicker LG, Adler S, Caggiula A, et al: Predictors of the progression of renal disease in the modification of diet in renal disease study. Kidney Intern 1997, 51:1908–1919.
8. The GISEN group (Gruppo Italiano di Studi Epidemiologici in Nefrologia): Randomized placebo-controlled trial of effect of ramipril on decline in glomerular filtration rate and risk of terminal renal failure in proteinuric, non-diabetic nephropathy. Lancet 1997, 349:1857–1863.
9. Kean WF, Eknoyan G. Proteinuria: Albuminuria, Risk Assessment, Detection, Elimination (PARADE): A position paper of the National Kidney Foundation. Am J Kidney 1999, 33:1004–1010.
10. Lewis EJ, Hunsicker LG, Bain RP, Rohde RD, for the Collaborative Study Group: The effect of angiotensin-coverting-enzyme inhibition on diabetic nephropathy. N Engl J Med 1993, 329:1456–1462.
11. The ACE Inhibitor Diabetic Nephropathy Trialist Group: Should all patients with Type I diabetes mellitus and microalbuminuria receive angiotensin-converting enzyme inhibitors? Ann Intern Med 2001, 134:370–379.
12. Ravid M, Savin H, Jutrin I, et al: Long-term stabilizing effect of angiotensin-converting enzyme inhibition on plasma creatinine and on proteinuria in normotensive type II diabetic patients. Ann Intern Med 1993, 118:577–581.
13. Giatras I, Lau J, Levey AS: Effect of angiotensin-converting enzyme inhibitors on the progression of nondiabetic renal disease: a meta-analysis of randomized trials. Ann Intern Med 1997, 127:337–345.
14. Kshirsagar AV, Joy MS, Hogan SL, et al: Effect of ACE inhibitors in diabetic and nondiabetic chronic renal disease: a systematic overview of randomized placebo-controlled trials. Am J Kidney Dis 2000, 35:695–707.
15. Maki DD, Ma JZ, Louis TA, Kasiske BL: Long-term effects of antihypertensive agents on proteinuria and renal function. Arch Intern Med 1995, 155:1073–1080.

16. Jafar TH, Schmid CH, Landa M, et al: Angiotensin-converting enzyme inhibitors and progression of nondiabetic renal disease. Ann Intern Med 2001, 135:73–87.

17. Gansevoort RT, Sluiter WJ, Hemmelder MH, et al: Antiproteinuric effect of blood-pressure-lowering agents: a meta-analysis of comparative trials. Nephrol Dial Transplant 1995, 10:1963–1974.

18. Maschio G, Alberti D, Janin G, and the Angiotensin-Converting Enzyme Inhibition in Progressive Renal Insufficiency Study Group: Effect of the angiotensin-converting enzyme inhibitor benazepril on the progression of chronic renal insufficiency. N Eng J Med 1996, 334:939–945.

19. Ruggenenti P, Perna A, Gherardi G, et al. on behalf of Gruppo Italiano di Studi Epidemiologici in Nefrologia (GISEN): Renal function and requirement for dialysis in chronic nephropathy patients on long-term ramipril: REIN follow-up trial. Lancet 1998, 352:1252–1256.

20. Ruggenenti P, Perna A, Gherardi G, et al: Renoprotective properties of ACE-inhibition in non-diabetic nephropathies with non-nephrotic proteinuria. Lancet 1999, 354:359–364.

21. Ruggenenti P, Perna A, Remuzzi G: ACE inhibitors to prevent end-stage renal disease: when to start and why possibly never to stop: a post hoc analysis of the REIN trial results. J Am Soc Nephrol 2001, 12:2832–2837.

22. Agodoa LY, Appel L, Bakris GL, et al: for the African American Study of Kidney Disease and Hypertension (AASK) Study Group: Effect of ramipril vs amlodipine on renal outcomes in hypertensive nephrosclerosis. JAMA 2001, 285:2719–2728.

23. The Heart Outcomes Prevention Evaluation Study Investigators: Effects of ramipril on cardiovascular and microvascular ourcomes in people with diabetes mellitus: results of the HOPE study and MICRO-HOPE substudy. Lancet 2000, 355:253–259.

24. Bakris GL, Siomos M, Richardson D, et al: ACE inhibition or angiotensin receptor blockade: impact on potassium in renal failure Kidney Int 2000, 58:2084–2092.

25. Brenner BM, Cooper ME, de Zeeuw D, et al: Effects of Losartan on renal and cardiovascular outcomes in patients with type 2 diabetes and nephropathy. N Engl J Med 2001, 345:861–869.

26. Lewis EJ, Hunsicker LG, Clarke WR, et al: Renoprotective effect of the angiotensin-receptor antagonist irbesartan in patients with nephropathy due to type 2 diabetes. N Engl J Med 2001, 345:851–860.

27. Parving Hans-Henrik, Lehnert H, Mortensen JB, et al: The effect of irbesartan on the development of diabetic nephropathy in patients with type 2 diabetes. N Engl J Med 2001, 345:870–878.

28. Russo D, Pisani A, Balletta MM, et al: Additive antiproteinuric effect of converting enzyme inhibitor and losartan in normotensive patients with IgA nephropathy. Am J Kidney Dis 1999, 33:851–856.

29. Ruiolope LM, Aldigier JC, Ponticelli C, et al: Safety of the combination of valsartan and benaepril in patients with chronic renal disease. J Hypertens 2000, 18:89–95.

30. Ruggenenti P, Perna A, Benini R, Remuzzi G: Effects of dihydropyridine calcium channel blockers, angiotensin-converting enzyme inhibition, and blood pressure control on chronic, nondiabetic nephropathies. J Am Soc Nephrol 1998, 9:2096–2101.

31. Moore MA, Epstein M, Agodoa L, Dworkin LD: Current strategies for management of hypertensive renal disease. Arch Intern Med 1999, 159:23–28.

32. Bakris GL, Weir MR, DeQuattro V, McMahon FG: Effects of an ACE inhibitor/calcium antagonist combination on proteinuria in diabetic nephropathy. Kidney Int 1998, 54:1283–1289.

33. Holman R, Turner R, Stratton I, et al: Efficacy of atenolol and captopril in reducing risk of macrovascular and microvascular complications in type 2 diabetes: UKPDS 39. Br Med J 1998, 317:713–720.

34. Wright JT, Bakris G, Greene T, et al. for the African American Study of Kidney Disease and Hypertension Group: effect of blood pressure lowering and antihypertensive drug class on progression of hypertensives kidney disease: results from the AASK trial. JAMA 2002, 288:2421–2431.

35. Bakris GL, Mangrum A, Copley JB, et al: Effect of calcium channel or B-blockade on the progression of diabetic nephropathy in African Americans. J Hypertens 1997, 29: 744–750.

36. Bakris GL, Copley JB, Vicknair N, et al: Calcium channel blockers versus other antihypertensive therapies on progression of NIDDM associated nephropathy. Kidney Int 1996, 50:1641–1650.

37. MacLeod MJ, Mc Lay J, Drug treatment of hypertension complicating diabetes mellitus. Drugs 1998, 56:189–202.

38. Fishbane S, Nissenson AR: Early referral of patients with kidney disease: overcoming the obstacles. J Chronic Kidney Dis 2002, 1:3–6.

39. Kinchen K Sadler J, Fink N, et al: Early nephrology evaluation for chronic kidney disease in CHOICE study: patient characteristics, comorbidity, and survival in Update on chronic kidney disease. News and expert analysis of findings presented at the ASN/ISN World Congress of Nephrology, October 13–17, 2001.

40. Tisher CC, Bastl CP, Bistrian BR, et al: Morbidity and mortality of renal dialysis: an NIH Consensus Conference Statement. Ann Intern Med 1994, 121:62–70.

41. Nissenson AR, Collins AJ, Hurley J, et al: Opportunities for improving the care of patients with chronic renal insufficiency: Current practice patterns. J Am Soc Nephrol 2001, 12:1713–1720.

42. Arora P, Obrador GT, Ruthazer R, et al: Prevalence predictors and consequences of late nephrology referral at a tertiary care center. J Am Soc Nephrol 1999, 10:1281–1286.

43. Nissensen AR, Pereira BJG: Current care of patients with chronic kidney disease: opportunities fro improvement. J Chronic Kidney Dis 2002, 1:7–10.

Supine Hypertension with Orthostatic Hypotension

chapter

30

Gary L. Schwartz, M.D.

Orthostatic hypotension, which is often combined with supine hypertension, is a relatively common medical condition that is likely to increase because the population is not only aging but also becoming more obese, and, therefore, more likely to be diabetic (Table 1). This chapter reviews the pathophysiology of orthostatic hemodynamic responses, which, in turn, provides the framework for the evaluation and management of patients with this condition, which is challenging to manage.

Blood pressure (BP) decreases in the upright position because of gravitational pooling of blood in the abdomen and lower extremities. This hemodynamic change is sensed by arterial baroreceptors principally in the carotid arteries and aortic arch, which act on the brain stem to alter sympathetic and parasympathetic activity, leading to several effects that limit the BP decrease.[1] Sympathetic stimulation leads to an immediate increase in catecholamine levels and delayed activation of the renin-angiotensin-aldosterone system. Immediately, arteriolar vasoconstriction increases peripheral vascular resistance. Reflex venous constriction and augmentation of respiration increase venous return to the heart, and increases in muscle tone in the legs and abdominal muscles further augments venous return. Increased venous return is coupled with an accelerated heart rate, reflecting mainly a decrease in vagal parasympathetic tone in the initial phases. With an intact autonomic nervous system, assumption of the upright position is usually associated with a brief decline in systolic BP of only 5 to 20 mm Hg, no change or a slight increase in diastolic BP, and an increase in heart rate of 5 to 25 bpm.

Orthostatic hypotension is defined as a decline in BP upon standing associated with symptoms of organ hypoperfusion.[2,3] Common causes are shown in Table 1.[4] Transient orthostatic hypotension may occur as a benign condition in otherwise healthy people. It can be caused by non-

TABLE 1.   Disorders that Cause Orthostatic Hypotension

Primary Autonomic Failure (Generalized)
Idiopathic orthostatic hypotension (pure autonomic failure, Bradbury-Eggleston syndrome)
Idiopathic orthostatic hypotension with somatic neurologic deficit (idiopathic orthostatic
    hypotension with multiple system atrophy, Shy-Drager syndrome)
Familial dysautonomia (Riley-Day syndrome)

Primary Autonomic Failure (Partial)
Dopamine-β hydroxylase deficiency
Postural orthostatic tachycardia syndrome
Monoamine oxidase deficiency

Central Nervous System Disorders
Tumors (parasellar, hypothalamic, posterior-fossa)
Multiple cerebral infarcts
Wernicke encephalopathy
Tabes dorsalis
Myelopathies
Parkinson's disease
Syringomyelia
Dysautonomia of advanced age
Multiple sclerosis

Systemic Diseases with Autonomic Neuropathy
Diabetes mellitus
Amyloidosis
Cancer (paraneoplastic syndrome)
Uremia
Vitamin B_{12} deficiency
Guillain-Barré syndrome

Endocrine and Metabolic Disorders
Adrenocortical insufficiency (Addison's disease)
Pheochromocytoma
Hypoaldosteronism
Hypothyroidism

Disorders with Impaired Cardiac Output
Volume depletion
Impaired venous return
    Poor postural adjustment
    Varicose veins
    Prolonged recumbency
    Cachexia
Intrinsic cardiac disease
    Heart failure
    Arrhythmias
    Restrictive pericarditis

(continued)

TABLE 1. Disorders that Cause Orthostatic Hypotension (*Continued*)

Iatrogenic Disorders
Drugs (antihypertensive, psychotropic, antiparkinsonian)
Injury to carotid baroreflexes (bilateral carotid endarterectomy, radical neck surgery, radiation therapy)

Miscellaneous Disorders
Hyperbradykinism
Anorexia nervosa
Mastocytosis
Reduced aortic compliance (isolated systolic hypertension with baroreflex dysfunction)
Hypokalemia

neurogenic factors that primarily influence vascular volume, venous return, or cardiac function. Most serious causes of chronic orthostatic hypotension involve primary or secondary disorders associated with injury to the autonomic nervous system: these causes are the focus of this chapter. It should be noted that some degree of dysautonomia often accompanies aging and can be a common cause for symptomatic orthostatic hypotension in elderly individuals in the absence of other recognized disorders.

Blood Pressure and Heart Rate Profile in Neurogenic Orthostatic Hypotension

Non-invasive 24-hour monitoring of BP and heart rate allows characterization of features of orthostatic hypotension caused by disorders of autonomic function (Fig. 1).[3,5] Standing, stooping, exercising, or ingesting food can cause significant declines in BP. Symptomatic declines in BP tend to be more frequent and severe in the morning (because of overnight dehydration). In contrast to non-neurogenic orthostatic hypotension, that caused by autonomic failure is not accompanied by an expected increase in heart rate. Assumption of the supine position removes gravitational effects on vascular pooling, increasing effective circulating vascular volume and BP. However, BP normally follows a circadian pattern, with a decline of 10% accompanying the supine position during sleep at night. This decline is influenced by baroreflex-mediated changes in sympathetic and parasympathetic activity. Thus, in automatic failure, the expected decline in BP fails to occur, and, in some instances, significant increases in BP are observed. Supine hypertension can cause

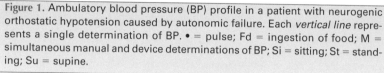

Figure 1. Ambulatory blood pressure (BP) profile in a patient with neurogenic orthostatic hypotension caused by autonomic failure. Each *vertical line* represents a single determination of BP. • = pulse; Fd = ingestion of food; M = simultaneous manual and device determinations of BP; Si = sitting; St = standing; Su = supine.

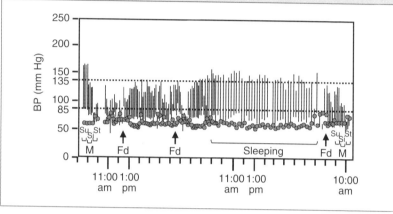

significant organ injury over time and must be monitored and treated along with management of hypotension.

Diagnosis of Orthostatic Hypotension and Supine Hypertension

Definition and Detection

A practical definition of orthostatic hypotension is a measured decrease in BP associated with symptoms of organ hypoperfusion. Formal definitions have required declines of at least 20 to 30 mm Hg in systolic BP or 10 to 15 mm Hg in diastolic BP.[2] A simple technique is to measure the patients' BP and heart rate after 2 minutes in the supine position and to repeat these measures after the patient stands for 2 minutes and after a brief period of exercise in the office. However, it is important to note that the degree of orthostatic change in BP may vary significantly throughout the day and in some patients, it may only be manifest after vigorous exercise or meals. Extended monitoring of BP by non-invasive ambulatory recording can provide essential diagnostic information.[5]

Evaluation

Many treatments for orthostatic hypotension are similar regardless of the cause. Nevertheless, treatment efficacy can be enhanced by knowledge of the specific cause. Thus, a diagnostic evaluation is important. This starts with a careful medical history, and medical and neurological examinations (Fig. 2).[4] Laboratory studies are often required. Medical laboratory tests exclude common secondary causes for orthostatic hypotension familiar to most physicians. Special tests are used to determine if the cause is autonomic nervous system dysfunction, and, if so, to determine if the predominant dysfunction is preganglionic or postganglionic, a factor that may be helpful in both making the correct diagnosis and in selecting specific treatment. Neurologic consultation is often helpful and necessary in the diagnostic evaluation.

Figure 2. Proposed diagnostic evaluation for orthostatic hypotension.

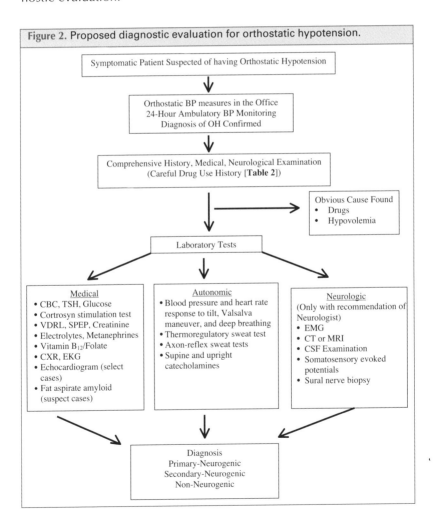

Management of Orthostatic Hypotension

Reversible Factors

In many instances of non-neurogenic orthostatic hypotension, reversal of the underlying cause is possible and may be curative. For most patients with neurogenic orthostatic hypotension, treatment involves a combination of lifestyle modifications and nonpharmacologic and pharmacologic therapy. Reversible factors that should be considered in all patients include drug use (Table 2), anemia, hypoxia, muscle deconditioning, electrolyte disturbances (hypokalemia), and hypovolemia.

Patient Education

Patient education is vital to the successful management of neurogenic orthostatic hypotension.[3] An ambulatory BP recording can serve as a useful instructional aid. Informed patients can avoid circumstances predisposing them to the risks of severe hypotension. Patients should be made aware that hypotension tends to be worse in the morning, in hot

TABLE 2. Drugs That May Cause Orthostatic Hypotension
Antihypertensives
Diuretics
Vasodilators (hydralazine, minoxidil, calcium antagonists, nitrates)
Adrenergic inhibitors (reserpine)
Alpha-adrenergic blockers (prazosin, doxazosin, terazosin, phenoxybenzamine)
Alpha-beta–adrenergic blockers (labetalol)
Central alpha-agonists (clonidine, guanfacine, methyldopa)
ACE inhibitors, ARBs
Antipsychotics
Phenothiazines, haloperidol
Antidepressants
Tricyclics
MAO inhibitors
CNS depressants
Narcotics
Benzodiazepines
Barbiturates
Alcohol
Bronchodilators
Beta-agonists
Anti-Parkinson drugs
Levodopa
Bromocriptine
Appetite suppressants
Amphetamine-like drugs
ACE = angiotensin-converting enzyme; ARB = angiotensin receptor blocker; CNS = central nervous system; MAO = monoamine oxidase inhibitor.

weather, and after meals. Prolonged upright activity at these times should be avoided. Patients with severe neurogenic orthostatic hypotension are susceptible to falls and serious injury when walking to the bathroom at night. In addition, the Valsalva maneuver that accompanies straining with defecation or urination may cause syncope attributable to an acute decline in venous return with reduction in cardiac output. Use of a bedside commode that has a reclining backrest and an adjustable footrest should be encouraged. Constipation should be prevented with a stool softener, if necessary. Autonomic failure is associated with impaired sweating; therefore, patients are susceptible to heat stroke. They should be advised to avoid prolonged heat exposure. If living in a hot climate, air conditioning is mandatory.

Because many drugs can aggravate hypotension, patients should be encouraged to seek approval before using any over-the-counter medications. Before use of medications, physicians need to contemplate the possible adverse effect of any prescribed drug on BP. For example, in patients with coronary artery disease, hypotension in the upright position may precipitate angina. Assumption of the supine position is the best initial treatment. Nitrates should be avoided initially and used only if angina persists despite assumption of the supine position. Because it is a vasodilator, alcohol use should generally be avoided or used judiciously because of its potential adverse effects on BP.[6]

Patients should sit before they stand and stand before they walk to assess for hypotensive symptoms. Heavy lifting, strenuous exercise (skeletal muscle vasodilatation), the ingestion of large meals (splanchnic vasodilatation), hot showers or baths (cutaneous vasodilatation), or working with the arms elevated should be avoided.

In more severe cases of chronic neurogenic orthostatic hypotension, limitations of lifestyle need to be honestly discussed with the patient. The goals of treatment are to protect patients from falls and syncope and to create a window of time during the day in which they can carry out essential tasks of living that require them to be in the upright position.

Nonpharmacologic Therapy

In patients with chronic orthostatic hypotension, the autoregulatory range of cerebral blood flow is shifted to lower levels of BP. Thus, many patients remain asymptomatic despite having low systemic BP. Because most treatments for orthostatic hypotension can be associated with side effects and can aggravate supine hypertension, therapy should be limited to symptomatic patients. Nonpharmacologic therapies are relatively low risk and should be considered first (Table 3).[7–12] They may be the only interventions needed in mildly symptomatic patients and provide a foundation for drug therapy for those with more severe disease.

TABLE 3. Nonpharmacologic Treatments for Orthostatic Hypotension
Diet
150 to 200 mEq sodium (4 g sodium)
2.0 to 2.5 L of fluid (400 mL water before each meal and 300 mL between meals)
High fiber (to prevent constipation)
Smaller but more frequent meals (lessens splanchnic blood pooling)
Avoid alcohol
Body Positions
Head-up tilt while sleeping at night (head of bed elevated 8 to 12 inches with blocks)
Sit at the edge of the bed for 2 to 5 minutes before standing
Stand for 1 minute before ambulating
Sleep in sitting position during the daytime (use a recliner)
Cross legs while standing
Equipment
Elastic, graded-pressure body garment
Thigh-high support stockings with abdominal binder
Derby chair
Exercise
Isotonic rather than isometric
Swimming
Aerobic water exercise
Rowing
Stationary bicycle

Diet

A high salt diet and adequate fluid intake increase vascular volume and dampen the decline in venous return that occurs with standing. Acute ingestion (< 5 minutes) of 400 to 500 mL of water increases BP by activating the sympathetic nervous system.[10] The effect of water ingestion occurs within minutes and may last for more than 1 hour. It may be particularly helpful in the management of patients with postprandial hypotension. Diet therapy is safe except for patients with impaired cardiac or renal function in whom vascular overload can be precipitated. High water intake can lead to water intoxication. Some patients have difficulty ingesting the required amount of salt through diet alone; such individuals are candidates for salt tablets given with meals (Table 4). Smaller meals lessen the degree of splanchnic pooling and are better tolerated by most patients.[9] To lessen constipation and the concomitant need to perform the Valsalva maneuver, high fiber intake is encouraged. A dietitian is often helpful in designing a diet that improves BP and is still healthy.

TABLE 4.	Drug Treatments for Orthostatic Hypotension	
Drug/Mechanism	**Dose**	**Comments**
Plasma Volume Expansion		
9α-fludrocortisone (Florinef) Mineralocorticoid increases vascular volume	0.1 mg/day; increase as needed to maximum of 1.0 mg /day given in one or two doses	Increase dose weekly until symptoms improve or mild peripheral edema occurs Monitor plasma potassium Caution if impaired cardiac or renal function
Sodium chloride tablets Indomethacin (Indocin) Blocks production of renal natriuretic prostaglandins	1–3 tablets TID w/ food 25 to 50 mg TID with meals	May cause nausea Discontinue after 6 weeks if no benefit Major concerns are gastric irritation and long-term renal effects
Ibuprofen (Motrin) Blocks production of renal natriuretic prostaglandins	200 to 600 mg TID with food	Discontinue after 6 weeks if no benefit Major concerns are gastric irritation and long-term renal effects
Desmopressin (DDAVP) Acts on vasopressin-2 renal tubular receptors to promote water reabsorption	Nasal spray (5 to 40 μg intranasally at bedtime) or 100 to 400 μg in tabletform at bedtime	Reduces nocturnal polyuria Can cause hyponatremia
Vasoconstriction		
Midodrine (Proamitine) Peripheral α-receptor agonist that acts on resistance vessels and venous capacitance vessels	2.5 to 10.0 mg TID; dose interval of 3 to 4 hours; do not give after evening meal or within 4 hours of bedtime	Do not use in setting of severe heart disease, urinary retention, or acute renal disease Side effects include scalp itching, piloerection, headache, urinary retention Do not use with cardiac glycosides
Methylphenidate (Ritalin) Indirect sympathomimetic agent	5 to 10 mg TID 15 to 30 minutes before meals; none after 6 pm	Side effects include CNS stimulation, tolerance, dependence
Ephedrine sulfate Indirect sympathomimetic	12.5 to 75.0 mg TID	Side effects include tremulousness, apetite suppression, urinary retention Useful in central autonomic disorders (Shy-Drager syndrome)
Yohimbine (Yohimex) α2-Adrenergic antagonist that acts centrally to enhance sympathetic outflow and potentiates norepinephrine release peripherally by blocking presynaptic receptors	2.0 to 6.0 mg BID or TID	Anxiety, nervousness, and diarrhea are side effects Useful in setting of partial adrenergic failure

(continued)

TABLE 4. Drug Treatments for Orthostatic Hypotension (*Continued*)

Drug/Mechanism	Dose	Comments
Vasoconstriction (*continued*)		
Clonidine (Catapres) α-agonist that acts peripherally to increase peripheral vascular resistance and venous return	0.1 to 0.8 mg BID or TID	Most effective in severe peripheral autonomic failure when norepinephrine level is low Also effective in baroreflex failure syndrome Side effects include sedation and dry mouth
Phenylephrine (Neo-Synephrine) Direct sympathomimetic agent	Nasal spray	Short-acting drug can be used as needed immediately before prolonged upright activity
Dihydroergotamine (DHE-45) Constriction of venous capacitance vessels	2.5 to 10.0 mg BID to QID	Can cause ergotism
Postprandial Hypotension		
Caffeine Adenosine receptor blocker Prevents adenosine-mediated splanchnic vasodilation	1 to 3 cups of coffee or caffeine tablets (No-Doz) given once daily in am	Helpful for postprandial hypotension Tolerance can develop with chronic use
Octreotide (Sandostatin) Prevents release of gut vasodilatory peptides	25 to 200 μg subcutaneously BID or TID	Very expensive
Impair Vasodilatation		
Metoclopramide (Reglan) Dopamine receptor blocker	5 to 10 mg TID before meals	Effective when dopamine levels are high Helpful for gastroparesis accompanying autonomic failure because it promotes gastric emptying
Propranolol (Inderal) β_2-adrenoreceptor blocker	10 to 40 mg QID	Side effects include hypotension and bradycardia Avoid in setting of bronchospastic lung disease
Pindolol (Visken) Partial beta-agonist activity; increases cardiac output	2.5 to 5.0 mg BID or TID	Most effective in severe peripheral autonomic failure when norepinephrine is low
Correct Anemia		
Erythropoietin (Procrit) Increases red cell mass and improves cerebral oxygenation.	50 μg/kg body weight three times weekly for 6–8 weeks	Use to correct anemia in absence of known reversible causes Give oral iron during treatment period

BID = twice a day; CNS = central nervous system; TID = three times a day; QID = four times a day

Sleeping Position

Sleeping at night with the head of the bed tilted to 45-degrees places patients in a semi-upright position.[8] The prolonged exposure to the associated lower BP may help shift cerebral autoregulation to lower levels of systemic BP and, therefore, decrease symptoms during the day even in the absence of BP changes. In addition, the renin-angiotensin-aldosterone axis may be stimulated, which may decrease the fluid and salt losses that often occur at night. Head-up tilt also decreases the frequency of nocturia and the concomitant need to get out of bed at night. For similar reasons, rest during the day should occur in a semi-upright position. This can be accomplished by using a recliner. Crossing the legs when standing improves venous return and is often helpful to decrease symptoms associated with prolonged standing.[12] Patients need to develop the habit of avoiding going from the supine to the standing position quickly. They should discipline themselves to sit at the bedside for several minutes and then stand at the bedside for at least 1 minute before walking. If symptoms of hypotension occur, patients can immediately put themselves into a safe position.

Anti-gravity Measures

Venous pooling when upright can be lessened with the use of an elasticized graded-pressure leotard available commercially.[11] These custom-fit garments produce a gradient of counter pressure that is maximal in the lower extremities. Waist-high leotards may be sufficient in milder cases, but in more severe cases, garments that fit under the costal margin provide the added benefit of reducing splanchnic pooling. Leotards should be put on first thing in the morning while the patient is supine and taken off before sleep at the end of the day. They can be fit with an open crotch to facilitate urination. Patients should buy two pairs so one can be worn while the other is being washed. Washing should be done by hand. An alternative to leotards is use of thigh-high graded support stockings designed to provide 30 to 40 mm Hg of maximum counter pressure. These can be used with or without an abdominal binder to reduce splanchnic pooling. A "derby chair" is a cane that can be quickly unfolded into a chair. This allows ambulating patients to get into a safe position wherever symptoms of hypotension occur.[13]

Exercise

Mild aerobic exercise is encouraged. Satisfactory leg muscle tone facilitates venous return. Symptomatic hypotension can be totally alleviated with immersion; therefore, swimming or other aerobic activities in the water are excellent forms of exercise. An alternative horizontal exercise is rowing. Vigorous exercise can aggravate hypotension by depleting catecholamines and inducing skeletal muscle vasodilation.[14]

Pharmacological Therapy

If nonpharmacologic interventions fail, drug therapy is the next step. Because drugs are often associated with side effects and can aggravate supine hypertension, they should be used initially as monotherapy; however, multiple drugs in combination are often required to achieve symptomatic improvement.

Midodrine (Proamitine) is the only drug currently approved by the Food and Drug Administration for the treatment of patients with orthostatic hypotension. The value of many of the drugs currently used to treat this disorder has not been definitively determined in prospective trials. Similar to the strategy of treating patients with essential hypertension, the effectiveness of a single drug should be assessed for a 6 to 8-week period. If it is partially effective and well tolerated, the dose should be increased or a second drug added to the program. If it is providing no symptomatic relief and is poorly tolerated, it should be discontinued and another agent tried. Available drugs are listed in Table 4. All of the drugs used to limit orthostatic hypotension can induce severe supine hypertension. Therefore, careful monitoring of supine BP is required when any of the available drugs is used. It is important to assess the effect of any drug on symptoms as well as BP. Many patients experience symptomatic relief without objective improvement in BP. In this regard, it should be remembered that the major goal of treatment is symptom relief. In general, first-step drugs are those that increase vascular volume.[15–17] Second-step drugs increase peripheral vascular resistance or decrease venous capacitance.[18–21] Other drugs are useful under selective conditions.[22–27] A proposed algorithm is outlined in Figure 3.

Management of Supine Hypertension

Treatment of patients with supine hypertension involves several strategies (Table 5). The most important first step is to recognize that it often accompanies neurogenic orthostatic hypotension and is aggravated by all pressor therapies. Careful monitoring of supine BP is mandatory. Noninvasive ambulatory BP monitoring may be helpful in this regard, especially if signs of hypertensive target organ injury (e.g., left ventricular hypertrophy, proteinuria) evolve. Body position is the most effective and consistent tool in the management of supine hypertension. This involves rest in the semi-upright position, both during the daytime (recliner) and at night (head-up tilt). Pressor therapies should be avoided before anticipated periods of prolonged rest in the supine position dur-

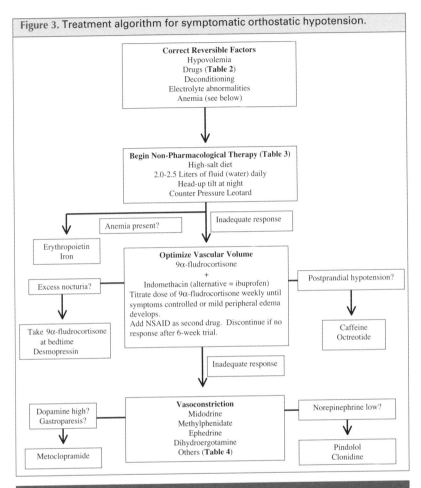

Figure 3. Treatment algorithm for symptomatic orthostatic hypotension.

TABLE 5. Treatments for Supine Hypertension

Monitor supine BP level
Periodically assess for evolving hypertensive target organ injury
Use the semi-upright body position during rest
Avoid pressor therapy before rest during the day or within 4 hours of bedtime
Adjust doses of pressor therapies
Mild exercise before bedtime
Have carbohydrate snack before bedtime
Drink small doses of alcohol at bedtime
Vasodilator drugs at bedtime:
   Nifedipine: 10 to –20 mg orally
   Diltiazem: 30 to 60 mg orally
   Verapamil: 80 mg orally
   Hydralazine: 10 to 25 mg orally

BP = blood pressure

ing the daytime or within 4 hours of bedtime. Severe supine hypertension may limit the use of pressor therapies and force a dosage reduction. Often this results in compromising the degree of symptomatic relief of standing hypotension. By causing muscle vasodilation, mild exercise before bedtime may be helpful. By causing splanchnic pooling and the release of vasodilatory peptides from the gut, a bedtime snack may also help lower supine BP. Also, because it acts as a vasodilator, a small amount of alcohol at bedtime may lessen supine hypertension. Finally, small doses of short-acting vasodilators given at bedtime may be useful.

References

1. Joyner MJ, Shepherd JT: Autonomic control of Circulation. In Low PA (ed): Clinical Autonomic Disorders. Boston, Little, Brown and Company, 1993, pp. 55–67.
2. Mathias CJ, Kimber JR: Postural hypotension: causes, clinical features, investigation, and management. Annu Rev Med 1999, 50:317–336.
3. Schwartz GL, Schirger A: Idiopathic orthostatic hypotension and supine hypertension. In Cook JP and Frolich ED (eds): Current Management of Hypertensive and Vascular Diseases. St. Louis, Mosby-Yearbook, Inc., 1994, pp 82–86.
4. Fealey RD, Robertson D: Management of orthostatic hypotension. In Low PA (ed): Clinical Autonomic Disorders. Boston, Little, Brown and Company, 1993, pp 731–743.
5. National High Blood Pressure Education Coordinating Committee: National High Blood Pressure Education Program Working Group report on ambulatory blood pressure monitoring. Arch Intern Med 1990, 150:2270–2280.
6. Chaudhuri KR, Maule S, Thomaides T, et al: Alcohol ingestion lowers supine blood pressure, causes splanchnic vasodilatation and worsens postural hypotension in primary autonomic failure. J Neurol 1994, 241:145–152.
7. Bachman DM, Youmans WB: Effects of posture on renal excretion of sodium and chloride in orthostatic hypotension. Circulation 1953, 7:413–421.
8. MacLean AR, Allen EV: Orthostatic hypotension and orthostatic tachycardia: treatment with the "head-up" bed. JAMA 1940, 115:2162–2167.
9. Mathias CJ, Holly E, Armstrong E, et al: The influence of food on postural hypotension in three groups with chronic autonomic failure: clinical and therapeutic implications. J Neurol Neurosurg Psychiatry 1991, 54:726–730.
10. Shannon JR, Diedrich A, Biaggioni I, et al: Water drinking as a treatment for orthostatic syndromes. Am J Med 2002, 112:355–360.
11. Sheps SG: Use of an elastic garment in the treatment of orthostatic hypotension. Cardiology 1976, 61(suppl 1):271–279.
12. Wieling W, van Lieshout JJ, van Leeuwen AM: Physical maneuvers that reduce postural hypotension. Clin Auton Res 1993, 3:57–65.
13. Smit AAJ, Hardjowijono MA, Wieling W: Are portable folding chairs useful to combat orthostatic hypotension? Ann Neurol 1997, 42:975–978.
14. Puvi-Rajasingham S, Smith GD, Akinola A, Mathias CJ: Abnormal regional blood flow responses during and after exercise in human sympathetic denervation. J Physiol 1997, 505(pt 3):841–849.
15. Chobanian AV, Volicer L, Tifft CP, et al: Mineralocorticoid-induced hypertension in patients with orthostatic hypotension. N Engl J Med 1979, 301:68–73.

16. Hickler RB, Thompson GR, Fox LM, Hamlin JT: Successful treatment of orthostatic hypotension with 9-alpha-fluorohydrocortisone. N Engl J Med 1959, 261:788–791.

17. Kochar MS, Itskowitz HD, Aolbers JW: Treatment of orthostatic hypotension with Indomethacin. Am Heart J 1979, 98:271–280.

18. Chobanian AV, Volicer L, Liang CS, et al: Use of propranolol in the treatment of idiopathic orthostatic hypotension. Trans Assoc Am Physicians 1977, 90:324–334.

19. Davies B, Bannister R, Sever P: Pressor amines and monoamine oxidase inhibitors for treatment of postural hypotension in autonomic failure: limitations and hazards. Lancet 1978, 1:172–175.

20. Jankovic J, Gilden JLD, Heine BC, et al: Neurogenic orthostatic hypotension: a double blind, placebo-controlled study with midodrine. Am J Med 1993, 95:38–48.

21. Low PA, Gilden JL, Freeman R, et al: Efficacy of midodrine vs placebo in neurogenic orthostatic hypotension: a randomized, double blind multicenter study. J Am Med Assoc 1997, 277:1046–1051.

22. Alam M, Smith GDP, Bleasdale-Barr K, et al: Effects of the peptide release inhibitor, octreotide, on daytime hypotension and on nocturnal hypertension in primary autonomic failure. J Hypertens 1995, 13:1664–1669.

23. Armstrong E, Mathias CJ: The effects of the somatostatin analogue, octreotide, on postural hypotension, before and after food ingestion in primary autonomic failure. Clin Auton Res 1991, 2:135–140.

24. Hoeldke RD, Streeten DH: Treatment of orthostatic hypotension with erythropoietin. N Eng J Med 1993, 329:611–615.

25. Mathias CJ, Fosbraey P, da Costa DF, et al: The effect of desmopressin on nocturnal polyuria, overnight weight loss, and morning postural hypotension in patients with autonomic failure. Br Med J 1986, 293:353–354.

26. Onrot J, Goldberg MR, Biaggioni I, et al: Hemodynamic and humeral effects of caffeine in human autonomic failure. N Engl J Med 1986, 313:549–554.

27. de Caestecker JS, Ewing DJ, Tothill P, et al: Evaluation of oral cisapride and metoclopramide in diabetic autonomic neuropathy: an eight week double-blind crossover study. Aliment Pharmacol Ther 1989, 3:69–81.

Management of Renovascular Hypertension

chapter
31

Michael J. Bloch, M.D., and
Jan Basile, M.D.

The true prevalence of renovascular hypertension (RVH) is unknown but probably accounts for between 0.2% and 5.0% of hypertension. The diagnosis is important because RVH contributes to uncontrolled hypertension and increases the risk of developing renal insufficiency.

There is probably no topic in hypertension management with less consensus than RVH. Lack of consensus exists because renovascular disease (RVD) is a complex disorder with various causes and presentations. The most common causes of RVD are *fibromuscular dysplasia* (FMD) and *atherosclerosis*. FMD tends to present in young women but many cases are not diagnosed until after age 40 years. Atherosclerotic disease is usually seen in older patients with traditional risk factors.

The diagnosis and management of patients with FMD is usually rather straightforward, and there is generally a good clinical response to interventions such as percutaneous renal artery angioplasty (PTRA). In contrast, patients with atherosclerotic disease can be extremely difficult to evaluate and manage. Patients with atherosclerotic RVD often have coexistent essential hypertension, progressive loss of renal function is common, and response to intervention is often suboptimal. Because they tend to have atherosclerosis in other vascular beds, patients with atherosclerotic RVD are also prone to complications such as stroke, myocardial infarction, and cardiovascular death. Because FMD and atherosclerotic RVD are two distinct diseases, their diagnostic and treatment strategies differ considerably.

The confusion associated with RVD comes from a lack of understanding concerning three terms: *renal artery stenosis* (RAS), a purely anatomic diagnosis of an obstructive lesion within the renal artery; *renovascular hypertension* (RVH), a clinical diagnosis referring to hypertension that occurs as the direct physiological result of a RAS; and *ischemic nephropathy,* progressive loss of renal function caused by an obstructive renal artery lesion. Ischemic nephropathy usually requires global renal ischemia (i.e., bilateral RAS, RAS in the artery to a single kidney, or unilateral RAS with a damaged contralateral kidney).

The mere demonstration of RAS in a patient with hypertension does not necessarily constitute RVH. Anatomically apparent renal artery lesions without physiologic significance are often found in patients with both essential hypertension and normal blood pressure (BP). This makes the diagnosis of clinical RVH more difficult and calls into question the controversial practice of routine "drive-by" renal angioplasty in patients undergoing coronary or peripheral angiography.

Moreover, especially in patients with atherosclerosis, many physicians are surprised with the lack of efficacy from renal arterial revasculation procedures. With the advent of agents that block the renin-angiotensin system, medical management has become a viable option for many patients. When reviewing the data, one theme is readily apparent: no one diagnostic and therapeutic approach is acceptable for all patients. Instead, a flexible, individualized approach, based on suspected cause and presentation, is necessary.

Diagnosis

The Importance of High Clinical Suspicion

As in most diseases, the most important factor in the treatment of patients with RVH is making the appropriate diagnosis. The relatively low prevalence of RVH makes inappropriate universal screening of all patients with hypertension or renal insufficiency. Limiting screening to patients with clinical clues suggestive of RVD (Table 1) leads to a higher positive and negative predictive value for diagnostic studies.

See Chapter 9 for a detailed outline of the approach to establishing the diagnosis of RVH.

General Issues in the Management of Renovascular Disease

The optimal management of patients with RVD is not well established given the limited number of high-quality randomized, controlled treatment trials. Management choices include medical management, percutanous interventions (PTRA and stenting), and surgical revascularization. The goals of management are to control BP, preserve renal function, and avoid complications and adverse effects of treatment.

Percutaneous or surgical intervention for renal artery disease should be undertaken only when there is evidence that the RAS has clinical consequence (RVH or ischemic nephropathy). Intervention should not be undertaken for isolated anatomic disease, and renal artery lesions do not usually attain functional significance until they obstruct at least 70% of the vessel lumen. Furthermore, the relief of stenosis does not always lead to clinical improvement.

The management of patients with RVD is made more difficult by the nature of the available data. Studies of management options suffer from striking differences in methodology, and many studies combine patients with FMD and atherosclerotic disease. Definitions of response also remain troublesome. In studies of RVH, BP is classified as "cured," "improved," "stable," or "worse," with little standardization of these definitions. Most studies define "improvement" as a decrease in the number of antihypertensive medications taken rather than normalization of BP. Also, "stabilization" of renal function (i.e., no change in serum creatinine level at follow-up) is usually presumed to be a beneficial result of intervention, but this may simply be a result of the natural history of the disease process.

Surgical Revascularization

For many years, surgical revascularization was the treatment of choice for patients with RVD. Given the significant morbidity and mortality associated with surgical revascularization in patients with atherosclerotic renal artery disease, this option is now usually reserved for patients with concomitant aortic aneurysms requiring repair or complex lesions that are not amenable to, or who have failed, previous PTRA and stenting. Surgical options include endarterectomy, aortorenal bypass, and extra-anatomic bypass (i.e., bypass from the celiac or mesenteric branches). Most studies of surgical revascularization have shown excellent long-term vessel patency, clinical improvement in hypertension, and preservation of renal function.[2,3] Perioperative mortality rates range from 1% to 6% and are generally higher with concurrent repair of aortic aneurysms.

Percutaneous Renal Artery Angioplasty and Stenting

Patients with FMD usually show an impressive clinical and anatomical response to percutaneous renal artery angioplasty (PTRA). Technical success approaches 100%, and there is a substantial hypertension "cure" rate of approximately 40% to 50%. BP is "improved" in an additional 40% to 50% of patients with FMD.[4–7] Based on these data, PTRA is generally considered to be the initial procedure of choice for patients with RVH caused by FMD.

In contrast, atheromatous disease, especially when occurring at the ostium, responds less well to PTRA as a result of elastic recoil of the renal artery and early restenosis. Endoluminal stent deployment was developed to overcome this obstacle, and its use has increased in recent years. Although the current indications for stenting include poor angiographic response to routine PTRA, early restenosis after PTRA, and renal artery dissection during PTRA, a number of centers have begun routinely stenting all ostial lesions. Figure 1 illustrates an example of a right ostial renal artery stenosis before and after stenting.

Reported technical success rates in contemporary studies using renal artery stenting are usually greater than 90%. Although little data directly compare stenting to PTRA alone, the reported BP responses with stenting are generally better. Table 1 illustrates the BP results from some of the largest and most recent trials of renal artery stenting.[8–15] Rates of "cure" vary from 0% to 16% to and "improvement" from 35% to 76%. Remember, however, that PTRA and stenting often reduce, but rarely eliminate, the need for antihypertensive medications in patients with atherosclerotic RVH.

Potential complications, which occur in approximately 10% to 20% of procedures, include groin hematoma or pseudoaneurysm, renal artery dissection or thrombosis, atheroembolism, and acute renal failure. Patients with atherosclerosis are more likely to have complications than those with fibromuscular disease. The presence of extensive aortic atherosclerosis, significant cardiovascular disease, chronic renal failure, and the use of stents also lead to increased risk.

Preservation of Renal Function with Percutaneous Renal Artery Angioplasty and Stenting

In recent years, the emphasis of renal artery intervention has shifted from BP control to preservation of renal function. In general, contemporary reports of percutaneous intervention, most using stents, show that approximately one third of patients show long-term improvement, one third show stability, and one third show worsening of renal function.[8–9,12,16–20] Clinical clues that suggest a poor clinical outcome even after intervention include long-standing hypertension or renal dysfunction, kidney size less than 8 cm, serum creatinine level greater than 3.5 or 4.0 mg/dl and another potential cause of renal dysfunction (e.g., diabetes).

Because RVD is presumed to be a progressive disease, many clinicians equate no change in renal function after a procedure with clinical benefit. Similarly, any worsening of renal function is presumed to be secondary to underlying disease progression rather than procedural complications such as atheroembolism, a process that is underdiagnosed. Although atheroembolism after a procedure may produce an acute reduction in renal function, the deterioration may also be progressive over a period of weeks. Although older anatomic studies of RAS

Figure 1. Conventional contrast angiogram showing a high-grade renal artery stenosis at the ostium of the right renal artery consistent with atherosclerotic disease (**A**) before and (**B**) after renal artery stent placement.

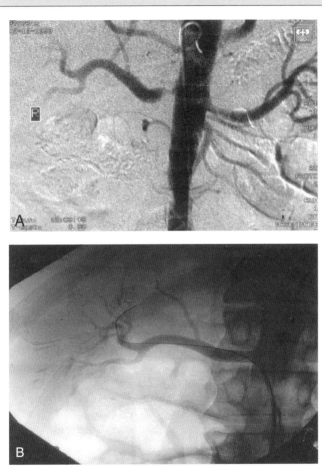

show that 36% to 63% of all lesions progress (8% to 16% to complete occlusion) over a 2- to 5-year period,[21–23] we have had little data about the risk of clinical disease progression.

A recent prospective study[24] of 122 subjects with RVD showed that only 20.8% of subjects with a lesion greater than 60% at baseline had a decrease in renal size on ultrasound over approximately 3 to 5 years of follow-up. A similar study[25] of 126 subjects with incidentally discovered RAS greater than 50% found that serum creatinine level remained stable over 10 years of follow-up, and none of these patients required renal replacement therapy (e.g., transplantation or dialysis). Although a subset of patients do require intervention to delay the progression of renal failure, a large group of patients do not progress to renal failure even without intervention.

			Mean				
Reference	Year	Patients, n	Follow-up, months	Cure, %	Improve, %	Stable, %	Worse, %
van de Ven et al.[8]	1995	22	9.0	0.0	72.7	22.7	4.5
Iannone et al.[9]	1996	63	10.2	3.7	35.2	53.7	7.4
Bosiclari et al.[15]	1997	33	13.4	6.0	61.0	33.0*	
White et al.[13]	1997	100	6.0		76†	24.0*	
Dorros et al.[10]	1998	106	24.0	1.0	52.0	47.0*	
Blum et al.[11]	1997	68	27.0	16.2	61.8	22.0*	
Tuttle et al.[12]	1998	129	24.0	0.0	55.0	32.0	13.0
Rodriguez-Lopez et al.[14]	1999	108	36.0	13.0	55.0	27.0	5.0

TABLE 1. Blood Pressure Response to Renal Artery Stent Placement

*No improvement (combined endpoint of stable + worse).
†Normalization of BP (< 150/90 mm Hg).

Medical Management

Medical management is an aggressive pharmacological approach, not simply watchful waiting. Because it is a systemic disease, aggressive medical management of patients with atherosclerotic RAS requires not only BP medications but also antiplatelet agents, lipid-lowering therapy, diabetes care (when appropriate), and smoking cessation, and other appropriate lifestyle changes. The most common cause of death in patients with atherosclerotic RVD is cardiovascular disease.

Several well-designed trials have reported good BP control using combinations of antihypertensive medications, including ACE inhibi-tors.[26,27] In one such study of 188 patients with RVH, 3 months of treatment with captopril-based therapy led to complete control of BP in 74% of subjects, partial control in 8%, and no improvement in only 5%. Although acute deterioration in renal function has been well documented in patients with bilateral RAS treated with ACE inhibitors and reluctance to use ACE inhibitors (and ARBs) in RVH continues to occur, the risk of worsening renal function has been overstated. When acute renal failure does occur from ACE inhibition, it is fully reversible by stopping the drug. For example, in one study[28] of 32 patients with RVH who were treated with captopril and a diuretic for a mean of 49 weeks, only six patients (19%) developed significant increases in serum creatinine even though 66% of these subjects had either bilateral disease or stenosis in the artery to a solitary kidney.

Medical Versus Interventional Therapy

In patients with FMD, percutaneous (or surgical) management is generally considered superior because it is associated with low risk and can offer a potential cure of hypertension.

In patients with atherosclerotic disease the question is more complex. Recently, prospective randomized trials[29-31] (Table 2) compared BP results in subjects treated medically versus PTRA. Although these studies have significant limitations, it appears that a substantial number of patients can achieve reasonable BP control with medication alone without significant deterioration in renal function.

TABLE 2. Prospective Randomized Trials Comparing Blood Pressure Control with Medical Management or PTRA				
	Patients	Length of	BP achieved, mm Hg	
Study	Randomized, *n*	Follow-up, months	Medical	PTR
Scottish and Newcastle Unilateral[29]	27	6 months	168/91	177/93
Scottish and Newcastle Bilateral[29]	28	12 months	171/91	155/80
EMMA[30]	49	6 months	141/85	140/81
DRASTIC[31]	106	3 months	176/101	169/99

DRASTIC = Dutch Renal Artery Stenosis Intervention Cooperative; EMMA = Essai Multicentrique Medicaments v. Angioplastie.

When reviewing the available data, it is clear that there is no one single ideal management option for all patients with RVD. However, it is clear that careful risk–benefit assessment should be undertaken with each patient. With our aging population, RVH is occurring in an older and generally sicker population than we saw a decade ago. These older patients, many with diffuse atherosclerosis, may have a greater risk of complications with percuataneous interventions.

Although it may not be appropriate for all patients (e.g., those with rapidly progressive disease or very high-grade lesions that have substantial risk for occlusion), a potential treatment algorithm is presented in Figure 2. No matter which initial course is taken, medical management of associated risk factors and close surveillance remain important. In order to monitor for renal function decline, it is necessary to measure serum creatinine level at least once every 3 months and renal sonography once a year or more frequently as guided by changes in renal function.

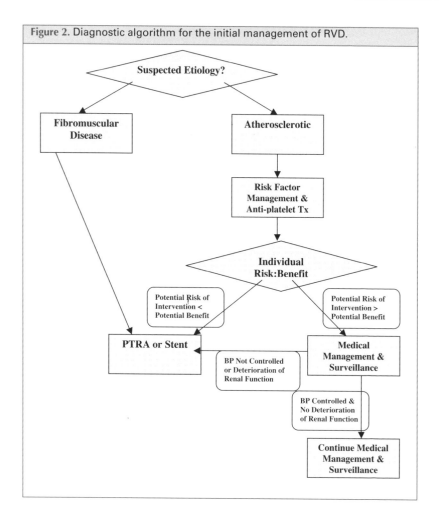

Figure 2. Diagnostic algorithm for the initial management of RVD.

References

1. Safian RD, Textor SC: Renal-artery stenosis. New Eng J Med 2001, 344:431–442.
2. Libertino JA, Bosco PJ, Ting CY: Renal revascularization to preserve and restore renal function. J Urol 1982, 145:1485–1487.
3. Hansen JF, Starr SM, Sands RE, et al: Contemporary surgical management of renovascular disease. Urol Clin North Am 1984, 11:435–449.
4. Sos TA, Pickering TG, Sniderman K, et al: Percutaneous transluminal angioplasty in renovascular hypertension due to atheroma or fibromuscular dysplasia. N Eng J Med 1983, 309:274–279.
5. Bonelli FS, McKusick MA, Textor SC, et al: Renal artery angioplasty: technical results and clinical outcome in 320 patients. Mayo Clin Proc 1995, 70:1041–1052.

6. Libertino JA, Beckmann CF: Surgery and percutaneous angioplasty in the management of renovascular hypertension. Urol Clin N Am 1994, 21:235–243.

7. Cluzel P, Raynaud A, Beyssen B, et al: Stenosis of renal branch arteries in fibromuscular dysplasia: results of percutaneous transluminal angioplasty. Radiology 1994, 193:227–232.

8. van de Ven PJG, Beutler JJ, Daatee R, et al: Transluminal vascular stent for ostial atherosclerotic renal artery stenosis. Lancet 1995, 346:672–674.

9. Iannone LA, Underwood PL, Nath A, et al: Effect of primary balloon expandable renal artery stents on long-term patency, renal function and blood pressure in hypertensive and renal insufficient patients with renal artery stenosis. Cathet Cardiovasc Diagn 1996, 37:243–250.

10. Dorros G, Jaff M, Mathiak L, et al: Four year follow-up of palmaz-shatz stent revascularization as treatment for atherosclerotic renal artery stenosis. Circulation 1998, 98:642–647.

11. Blum U, Flugel P, Gabelmann A, et al: Treatment of ostial renal artery stenoses with vascular endoprosthesis after unsuccessful balloon angioplasty. N Eng J Med 1997, 337:459–465.

12. Tuttle KR, Chouinard RF, Webber JT, et al: Treatment of atherosclerotic ostial renal artery stenosis with intravascular stent. Am J Kidney Dis 1998, 32:611–622.

13. White CJ, Ramee SR, Collins TJ: Renal artery stent placement: utility in lesions difficult to treat with balloon angioplasty. 1997, 30:1445–1450.

14. Rodriguez-Lopez JA, Werner A, Ray LI, et al: Renal artery stenosis treated with stent deployment: indications technique and outcome for 108 patients. J Vasc Surg 1999, 29:617–624.

15. Bosiclair C, Therasse E, Oliva VL, et al: Treatment of renal angioplasty failure by percutaneous renal artery stenting with palmaz stents: mid-term technical and clinical results. Am J Roentgenol 1997, 168:245–251.

16. Rees CR, Palmaz JC, Becker GJ, et al: Palmaz stent in atherosclerotic stenosis involving the ostia of the renal arteries: preliminary report of a multicenter study. Radiology 1991, 181:507–514.

17. Hennequin LM, Joffre FG, Rousseau HP, et al: Renal artery stent placement: long term results with the wallstent endoprosthesis. Radiology 1994, 191:713–719.

18. Raynaud AC, Beyssen BM, Turmel-Rodigues LE, et al: Renal artery stent placement: intermediate and mid-term results. J Vasc Surg Intervent Radiol 1994, 5:849–858.

19. Watson PS, Hadjipetrou P, Cox SV, et al: Effect of renal artery stenting on renal function and size in patients with atherosclerotic renovascular disease. Circulation 2000, 102:1671–1677.

20. Taylor A, Sheppard D, MacLeod MJ: Renal artery stent placement in renal artery stenosis: technical and early clinical results. Clin Radiol 1997, 52:451–457.

21. Novick AC: Atherosclerotic ischemic nephropathy: epidemiology and clinical considerations. Urol Clin North Am 1994, 21:195–200.

22. Stewart BH, Dustan HP, Kiser WS, et al: Correlation of angiography and natural history in evaluation of patients with renovascular hypertension. J Urol 1970, 104:231–238.

23. Tollefson DE, Ernst CB: Natural history of atherosclerotic renal artery stenosis associated with aortic disease. J Vasc Surg 1991, 14:327–331.

24. Caps MT, Zierler E, Polissar NL, et al: Risk of atrophy in kidneys with atherosclerotic renal artery stenosis. Kidney Int 1998, 53:735–742.

25. Leertouwer TC, Pattynama PMT, Van Den Berg-Hysmans A: Incidental renal artery stenosis in peripheral vascular disease: a case for treatment? Kidney Int 2000, 59:1480–1483.

26. Hollenberg NK: Medical therapy of renovascular hypertension: efficacy and safety of captopril in 269 patients. Cardiovasc Review and Reports 1983, 4:852–876.

27. Franklin SS, Smith RD: Comparison of effects of enalapril plus hydrochlorothiazide versus standard triple therapy on renal function in renovascular hypertension. Am J Med 1985, 79(suppl):14–23.

28. Jackson B, Matthews PG, McGrath BP, Johnston CI: Angiotensin converting enzyme inhibition in renovascular hypertension: frequency of reversible renal failure. Lancet 1984, 28:225–226.

29. Webster J, Marshall F, Abdalla M, et al: Randomized comparison of percutaneous angioplasty vs continued medical therapy for hypertensive patients with atheromatous renal artery stenosis. J Human Hypertens 1998, 12:329–335.

30. Plouin PF, Chatellier G, Darne B, Raynaud A: Blood pressure outcome of angioplasty in atherosclerotic renal artery stenosis: a randomized trial. Hypertension 1998, 31: 823–829.

31. van Jaarsveld BC, Krijnen P, Pieterman H et al: The effect of balloon angioplasty on hypertension in atherosclerotic renal-artery stenosis: Dutch Renal Artery Stenosis Intervention Cooperative Study Group. N Engl J Med 2000, 342:1007–1014.

HOT TOPICS

Management of Transplant Hypertension

chapter
32

C. Venkata S. Ram, M.D. and
Pedro Vergne-Marini, M.D.

Systemic hypertension is an important and a common complication after organ transplantation.[1–5] Hypertension in organ transplant recipients is a major cause of cardiovascular morbidity and mortality; cardiovascular disease is the principal cause of mortality in renal transplant patients.[5] Furthermore, hypertension is an independent, powerful risk factor for graft failure.[6–8] The universal development of hypertension among transplant recipients requires aggressive treatment. The manifestations of hypertension such as left ventricular hypertrophy, congestive heart failure, coronary artery disease, and strokes also occur in transplant recipients, just as in the nontransplant population. Thus, early and vigorous blood pressure (BP) control in transplant recipients is mandatory. It has been suggested that proper control of hypertension is the only consistent predictor of long-term graft survival.[9]

Causes and Mechanisms of Hypertension in Transplant Patients

Most patients with renal failure who undergo organ transplantation are already receiving multiple antihypertensive drugs. However, the severity of hypertension before transplantation does not predict posttransplant hypertension because of the variable success of allograft (insertion), steroid, and cyclosporine usage. A large number of renal transplant patients develop hypertension. Although the introduction of cyclosporine has had a significant impact on allograft (and patient) survival, it is also responsible for the development and sustenance of hypertension in the transplant population.[10,11] Cyclosporine therapy not only causes significant hypertension but has also changed the pathophysiology of BP control mechanisms in the transplant population. Because of the dynamic and aggressive vascular pathophysiological mechanisms (Table 1)

TABLE 1.   Possible Vascular Abnormalities in Posttransplantation Hypertension

Condition	Mechanism
Chronic rejection	Intrarenal narrowing of small blood vessels
Renal artery stenosis	Obstruction of major vessel
Cyclosporine	Predominantly preglomerular vasoconstriction or sympathetic activation
Native kidneys	Angiotensin-induced vasoconstriction

causing posttransplantation hypertension, treatment should be directed against the underlying causes, including adjustment in the dosages of immunosuppressive drugs.

Until the availability of cyclosporine, posttransplant hypertension was mainly by a renin-mediated mechanism[12,13], but with immunosuppressive drugs, several mechanisms may be operational independently or via several interacting causes. In evaluating patients with posttransplantation hypertension, certain possible causes (Table 2) should be carefully considered before initiating antihypertensive drug therapy. Among the important etiological factors, use of cyclosporine, steroids, and tacrolimus should be considered. During the pre-cyclosporine era, chronic rejection frequently caused hypertension in transplant recipients. Other nephrotoxic agents such as amphotericin, aminoglycosides, and nonsteroidal anti-inflammatory drugs can also lead to significant hypertension in the transplant patients. Despite therapeutic advances in immunosuppression, corticosteroids are needed for most transplant patients, and these drugs often elevate systemic BP.[14,15] Fortunately, corticosteroid dosage can be reduced with use of newer immunosuppressive regimens. Discontinuation of corticosteroids in stable patients may alleviate hypertension.[5]

Calcineurin inhibitors (e.g., cyclosporine or tacrolimus), which are essential for transplant recipients, cause a number of vascular and renal

TABLE 2.   Causes of Hypertension in Transplant Recipients

- Cyclosporine or tacrolimus toxicity
- Renal dysfunction
    Chronic allograft rejection
    Drug-induced (immunosuppressive drugs, antibiotics)
- Transplant renal artery stenosis
- Native renal artery stenosis
- Recurrent primary hypertension
- High renin output from native kidneys
- Endocrine causes
    Aldosteronism
    Pheochromocytoma
    Hypercalcemia

aberrations, culminating in the development of hypertension. Calcineurin, a protein phosphatase, is extensively distributed in the kidney, vascular smooth muscle, and nervous system, all of which are targets for BP control. Calcineurin inhibition in these pivotal tissues causes sympathetic activation, powerful vasoconstriction, and sodium and water retention, all of which serve to elevate BP.[16] Cyclosporine and tacrolimus can cause acute as well as chronic nephrotoxicity; these drugs cause intense systemic and renal (afferent pre-glomerular) vasoconstriction either directly or via activating other pressor systems[17,18]; vascular regulators such as thrombaxane, prostacyclines, and nitrate oxide may also participate in the prohypertensive effects of calcineurin inhibition. Endothelin, a potent vasoconstrictor, may be involved because endothelin antagonists reverse cyclosporine-induced hypertension.[19]

Although there was speculation that tacrolimus may cause a lesser degree of hypertension than cyclosporine,[20] prospective studies comparing these drugs showed no such difference in their hypertensinogenic effects.[21] In the European experience, tacrolimus appeared to cause less hypertension compared with cyclosporine.[22] It has been reported that substituting tacrolimus for cyclosporine[23] decreases BP. In another observation,[24] the nighttime mean arterial BP was lower on tacrolimus compared to cyclosporine. The clinical, pathological, and therapeutic significance of these observations remains to be elucidated and confirmed by long-term follow-up of transplant patients receiving different combinations of immunosuppressive regimens.

Renal artery stenosis of transplanted kidney can cause hypertension, and this possibility should always be included in the assessment of patients with transplant hypertension. Transplant renal artery stenosis can also cause acute deterioration of renal function. Detection of a new bruit over the transplanted kidney may be a clue to renal artery stenosis. Similarly, renal artery stenosis of the native kidney should also be considered. Uncontrolled hypertension in a transplant patient should arouse the suspicion of renin release from the native kidneys. If this mechanism is confirmed by renal vein rein measurements and if the BP cannot be controlled, nephrectomy (of native kidneys) might be necessary.[25] With the relative ease of laparascopic nephrectomy, we anticipate this procedure to be applied more widely in properly selected patients. Other causes of hypertension in transplant recipients are listed in Table 2.

New Immunosuppressive Drugs and Posttransplantation Hypertension

In view of the hemodynamic and renal adverse effects of routinely used immunosuppressive drugs, newer therapeutic agents are of considerable

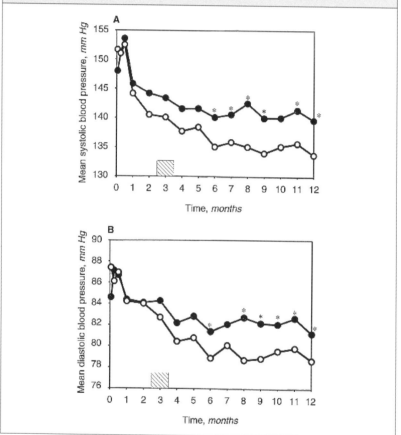

Figure 1. Influence of the new immunosuppressive combinations on hypertension after renal transplantation. *Solid circles* = steroids, sirolimus, and cyclosporine; *open circles* = steroids and sirolimus only after discontinuing cyclosporine. (From Morales, J.M. Kidney Internat 2002, 62(suppl)81–87; with permission).

interest and serve to complement the current therapeutic options; although these newer drugs cannot be entirely substituted for cyclosporine or steroids, they are emerging as attractive choices. Mycophenolate mofetil (MMF) is one such option; it inhibits T and B cell proliferation and B cell–mediated antibody production. MMF is a useful option for immunosuppression, since it does not alter lipid or glucose metabolism. Furthermore, MMF does not appear to induce nephrotoxicity or hypertensive effects.[26–28] Thus, MMF may be an alternative to cyclosporine in serving as an effective immunosuppressive drug but without provoking significant renal toxicity or raising BP.

Sirolimus is structurally similar to tacrolimus but may have different mechanism of action (does not inhibit calcinerin). Thus, it may not cause much renal toxicity or hypertension (Fig. 1).[29,30] Sirolimus also inhibits smooth muscle cell proliferation and migration. Although by itself, sirolimus does not cause significant hypertension, it may potentiate the adverse effects of cyclosporine.[31] Although the preliminary experience with MMF and sirolimus is encouraging, further studies are necessary to assign a definite role for these agents as an alternative to corticosteroids and calcineruin inhibitors.

Clinical Assessment and Management of Posttransplantation Hypertension

Nearly 125,000 patients in the United States have undergone organ transplantation in the past 10 to 12 years. With the increased use of organ transplantation and concomitant immunosuppressive drugs, systemic hypertension is not only common among transplant recipients, but it can also be severe. Uncontrolled hypertension can cause progressive target organ damage and allograft failure. Thus, effective treatment of hypertension is mandatory. Although antihypertensive drugs are routinely used, causes of hypertension in the transplant patient should be considered. Appropriate work-up should be undertaken based on clinical and laboratory evaluation. If a correctible cause is not identified, effective antihypertensive therapy should be initiated without delay and with close monitoring of the patient.

In view of multiple mechanisms that cause hypertension after organ transplantation, several classes of antihypertensive drugs are often required to achieve goal levels of BP ($< 140/90$ mm Hg; preferably $< 130/80$ mm Hg). The scope of this chapter does not permit a detailed description of antihypertensive drugs, but it does include certain salient remarks pertinent to the care of transplant patients. Loop diuretics may be needed but should be used with caution to avoid volume depletion and because cyclosporine may interfere with renal autoregulation.[32] Calcium channel blockers (CCBs) are particularly effective because they reverse the vasoconstrictive and other hemodynamic consequences of cyclosporine.[33,34] Dihydropyridine CCBs are extensively used to treat posttransplant hypertension. They are used alone or frequently in combination with other antihypertensive drugs. Verapamil, a nondihydropyridine CCB also has notable, favorable effects on immune function.[35] The clinical implications of this finding on graft function are not known. The effects of CCBs on cyclosporine metabolism are highly variable. DHPs do not affect cyclosporine metabolism consistently. Diltiazem[36] and, to some extent, verapamil[37] may increase blood cyclosporine levels. The effects of CCBs on tacrolimus blood levels are not conclusively characterized, but diltiazem can increase tacrolimus levels.[38] CCBs remain a practical and necessary ingredient in antihypertensive therapy for transplant patients.

Angiotensin-converting enzyme (ACE) inhibitors are an attractive option because of their important renal and cardiac effects. There is some concern that ACE inhibitors may decrease GFR even in the absence of renal artery stenosis,[39] but in the long-term management of transplant hypertension, ACE inhibitors are well tolerated.[40] Because the blood supply to the renal allograft is distinctive, ACE inhibitor therapy should be monitored carefully; a sudden deterioration in renal function may necessitate work-up to exclude renal artery stenosis. If the hypertension is solely caused by cyclosporine, ACE inhibitors may be less effective because of the low renin state. This disadvantage can be offset by concomitant administration of a diuretic. Whether the occasional occurrence of posttransplantation erythrocytosis is a risk factor for BP elevation is not established; nonetheless, ACE inhibitors, by inhibiting erythroprotein production,[41] may provide an added benefit.

Because hypertension is often severe in the transplant population, it is a common necessity to add a second or a third antihypertensive drug. Beta-blockers can be used in a combination with other drugs because of their safety in renal patients and because of their favorable cardiac effects. The combined α- and β-blockers such as labetalol or carvedilol can be used to treat transplant hypertension.[42]

Virtually all transplant recipients develop hypertension. All antihypertensive drugs can be effective in controlling transplant hypertension. Although CCBs are extremely effective in the transplant patients, multiple drugs are often combined to reach the goal BP levels. Renal function and potassium levels should be closely monitored. If possible, the dosages of calcineurin inhibitors and steroids should be optimally lowered without sacrificing graft protection. There is considerable hope that the new immunosuppressive drugs such as MMF and sirolimus may not exert hypertensive effects and may be a useful consideration in the management of transplant hypertension; these drugs may permit steroid withdrawal and offer an alternative to cyclosporine and tacrolimus. In the overall approach to patients with posttransplant hypertension, other corrective causes such as native kidney hypertension, renal artery stenosis of the transplanted kidney, hypercalcemia, and recurrent disease should be considered. Provided that all medical options are exhausted, native nephrectomy should be considered. Systemic hypertension is a major problem in transplant patients. Uncontrolled hypertension is a powerful risk factor, not only for graft failure but also for stroke and cardiac disease. Aggressive BP control embracing the etiologic, diagnostic, and therapeutic principles discussed in this chapter should permit optimal management of patients with posttransplantaion hypertension.

References

1. First MR, Neylan JF, Rocher LL, Tejani A: Hypertension after renal transplantation. J Am Soc Nephrol 1994, 4(suppl 1):30–38.
2. Morales JM, Andres A, Rengel M, Rodicio JL: Influence of cyclosporin, tacrolimus and rapamycin on renal function and arterial hypertension after renal transplantation. Nephrol Dial Transplant 2001, 16(suppl 1):121–124.
3. Textor SC, Canzanello VJ, Taler SJ, et al: Cyclosporine-induced hypertension after renal transplantation. Mayo Clin Proc 1994, 69:1182–1193.
4. Zeier M, Mandelbaum A, Ritz E: Hypertension in the transplanted patient. Nephron 1998, 80:257–268.
5. Kasiske BL, Ballantyne CM: Cardiovascular risk associated with immunosuppression in renal transplantation. Transplant Rev 2002, 16:1–21.
6. Frei U, Schindler R, Wieters D, et al: Pre-transplant hypertension: A major risk for chronic progressive renal allograft dysfunction. Nephrol Dial Transplant 1995, 10:1206–1211.
7. Opelz G, Wujciak T, Ritz E: The Collaborative Transplant Study Group: association of kidney graft failure with recipient blood pressure. Kidney Int 1998, 53:217–222.
8. Mange KC, Cizman B, Joffe M, Feldman HL: Arterial hypertension and renal allograft survival. JAMA 2000, 283:633–638.
9. Vianello A, Mastrosinone S, Cadcom G, et al. The role of hypertension as a damaging factor for kidney grafts under cyclosporine therapy. Am J Kidney Dis 1993, 21:79–83.
10. Curtis JJ: Hypertension following kidney transplantation. Am J Kidney Dis 1994, 23:471.
11. First MR, Neylan JF, Rocher LL, et al: Hypertension after renal transplantation. J Am Soc Nephrol 1994, 4(suppl):30.
12. Luke RG: Pathophysiology and treatment of post-transplant hypertension. J Am Soc Nephrol 1991, 2(suppl):37–44.
13. Porter GA, Bennett WM, Sheps SG: Cyclosporine-associated hypertension. Arch Intern Med 1990, 160;280–283.
14. Taler SJ, Textor SC, Canzanello VJ, et al: Role of steroid dose in hypertension early after liver transplantation with tacrolimus and cyclosporine. Transplantation 1996, 62:1588–1592.
15. Fryer JP, Granger DK, Leventhal JR, et al: Steroid-related complications in the cyclosporine era. Clin Transplant 1994, 8:224–228.
16. Sander M, Lyson T, Thomas GD, et al: Sympathetic neural mechanism of cyclosporine induced hypertension, Am J Hypertension 1996, 9(suppl):121–127.
17. Taler SJ, Textor SC, Canzanello VJ, et al: Cyclosporine-induced hypertension: Incidence, pathogenesis and management. Drug Safety 1999, 20:437–457.
18. Haas M, Mayer G: Cyclosporin A-associated hypertension: pathomechanisms and clinical consequences. Nephrol Dial Transplant 1997, 12:395–397.
19. Takeda Y, Mitamori I, Wu P, et al: Effects of an endothelin receptor antagonist in rats with cyclosporine-induced hypertension. Hypertension 1995, 26:932–937.
20. Textor SC, Weisner R, Wilson DJ, et al: Systemic and renal hemodynamic differences between FK506 and cyclosporine in liver transplant recipients. Transplantation 1993, 55:1332–1337.

21. Mayer AD, Dmitrewski J, Squifflet J-P, et al: Multicentre randomized trial comparing tacrolimus (FK506) and cyclosporine in the prevention of renal allograft rejection. Transplantation 1997, 64:436–443.

22. Margreiter R: Efficacy and safety of tacrolimus compared with cyclosporin microemulsion in renal transplantation: a randomized multicentre study. The European Tacrolimus vs Cyclosporin-Micro-emulsion Renal Transplantation Study Group. Lancet 2002, 359:741–746.

23. Copley JB, Staffeld C, Lindberg J, et al: Cyclosporine to tacrolimus: effect on hypertension and lipid profile in renal allografts. Transplant Proc 1998, 30:1254–1257.

24. Ligtenberg G, Hene RJ, Blankeston PJ, Koomans HA: Cardiovascular risk factors in renal transplant patients: cyclosporin A versus tacrolimus. J Am Soc Nephrol 2001, 12:368–373.

25. Curtis JJ, Diethelm AG, Jones P, et al: Benefits of removal of native kidney in hypertension after renal transplantation. Lancet 1985, 2:739–742.

26. Platz DP, Sollinger HW, Hullet DA, et al: RS-61443, a new potent immunosuppressive agent. Transplantation 1991, 51;27–31.

27. European Mycophenolate Mofetil Cooperative Study Group: Placebo-controlled study of mycophenolate mofetil combined with cyclosporin and corticosteroids for prevention of acute rejection. Lancet 1995, 345:1321–1325.

28. Ojo AO, Meier-Kriesche HU, Hanson JA, et al: Mycocphenolate mofetil reduces late renal allograft loss independent of acute rejection. Transplantation 2000, 69:2405–2409.

29. Andoh TF, Burdmann EA, Fransechini N, et al: Comparison of acute rapamycin nephrotoxicity with cyclosporine and FK506. Kidney Int 1996. 50:1110–1117.

30. Murgia MG, Jordan S, Kahan BD: The side effect profile of sirolimus: a phase I study in quiescent cyclosporine-prednisone-treated renal transplant patients. Kidney Int 1996, 49:209–216.

31. Kahan BD, Camardo JS: Rapamycin: clinical results and future opportunities. Transplantation 2001, 72:1181–1193.

32. Laskow DA, Curtis J, Luke R, et al: Cyclosporine impairs the renal response to volume depletion. Transplant Proc 1988, 20:568–571.

33. Morales, JM, Rodriquez-Paternina E, Araque A, et al: Long-term protective effect of a calcium antagonist on renal function in hypertensive renal transplant patients on cyclosporine therapy: a 5-year prospective randomized study. Transplant Proc 1994, 26:2598–2599.

34. Hauser AC, Derler K, Stockenlauber F, et al: Effect of calcium channel blockers on renal function in renal graft recipients created with cyclosporine. N Eng J Med 1991, 324:517.

35. Weir MR: Therapeutic benefits of calcium channel blockers in cyclsporine treated organ transplant recipients: blood pressure control and immunosuppression. Am J Med 1991, 90(suppl A):32–36.

36. Smith CL, Hampton EM, Pederson JA, et al: Clinical and medicoeconomic impact of the cyclosporine-diltiazem interaction in renal transplant recipients. Pharmacotherapy 1994, 14:417–481.

37. Henricsson S, Lindholm A: Inhibition of cyclosporine metabolism by other drugs in vitro. Transplant Proc 1983, 20(suppl 2):569–571.

38. Xloshan R, Flowers J, Warry SW, Venkatamanahn R: Drug interactions with FK506. Pharm Res 1992, 9(suppl 10):314.

39. Curits JJ, Laskow DA, Jones PA, et al: Captopril induced fall in glomerular filtration rate in cyclosporine treated hypertensive patients. J Am Soc Nephrol 1993, 3:1570–1574.

40. Mourad G, Ribstein J, Mimran A: Converting enzyme inhibitor versus calcium antagonist in cyclosporine treated renal transplants. Kidney Int 1993, 43:419–425.

41. Gaston RS, Julian BA, Diethelm AG, et al: Effects of enalapril on erythrocytosis after renal transplantation. Ann Intern Med 1991, 115:954–955.

42. Leeman M, Vereerstraeten P, Uytdenhoef M, Degaute JP. Systemic and renal hemodynamic responses to carvedilol and metoprolol in hypertensive renal transplant patients. J Cardiovasc Pharmacol 1993, 22:706–710.

Management of Hypertensive Patients with Sexual Dysfunction

chapter

33

Carlos M. Ferrario, M.D.

Sexual dysfunction in patients with hypertension is a frequently encountered yet often neglected problem in the clinical practice setting. Studies indicate that as many as 68% of hypertensive men experience one or more symptoms of sexual dysfunction, a percentage that is likely an underestimate because of the reluctance of patients and physicians to openly discuss this issue.[5,7,12,23] Often perceived as a problem in men, sexual dysfunction may also develop in hypertensive women, particularly with respect to orgasm and vaginal lubrication. However, detailed research in this area is lacking.[21]

This chapter discusses the frequency and spectrum of sexual problems in hypertensive men and women; considers the impact of common concurrent diseases such as diabetes; reviews the cause of sexual dysfunction in these patients, including the emerging role of angiotensin II as an important mediator of sexual dysfunction; and describes the potential clinical benefits of angiotensin II antagonists (AIIAs) in treating patients with hypertension and sexual dysfunction.

The underlying cause of sexual dysfunction in hypertensive patients may encompass a variety of factors (Fig. 1).[16,29] A number of classes of antihypertensive agents, especially diuretics and beta-blockers, cause sexual problems or exacerbate existing problems in both men and women. Development of sexual dysfunction can limit patient adherence to therapy and impair quality of life.[28,29] High BP itself may also be responsible for sexual dysfunction, possibly as a result of arteriosclerosis and the evolution of hypertension-related vascular disease.[16] Increasingly, erectile dysfunction (ED) is seen as a vasculopathy attributable to endothelial cell dysfunction that is remediable by enhancing cyclic guanosine monophosphate levels with phosphodiesterase inhibitors and nitric oxide (NO) donors.[24] Concomitant diabetes may increase hyper-

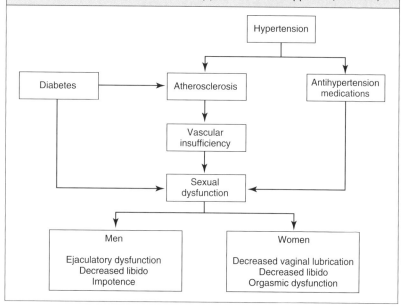

Figure 1. Possible causes of sexual dysfunction in patients with hypertension. Development of sexual dysfunction in hypertensive men and women may result from several factors, including the effects of some antihypertensive medications, vascular insufficiency caused by atherosclerotic disease, and ancillary factors (e.g., diabetes). (Adapted from Rosen RC: Sexual dysfunction as an obstacle to compliance with antihypertensive therapy. Blood Press Suppl 1997, 1:47–51.)

tensive patients' susceptibility for sexual dysfunction related to cavernosal artery insufficiency, corporal veno-occlusive dysfunction, and autonomic neuropathy.[13]

Prevalence and Spectrum of Sexual Problems in Hypertensive Patients

A number of studies published in the past 30 years show a high prevalence of sexual dysfunction in hypertensive men, with between 15% and 58% of patients experiencing one or more sexual problems with varying degrees of severity.[5,7,12,23] The most common expression of sexual dysfunction in hypertensive men is ED, although decrease in sexual desire and ejaculatory problems are also common.[7]

Limited research on hypertensive women suggests that roughly 50% of hypertensive women age 60 years or older also experience sexual dysfunction, including difficulty achieving orgasm (25%), decreased vaginal lubrication (23%), and diminished sexual desire (15%).[21]

In general, the frequency of sexual problems is higher in patients taking antihypertensive medication than in patients with untreated hypertension or in normotensive subjects (Fig. 2).[7] The coexistence of diabetes mellitus and hypertension markedly increases the risk of developing sexual problems in both men and women.[13] In the Massachusetts Male Aging Study,[9] men with treated diabetes were more than three times as likely to have ED than men without diabetes. Women with diabetes are at double the risk of women without diabetes for developing problems with sexual arousal,[26] demonstrate poorer levels of psychosexual functioning, and tend to be less satisfied with their relationships than their counterparts without diabetes.[17] In women, diabetes tends to have a greater impact on vaginal lubrication during arousal than on orgasm itself.[35]

Causes of Erectile Dysfunction in Hypertensive Men

High arterial blood pressure may affect penile vascular function and cause sexual dysfunction in hypertensive men.[13] High BP is frequently associated with coagulation disorders, increased platelet aggregability,

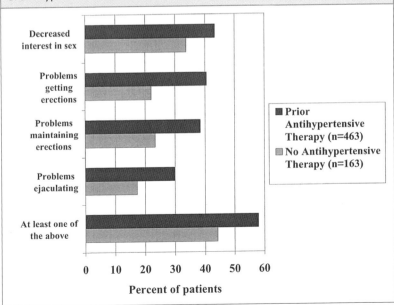

Figure 2. Impact of antihypertensive therapy on sexual function. Male patients who had previously received antihypertensive therapy had a higher incidence of distress over sexual symptoms than those who had not received antihypertensive therapy. The sexual symptoms distress index was assessed on a five-point scale as part of a questionnaire. (Adapted from Croog SH, Levine S, Sudilovsky A, et al: Sexual symptoms in hypertensive patients: a clinical trial of antihypertensive medications. Arch Intern Med 1988, 148:788–794.)

and vascular endothelial dysfunction—effects that are consistent with the recent concept of a dysmetabolic syndrome of hypertension.[22]

Vasculogenic Mechanism of Erectile Dysfunction

The anatomical and hemodynamic characteristics of penile circulation inextricably link the process of penile tumescence to BP and perfusion pressure. By affecting shear stress, high BP can potentially induce vascular endothelial abnormalities, including synthesis and secretion of vasoactive substances and increased permeability of the intimal layer—effects that ultimately lead to vascular smooth muscle cell (SMC) proliferation and collagen deposition in the vessel wall. Cavernous tissue vascular fibrosis is present in rats with spontaneous hypertension, and the degree of vascular sclerosis in the rat penis is highly correlated with the level of arterial pressure.[34]

These intriguing observations suggest a vasculogenic mechanism of ED in hypertensive patients. Indeed, according to a recent study on the prevalence and cause of ED in hypertensive men, penile arterial vascular changes, which were related to severity of hypertension and target-organ damage, appear to be a principal cause of ED.[13] However, further research is needed to more clearly delineate the link between BP elevation and ED, especially because endothelial dysfunction may occur before a substantial increase in BP. On the other hand, no data exist correlating the degree of BP elevation with severity of sexual dysfunction in men.

Although the physiology of erection is a complex, neurovascular event regulated by psychological and hormonal factors, corporal and vascular SMC tone and contractility play a key role in the erectile process by modulating penile blood flow. Both sympathetic and parasympathetic nerves regulate penile blood flow during erection and detumescence.[24] Parasympathetic activation is thought to relax trabecular muscle and dilate the pudendal arteries, although the neurotransmitters involved have not been conclusively identified. The principal mediator of erection appears to be NO, released from the endothelium and from nonadrenergic, noncholinergic cavernous nerves during sexual stimulation, although vasoactive polypeptide and prostaglandins may also be involved (Fig. 3).

Angiotensin II and Erectile Dysfunction

Recent studies indicate that angiotensin II plays a pivotal role in detumescence and possibly ED.[18,27] Angiotensin II was found in high concentrations in human corpus cavernosa, primarily in endothelial cells lining blood vessels and SMC bundles. Superfused cavernosal tissue from human subjects undergoing penile prosthesis implantation synthe-

Figure 3. Role of angiotensin II (ANG II) agonists in penile erection. ANG II as a regulator of penile erection through contractile effects on corporal and vascular smooth muscle. ANG II may play an important role in detumescence and erectile dysfunction by contracting corporal and vascular smooth muscle via an angiotensin II receptor. Local angiotensin-converting enzyme (ACE) may regulate smooth muscle tone by production of ANG II, which constricts blood flow through the penile arteries and reopens the penile venous plexus, thereby allowing flaccidity to return. By blocking the ANG II effects, the angiotensin II antagonist (AIIA) produces a dose-dependent increase in cavernosal pressure and relaxation of smooth muscle and, hence, development of an erection. cGMP = cyclic guanosine monophosphate. (Data from references 18, 24, and 27. Drawing courtesy of VMF Designs, Wilmington, NC.)

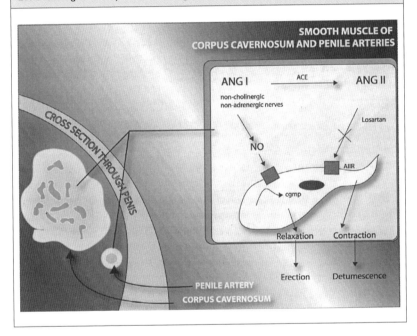

sizes and spontaneously secretes angiotensin II, which may subsequently modulate corporal and vascular SMC tone via an angiotensin II receptor. This process constricts penile arterial blood flow and reopens the venous plexus, thereby allowing penile flaccidity to return. The involvement of angiotensin II in the erection process is corroborated by findings that the angiotensin-converting enzyme (ACE) DD genotype, a polymorphism associated with high circulating and tissue ACE levels, may represent a risk factor for ED.[27]

Further evidence pointing toward a role for angiotensin II in ED comes from findings obtained in a canine model of penile erection.[18] Intracavernosal administration of angiotensin II terminated spontaneous erections in anesthetized dogs, an effect similar to that obtained with epinephrine. In contrast, administration of losartan, an AIIA, resulted in a dose-dependent increase in cavernosal pressure, relaxation of SMCs, and development of an erection. These intriguing data indicate that angiotensin II may represent an important mediator of erectile function and may serve to explain its improvement, as well as satisfaction and frequency of sexual activity, observed during clinical studies in hypertensive men with sexual dysfunction.[23]

Antihypertensive Agents as Cause for Sexual Dysfunction

Sexual dysfunction in men and women may result from the side effects of certain antihypertensive medications (Tables 1 and 2).[24,29] On the basis of clinical studies alone, it is difficult to assess the effects of antihypertensive agents because comparisons with baseline rates of sexual dysfunction were not made. However, not all antihypertensive agents are equivalent in their association with sexual problems.[11,29]

A high prevalence of male sexual dysfunction has been reported with the use of diuretics, including spironolactone, which inhibits dihydrotestosterone binding, and the thiazides, such as chlorthalidone, as well as beta-blockers (see Table 2).[5,7,12,20,25,31] Beta-blockers, such as atenolol and propranolol, may potentially affect sexual function through a variety of mechanisms, including a reduction in central sympathetic outflow; impairment of vasodilation of the corpora cavernosa; reduction in luteinizing hormone and testosterone secretion; and a tendency to produce sedation or depression, thereby causing a loss of libido.[11,19]

Centrally acting antiadrenergic agents such as methyldopa and clonidine may induce sexual dysfunction in men by attenuating sympathetic nerve outflow and diminishing libido, emission, and ejaculation. Direct vasodilators such as hydralazine and minoxidil have been associated with sexual problems, including ED and priapism, but this appears to be infrequent. Limited evidence indicates an association between calcium channel blockers and ED; at least, in comparison with ACE inhibitors (generally considered ED neutral), calcium channel blockers may have detrimental effects on erectile function and ejaculation.[23,32]

Angiotensin II Antagonists—Limited Impact on Sexual Function

AIIAs and ACE inhibitors do not usually cause sexual dysfunction (see Tables 1 and 2).[11,29,31] Indeed, antihypertensive agents that involve blockade of the renin-angiotensin system appear to be associated with improvements in sexual distress scores and are less likely to lead to a deterioration in sexual function compared with other antihypertensive agents.[29] This point is illustrated by the findings of two studies comparing beta-blockers and either an ACE inhibitor or the AIIA valsartan on

TABLE 1. Sexual Side Effects Reported During Therapy with Antihypertensive Agents

Drugs	Erectile Dysfunction	Decreased Desire	Impaired Ejaculation	Gyneco-mastia	Priapism
ACE inhibitors					
Angiotensin II antagonists					
Antiadrenergics					
Centrally acting	X	X	X	X	X
Peripherally acting	X		X	X	
Beta-blockers	X	X		X	
Calcium channel blockers			X	X	
Diuretics					
Thiazides	X	X	X		
Spironolactone	X	X		X	
Vasodilators	X				X

Suzuki H, Tominaga T, Kumagai H, Saruta T: Effects of first-line antihypertensive agents on sexual function and sex hormones. J Hypertens 1988, 6:649–651.
Kochar MS, Mazur LI, Patel A: What is causing your patient's sexual dysfunction? Uncovering a connection with hypertension and antihypertensive therapy. Postgrad Med 1999, 106:149–152, 155–57.

sexual function in hypertensive patients.[10,11] These studies show that whereas beta-blocker therapy increases sexual dysfunction, both the ACE inhibitor and AIIA had no long-term effect; in fact, the AIIA improved sexual activity.

In a double-blind, crossover study,[11] 160 hypertensive patients with newly diagnosed hypertension were randomized to receive valsartan 80 mg once daily or carvedilol 50 mg once daily for 16 weeks. Sexual activity was assessed using a self-administered questionnaire. Despite similar effects of the two agents on BP, AIIA therapy tended to increase sexual activity (8.3 at baseline to 10.2 sexual intercourse episodes per month), but beta-blocker therapy decreased sexual activity compared with baseline (8.2 to 3.7 episodes per month; $P < 0.01$) and compared with AIIA ($P < 0.01$).[11] Erectile dysfunction was reported by 15 patients receiving carvedilol (13.5%) and one patient receiving valsartan.

In another study of hypertensive patients, [23] the effect of the AIIA losartan on erectile function, sexual satisfaction, frequency of sexual activity, and perceived quality of life was evaluated in hypertensive men either with ($n = 82$) or without ($n = 82$) a diagnosis of sexual dysfunction. Eligible subjects, consecutively selected from primary care clinics, were diagnosed with sexual dysfunction according to a self-administered questionnaire, which was independently revalidated. Of the 323 hypertensive men and women in the initial sample, 82 men with sexual dysfunction (prevalence, 42.3%; 95% confidence interval, 35.3–49.3; age range, 30 to 65 years) received losartan 50 mg daily for 12 weeks. Before randomization, ACE inhibitors and calcium channel blockers

TABLE 2.	**Comparison of Effects of Antihypertensive Agents on Sexual Function in Hypertensive Men**		
Study	Study Design (*n*)	Antihypertensive Agent	Patients with Sexual Dysfunction (%)*
Bulpitt and Dollery[4]	Questionnaire (*n* = 373)	Diuretic	31.8
		Methyldopa + diuretic	35.7
		Bethanidine + diurectic	66.7
		Guanethidine + diuretic	54.5
		Reserpine + diuretic	33.3
		Methyldopa + bethanidine + diuretic	47.4
Hogan et al.[14]	Questionnaire (*n* = 861)	Hydrochlorothiazide	9[+]
		Methyldopa + diuretic	13[+]
		Clonidine + diuretic	15[+]
		Propranolol + hydralazine + diuretic	23[+]
		Control (no hypertension, no medication	4
Curb et al.[8]	(*n* = 5485)	Chlorthalidone	5
		Spironolactone	1.8
		Reserpine	5.6
		Methyldopa	5.5
		Hydralazine	1.2
		Guanethidine	10.8
		Other	2.3
Scharf and Mayleben[30]	R, CO (*n* = 12)	Hydrocholorothiazide	67
		Prazosin	42
Wassertheil-Smoller et al.[36]	R, PC, MC 6 mo, ED (*n* = 697)	Chlorthalidone	28[++]
		Atenolol	11
		Placebo	3
Chang et al.[6]	R, PC, 2 mo (*n* = 176)	Thiazide diurectic	14
		Placebo	5

Grim et al.[12]	DB, R, PC, 4 years, ED (*n* = 557)		24 mo	48 mo
		Acebutolol	9.2	11.8
		Amlodipine	8.3	15.0
		Chlorthalidone	17.1[+]	18.3
		Doxazosin	5.6	11.1
		Enalapril	9.7	14.1
		Placebo	8.1	16.7

Fogari et al.[10]	DB, R, 16 wk, men without ED (*n* = 90)	Lisinopril	3
		Atenolol	17.3**
Fogari[11]	DB, R, CO, 16 wk (*n* = 148)	Carvedilol	135.***
		Valsartan	0.9
		Placebo	0.9
Burchardt et al.[5]	Questionnaire, ED (*n* = 476)	Thiazide diuretics	27.9
		Beta-blockers	31.7
		ACE inhibitors	26.9

(continued)

TABLE 2.   Comparison of Effects of Antihypertensive Agents on Sexual Function in Hypertensive Men (Continued)

Study	Study Design (n)	Antihypertensive Agent	Patients with sexual dysfunction (%)*
		K+-sparing diuretics	23.1
		Calcium channel blockers	18.3
		Alpha blockers	13.5
		Angiotensin II antagonists	8.7
		Loop diuretics	5.8
		Direct vasodilators	2.9
Llisteri Caro et al.[23]	Questionnaire, prospective, 12 wk, ED (n = 82)	ACE Inhibitors	40.2
		Calcium channel blockers	19.5
		Beta-blockers	15.9
		Diuretics	13.4
		Others	6.1
		Alpha blockers	2.4
		Angiotensin II antagonists	2.4

*Includes one or more of the following problems: getting or maintaining erections, ejaculatory dysfunction, reduced libido, reduced sexual activity, orgasmic dysfunction.
+$P < 0.05$ vs. placebo or control
++$P = 0.009$ vs. placebo.
**$P < 0.05$ vs. lisinopril.
***$P < 0.001$ vs. valsartan
CO = crossover; DB = double-blind; ED = erectile dysfunction; K+ = potassium; MC = multicenter; PC = placebo controlled; R = randomized.

were the most common medications prescribed in patients with or without a diagnosis of sexual dysfunction (Table 3).

Compared with baseline values, losartan was associated with significantly increased sexual satisfaction (Table 4), frequency of sexual activ-

TABLE 3.   Medications Used by Subjects Before Initiation of Therapy with Losartan*

Presence of Sexual Dysfunction	Drug Class, % of Patients (n)						
	ACEIs	AllAs	CCBs	Diuretics	Alpha-blockers	Beta-blockers	Others
Yes	40.2% (n = 33)	2.4% (n = 2)	19.5% (n = 16)	13.4% (n = 11)	2.4% (n = 2)	15.9% (n = 13)	6.01% (n = 5)
No	58.5% (n = 48)	9.8% (n = 8)	14.6% (n = 12)	7.3% (n = 6)	0 (n = 0)	1.2% (n = 1)	8.5% (n = 7)

*In patients with or without a diagnosis of sexual dysfunction, ACE inhibitors and calcium channel blockers were the most commonly used medications at baseline in Europe, particularly in Spain, where the study was conducted. ACEIs = ACE inhibitors, AllAs = angiotensin II antagonists, CCBs = calcium channel blockers (Adapted from Llisteri Caro JL, Vidal JVL, Vincente JA, et al: Sexual dysfunction in hypertensive patients treated with losartan. Am J Med Sci 2001, 321:336–341.)

TABLE 4.   Effects of Losartan on Sexual Dysfunction and Satisfaction with and Frequency of Sexual Activity in Hypertensive Men

Parameter*	Patients, % (Baseline → 12 weeks)		P
Satisfied with sexual activity	7.3	→ 58.5	0.001
High frequency of sexual activity	40.5	→ 62.3	< 0.001
Erectile dysfunction	73.0	→ 11.8	—
Quality of life			—
Improved		73	
No change		25.5	
Worse		0.8	

*Assessed by a validated, self-administered, symptom-finding questionnaire.
Adapted from Llisterri Caro JL, Vidal JVL, Vincente JA, et al: Sexual dysfunction in hypertensive patients treated with losartan. Am J Med Sci 2001, 321:336–341.

ity, and quality of life with fewer patients reporting ED.[23] Only 11.8% of patients did not report an improvement in sexual function with losartan. In hypertensive patients without sexual dysfunction (control group), losartan did not change ED, sexual satisfaction, frequency of sexual activity, or perceived quality of life ($P > 0.05$). Improvements in sexual dysfunction indices were unrelated to age, duration of hypertension, educational level, marital status, BP levels, or the class of antihypertensive agent before entering the study.

Taken together, these findings suggest that AIIAs may offer a therapeutic option to prevent or correct ED in hypertensive patients. It is unclear whether the impact of AIIAs on sexual function represents a class effect or whether differences exist among the various AIIAs currently available. The favorable effects of AIIAs on sexual function may be related, in part, to their ability to block angiotensin II, a modulator of erectile function.[18]

Clinical Implications

Quality of Life

Sexual dysfunction associated with antihypertensive agents affects the ability of patients to stay on therapy and impairs patients' quality of life, especially with respect to sexual functioning or distress.[28,29,37] Sexual dysfunction in hypertensive patients treated with diuretics, beta-blockers, or methyldopa is also strongly associated with an impaired quality of life.[15] Approximately 78% of patients who had severe quality-of-life impairment (according to spouses' ratings) had a reduction in or no sexual interest. In contrast, only 38% of patients with mild impairment of quality of life had reduced sexual function.[15]

Drug Compliance

In the clinical trial setting, drug withdrawal caused by ED occurs at a significantly higher rate in patients receiving a thiazide diuretic ($P <$ 0.001) or beta-blocker ($P <$ 0.001) than in placebo-treated patients (12.6, 6.3, and 1.3 per 1000 patient years, respectively).[1] With respect to the AIIAs, the overall adverse event profile is similar to that of placebo in both short- and long-term clinical trials.[2] The more favorable overall side effects profile of AIIAs compared with other principal classes of antihypertensive agents may enhance patient adherence with therapy. In fact, a recent analysis[3] of prescription refill behavior of 21,000 hypertensive patients found that hypertensive patients receiving AIIAs as initial therapy were most likely to stay on therapy after 1 year compared with patients receiving other agents.

Timing

It is important to note that development of sexual dysfunction is usually evident within the first few months of initiating a particular antihypertensive regimen. Occurrence of sexual problems several years after starting therapy is unlikely to be the result of a particular medication, and, in this situation, the clinician should consider other causes for sexual problems rather than immediately discontinuing or switching therapeutic agents. However, when an antihypertensive agent is suspected of inducing sexual problems, it is appropriate to switch to another agent (e.g., an AIIA or ACE inhibitor) and follow-up with the patient for a period of 2 to 3 months.

Key Points

- Hypertensive patients often experience a variety of sexual problems; clinicians should be familiar with the causes, presentation, and management of sexual dysfunction in these patients.
- In addition to the effects of BP on vascular function, sexual dysfunction can occur as a side effect of antihypertensive agents.
- Evidence from various sources implicates a role of angiotensin II in ED and suggests that antihypertensive agents that interrupt the renin-angiotensin system are associated with less sexual dysfunction.
- Further research is required to more fully define the actions of AIIAs on the penile circulation and the process of penile tumescence, but it appears these agents may correct the underlying vascular pathophysiology in hypertensive patients that contributes to erectile dysfunction.

Acknowledgment

The authors wish to document their gratitude to Kala-Jyoti Redfern, Ph.D., for her valuable contribution in the preparation of this manuscript.

References

1. Anonymous: Medical Research Council trial of treatment of hypertension in older adults: principal results. Br Med J 1992, 304:405–412.
2. Benedict CR: Safe and effective management of hypertension with fixed-dose combination therapy: focus on losartan plus hydrochlorothiazide. Int J Clin Pract 2000, 54:48–54.
3. Bloom BS: Continuation of initial antihypertensive medication after 1 year of therapy. Clin Ther 1998, 20:671–681.
4. Bulpitt CJ, Dollery CT: Side effects of hypotensive agents evaluated by a self-administered questionnaire. Br Med J 1973, 3:485–490.
5. Burchardt M, Burchardt T, Baer L, et al: Hypertension is associated with severe erectile dysfunction. J Urol 2000, 164:1188–1191.
6. Chang SW, Fine R, Siegel D, et al: The impact of diuretic therapy on reported sexual function. Arch Intern Med 1991, 151:2402–2408.
7. Croog SH, Levine S, Sudilovsky A, et al: Sexual symptoms in hypertensive patients: a clinical trial of antihypertensive medications. Arch Intern Med 1988, 148:788–794.
8. Curb JD, Borhani NO, Blaszkowski TP, et al: Long-term surveillance for adverse effects of antihypertensive drugs. JAMA 1985, 253:3263–3268.
9. Feldman HA, Goldstein I, Hatzichristou DG, et al: Impotence and its medical and psychosocial correlates: results of the Massachusetts Male Aging Study. J Urol 1994, 151:54.
10. Fogari R, Zoppi A, Corradi L, et al: Sexual function in hypertensive males treated with lisinopril or atenolol: a cross-over study. Am J Hypertens 1998, 11:1244–1247.
11. Fogari R, Zoppi A, Poletti L, et al: Sexual activity in hypertensive men treated with valsartan or carvedilol: a crossover study. Am J Hypertens 2001, 14:27–31.
12. Grimm RH Jr, Grandits GA, Prineas RJ, et al: Long-term effects on sexual function of five antihypertensive drugs and nutritional hygienic treatment in hypertensive men and women. Treatment of Mild Hypertension Study. Hypertension 1997, 29:8–14.
13. Hakim LS, Goldstein I: Diabetic sexual dysfunction. Endo Metab Clin N Am 1996, 25:379–400.
14. Hogan MJ, Wallin JD, Baer RM: Antihypertensive therapy and male sexual dysfunction. Psychosomatics 1980, 21:234–237.
15. Jachuck SJ, Brierley H, Jachuck S, Wilcox PM: The effect of hypotensive drugs on the quality of life. J R Coll Gen Pract 1982, 32:103–105.
16. Jensen J, Lendorf A, Stimpel H, et al: The prevalence and etiology of impotence in 101 male hypertensive outpatients. Am J Hypertens 1999, 12:271–275.
17. Jenson SB: Sexual relationships in couples with a diabetic partner. J Sex Marital Ther 1985, 11:259–270.
18. Kifor I, Williams GH, Vickers MA, et al: Tissue angiotensin II as a modulator of erectile dysfunction. I. Angiotensin peptide content, secretion, and effects in the corpus cavernosum. J Urol 1997, 157:1920–1925.
19. Kochar MS, Mazur LI, Patel A: What is causing your patient's sexual dysfunction?

Uncovering a connection with hypertension and antihypertensive therapy. Postgrad Med 1999, 106:149–152, 155–57.

20. Kroner BA, Mulligan T, Briggs GC: Effect of frequently prescribed cardiovascular medications on sexual function: a pilot study. Ann Pharmacotherapy 1993, 27:1329.

21. Leiblum SR, Baume RM, Croog SH: The sexual functioning of elderly hypertensive women. J Sex Marital Ther 1994, 20:250–270.

22. Levy PJ, Yunis C, Owen J, et al. Inhibition of platelet aggregability by losartan in essential hypertension. Am J Cardiol 2000, 86:1188–1192.

23. Llisteri Caro JL, Vidal JVL, Vincente JA, et al: Sexual dysfunction in hypertensive patients treated with losartan. Am J Med Sci 2001, 321:336–341.

24. Lue TF. Erectile dysfunction. N Engl J Med 1997, 157:1920–1925.

25. Muller SC, el-Damanhoury H, Ruth J, et al: Hypertension and impotence. Eur Urol 1991, 19:29–34.

26. Newman A, Bertelson A: Sexual dysfunction in diabetic women. J Behavioral Med 1986, 9:261–270.

27. Park JK, Kim W, Kim SW, et al: Gene-polymorphisms of angiotensin converting enzyme and endothelial nitric oxide synthase in patients with erectile dysfunction. Int J Impot Res 1999, 11:271–276.

28. Prisant LM, Carr AA, Bottini PB, et al: Sexual dysfunction with antihypertensive drugs. Arch Intern Med 1994, 154:730–736.

29. Rosen RC: Sexual dysfunction as an obstacle to compliance with antihypertensive therapy. Blood Press Suppl 1997, 1:47–51.

30. Scharf MB, Mayleben DW. Comparative effects of prazosin and hydrochlorothiazide on sexual function in hypertensive men. Am J Med 1989, 86:110–112.

31. Suzuki H, Tominaga T, Kumagai H, Saruta T: Effects of first-line antihypertensive agents on sexual function and sex hormones. J Hypertens 1988, 6:649–651.

32. Tanner LA, Bosco LA: Gynecomastia associated with calcium channel blocker therapy. Arch Intern Med 1988, 148:379–380.

33. Tedesco MA, Ratti G, Mennella S, et al: Comparison of losartan and hydrochlorothiazide on cognitive function and quality of life in hypertensive patients. Am J Hypertens 1999, 12:1130–1134.

34. Toblli JE, Stella I, Inserra F, et al: Morphological changes in cavernous tissue in spontaneously hypertensive rats. Am J Hypertens 2000, 13:686–692.

35. Tyrer G, Steel JM, Ewing DJ, et al: Sexual responsiveness in diabetic women. Diabetologica 1983, 24:166–171.

36. Wassertheil-Smoller S, Blaufox MD, Oberman A, et al: Effect of antihypertensives on sexual function and quality of life:the TAIM Study. Ann Intern Med 1991, 114:613–620.

37. Weinberger MH: Lowering blood pressure in patients without affecting quality of life. Am J Med 1989, 86:94–97.

Novel Cardiovascular Risk Factors and Their Use in Clinical Practice

chapter

34

Peter W. F. Wilson, M.D.

There is great interest to move beyond the established risk factors and consider the usefulness of newer or novel markers of cardiovascular disease (CVD) risk in the prediction of CVD events. Data for a variety of factors are now available, and three general arenas are involved—lipoprotein particles, inflammatory markers, and other metabolic issues. This brief review highlights some of the leading candidates from each of these domains. For lipoproteins, the chapter discusses the low-density lipoprotein (LDL) subparticles, remnant particles, lipoprotein (a) [Lp(a)] and oxidized LDL. For inflammation, the chapter considers some of the endothelial and clotting proteins but concentrates on the findings related to C-reactive protein (CRP). Finally, the chapter briefly discusses homocysteine and coronary heart disease (CHD) risk.

Considerations for a New Risk Factor

New factors associated with increased risk for CHD arouse great interest and kindle the hope that these factors may enhance our ability to identify individuals at risk for CHD. Important concerns are that such metabolic factors be biologically plausible, measurable, repeatable, strong, graded, and treatable.[1] Measurement issues include accuracy and precision for the factor in the laboratory and evidence of low or modest variability in the clinical setting. If the laboratory or biological variability is very high, then the utility of the measurement for predictive purposes is seriously reduced. For markers such as total cholesterol, with which there are many years of experience and standardization of measurements has been underway for more than two decades, many of these characteristics are known. The biological and analytical variability of cholesterol determinations are typically < 3%, leading to an overall variability of approximately 6%.[2] Much greater variability can be expected with other lipid measurements.

New risk factors may provide clues to pathogenesis and, in some instances, may improve our ability to predict disease. The ability of the novel risk factor to predict new CHD events should be demonstrated after consideration of the core set of factors that are currently available, including age, gender, blood pressure (BP), cholesterol or LDL cholesterol (LDL-C), high-density lipoprotein (HDL) cholesterol (HDL-C), smoking, and diabetes mellitus. This criterion is often not met in new investigations, and considerable experience and relatively large datasets and follow-up may be necessary to ensure that a new factor has added utility.

Lipids

The concentration of cholesterol in the blood has been shown to be related to greater risk of CHD mortality in classic investigations such as the Seven Countries Study and men screened for the Multiple Risk Factor Intervention Trial.[3,4] Ultracentrifugation techniques allowed the estimation of LDL-C and precipitation techniques led to the measurement of HDL-C. Each of these moieties is highly related to the development of CHD, but if the measurements are used for screening purposes, the utility of LDL-C is very similar to that for total cholesterol, as shown in Framingham analyses.[5] Greater concentrations of apolipoprotein B, the major lipid protein in the LDL and very low-density lipoprotein (VLDL) particles, is related to increased risk for heart disease, but its utility is probably not much different from LDL measurements alone.[6] Similar statements can be made for apolipoprotein A, the key lipid protein in HDL particles.

Further differentiation of the major lipoprotein particles is an area of active research. Subclasses of LDL particles have gotten the most attention, and a greater concentration of smaller, denser LDL particles has been associated with an increased risk of CHD in cross-sectional, case-control, and prospective studies. The concentration of small, dense LDL particles was typically no longer statistically related to CHD outcomes after adjustment for traditional lipid risk factors such as HDL-C and LDL-C in these studies.[7,8]

Lipoprotein (a) is composed of a LDL particle that is bound to apoprotein (a), a protein that is similar in structure to the coagulation factor plasminogen. Characteristic repeating amino acid sequences, called kringles, are found in each of these molecules. One copy of kringle IV occurs in plasminogen, and the number of kringle IV repeats in apoprotein (a) are heritable. Typically, 15 to 40 copies of kringle IV are present in the apoprotein (a). High levels of Lp(a) (especially > 30 mg/dL) are associated with with presence of sinking prebeta lipoproteins on electrophoresis of the plasma, and the presence of either abnormality has been associated with greater relative odds for CHD in most,[9] but not all, studies.[10,11] Concentration of Lp(a) are typically only a few mg/dL in plasma from white population groups,[12] and recent data have demonstrated that the plasma concentration of Lp(a) is highly heritable. Greater concentration of Lp(a) are found in persons of African ancestry and in association with fewer kringle IV repeats in apoprotein (a).[13] Lower levels of Lp(a) are also found in women menopause and in association with the use of estrogens.[14]

Blood triglyceride concentration continues to be debated as a CHD risk factor. Both fasting and nonfasting triglyceride levels have been associated with increased CHD risk in Framingham and other investigations.[15–18] Controversy surrounds the importance of total triglycerides in CHD prediction after levels of HDL-C are already known. Analyses from the Lipid Research Clinic Program data and Framingham show a significant effect of triglyceride levels after HDL-C adjustment, and a significant relationship between triglyceride and CHD is more easily demonstrable if a logarithmic transformation of the triglyceride values is made before incorporation into prediction models. *Meta-analyses have demonstrated a statistically significant residual effect of triglycerides after consideration of HDL-C, and the effect appears to be greater in women than in men.*[17] The utility of triglyceride levels in overall prediction of CHD appears to be limited, but it may be relevant and useful in specific subgroups. Excessive risk for CHD was present when HDL-C levels were low, the ratio of LDL-C to HDL-C was elevated, and triglycerides were high, as reported by investigators from the Helsinki Heart Study and others.[19]

Oxidation of LDL particles has been related to a greater risk of atherosclerosis in animal models,[20] and there is growing interest to study the phenomenon in humans. Data on CHD and oxidation in population have largely focused upon the role of oral antioxidants, particularly intake of vitamin E and beta-carotene. Ingestion of these nutrients, particularly vitamin E, has been related to lower rates of CHD in the Nurses Health Study and the Health Associates Study.[21,22] Each report was based on observational data, and clinical trials to test the hypothesis that antioxidant vitamins protect against CHD have generally shown no effects.[23,24] Measurement of oxidized LDL has been problematic, because only a small fraction of LDL molecules are oxidized in the plasma. A variety of techniques have been considered, including measurement of the oxidizability of LDL, ratio of antibodies to LDL epitopes, and determination of vitamin E levels.[25]

Inflammation

Historically, simple markers of inflammation such as the white blood cell count were related to CHD risk. In the 1970s, elevated fibrinogen levels were shown to be a major independent risk factor for various heart disease and stroke outcomes in population studies.[26] Cardiovascular disease, CHD, and all-cause mortality were all increased in those with higher fibrinogen concentrations in both genders, and this excess risk persisted after adjustment for the standard risk factors. Higher fibrinogen levels enhanced CHD risk of hypertensive patients, cigarette smokers, and diabetic individuals. In Danesh et al.'s meta-analysis of 18 studies, the top third of the fibrinogen distribution was related to a greater relative risk of CHD with a relative odds of 1.8 (95% C.I 1.6 to 2.0)[26] (Fig. 1).

C-reactive protein (CRP), a pentameric protein associated with inflammation, has been traditionally used to monitor rheumatologic conditions. The protein is produced in the liver and found to be elevated when a variety of cytokines such as interleukin-6 and interleukin-1 are increased. A meta-analysis of 11 prospective studies in asymptomatic individuals compared persons in the bottom third of the CRP distribu-

Figure 1. Relative risk of CHD according to study-specific tertile of fibrinogen in primary and secondary occurrence studies. (Adapted from Danesh J, Collins R, Appleby P, Peto R: Association of fibrinogen, C-reactive protein, albumin, or leukocyte count with coronary heart disease: Meta-analyses of prospective studies. JAMA 279:1477–1482, 1998.)

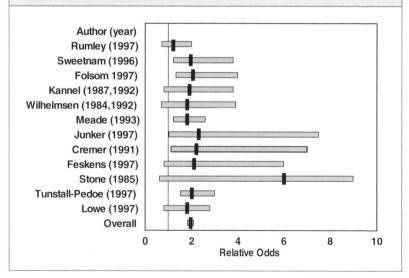

TABLE 1. C-Reactive Protein and Coronary Heart Disease Risk Results of Meta-Analysis	
Type of Cohort	**Risk Ratio (top third vs. bottom third)**
Population based ($n = 11$ studies)	2.0 (95% CI 1.6 to 2.5)
Preexisting vascular disease ($n =$ three studies)	1.5 (95% CI 1.1 to 2.1)
Total	1.9 (95% CI 1.5 to 2.3)
Adapted from Danesh J, Whincup P, Walker M, et al: Low grade inflammation and coronary heart disease: Prospective study and updated meta-analyses. Br Med J 321:199–204, 2000.	

tion with those in the top tertile. The authors reported an odds ratio of 2.0 (95% confidence interval [CI] 1.6 to 2.5) for CHD among persons in the top tertile of CRP (Table 1).[26] These results are among the strongest assembled thus far to recommend incorporating newer biomarkers into CHD risk estimation algorithms. Evidence has linked higher CRP levels to various risk factors such as obesity; cigarette smoking; estrogen use; and several vascular outcomes, including cerebrovascular and peripheral vascular disease.[26–28]

Other markers, such as serum amyloid A (SAA), soluble intracellular adhesion molecules (sICAM), and interleukins, have also been linked to initial and recurrent CHD, but data have not been uniformly convincing, and CRP appears to be the most predictive of CHD events of the markers that have been studied.[29] A review has presented the published evidence for SAA and risk of vascular disease, and Danesh et al.[26] reported that higher SAA levels were related to greater CHD risk; however, the effects were not as strong as for CRP (Fig. 2).[30] The current recommendation for screening with inflammatory markers to improve CHD risk assessment is "to measure high sensitivity CRP as an adjunct to the major risk factors to further assess absolute risk for coronary disease primary prevention. At the discretion of the physician, the measurement is considered optional, based on the moderate level of evidence."[31]

Homocysteine

Cross-sectional, case-control, and prospective studies linked high levels of homocysteine to greater risk for CHD (Fig. 3).[32,33] Meta-analyses and reviews noted that the associations with CHD have been smaller in prospective studies and after folate fortification, suggesting that homocysteine elevations may identify persons with existing atherosclerosis and could reflect metabolic and inflammatory responses that are not predictive of subsequent vascular events.[32]

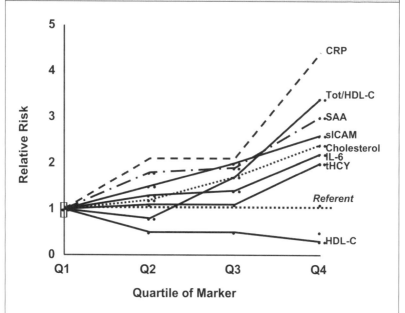

Figure 2. Relation between quartiles of inflammatory markers and CVD in the Women's Health Study. N = 122 cases and 244 controls. (Adapted from Ridker PM, Hennekens CH, Buring JE, Rifai N: C-reactive protein and other markers of inflammation in the prediction of cardiovascular disease in women. N Engl J Med 342:836–843, 2000.)

CRP = C-reactive protein, Tot/HDL-C = total/HDL cholesterol ratio, SAA = serum amyloid A, SICAM = soluble intercellular adhesion molecule, IL-6 = interleukin 6, tHcy = total homocysteine, HDL-C = high density lipoprotein cholesterol

Elevated homocysteine levels may be accompanied by decreased blood levels and intake of folate, vitamin B_6, or vitamin B_{12}.[34] These vitamins are important cofactors in the metabolism of homocysteine, and borderline deficiencies may be relatively common, especially in elderly individuals. Greater intake of these vitamins in the diet, with vitamin supplements, or with fortification of foods may lead to less vitamin deficiency and a decrease in the prevalence of elevated homocysteine levels.[35] Fortification of the U.S. food supply with folate was announced in early 1996 and was enacted before January 1, 1998. Analyses of homocysteine and folate levels before and after fortification demonstrated a dramatic decline in the prevalence of low folate levels, a reduction in the prevalence of elevated homocysteine from approximately 20% to 10%, and a decrease in mean homocysteine levels from approximately 10 to 9 umol/L. Concern has been expressed that case-control investigations with stronger findings have been more likely to reach publica-

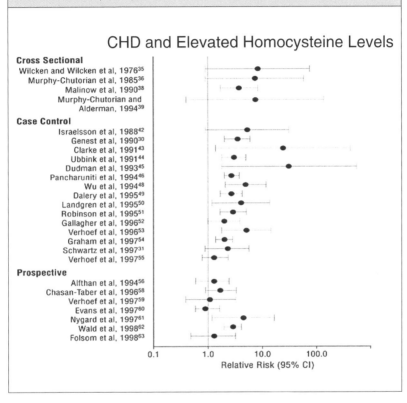

Figure 3. Relative risk of CHD according to study specific tertile of serum homocysteine in primary and secondary occurrence studies. (Adapted from Christen WG, Ajani UA, Glynn RJ, Hennekens CH: Blood levels of homocysteine and increased risks of cardiovascular disease: Causal or casual? Arch Intern Med 160:422–434, 2000.)

tion and that the effect of homocysteine on vascular disease risk in prospective studies and in the postfolate fortification era may be less than previous estimates.

Incorporation of New Risk Factors into Prediction of Coronary Heart Disease

As noted, the ability to predict new CHD events should be shown after consideration of the core set of established factors, including age, gender, BP, cholesterol or LDL-C, HDL-C, smoking, and diabetes mellitus. This criterion is often not met.

It is advantageous if most concepts discussed in the preceding sections are satisfied as prediction equations are developed to incorporate newer factors into CHD risk estimation equations. Many candidate factors are highly correlated with existing prediction variables, and these characteristics are important. For instance, after total cholesterol (or LDL-C) and HDL-C are included in a prediction equation, the added utility found for triglyceride information, used as a crude variable or after mathematical transformations, is relatively small.[16]

Strategies have been developed for the use of newer diagnostic tests (Fig. 4). The abscissa and the ordinate in Figure 4 represent prior probability and posterior probability of disease. If a screening test is performed and a second test is applied afterward but the probability of disease did not change, the result is a line of unity.[36] Such results occur rarely, and lenticular "envelope" around the estimation line is the typical result. Positive results with a second test, shown by arrows pointing up, leads to an increased risk of disease, and the posterior probability is greater than the prior probability. Conversely, a negative result with a second test, denoted by arrows pointing down, reduces the chance of, and the posterior probability is less than the initial probability of disease.

The utility of the newer inflammatory markers to improve risk estimation should be tested across a wide range of prior probabilities of CHD. The appropriate datasets to test are those for which we wish to apply the test, namely across several age groups, in both genders, and

Figure 4. Serial testing and risk of CHD. Prior and posterior probability of disease occurrence. *Straight line* shows the unity line; the *curve above* shows the utility of a positive test result; and the *curve below the line* shows the utility of a negative test result. (Adapted from Diamond GA, Hirsch M, Forrester JS, et al: Application of information theory to clinical diagnostic testing. The electrocardiographic stress test. Circulation 63:915–921, 1981.)

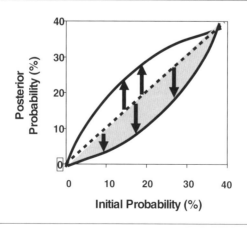

for different ethnic groups in population samples free of CHD at baseline. This approach will help to define not only the utility of positive test results, but also the potential use of negative test results that may be related to reduction in CHD risk because of new information that has not been contained in existing estimators of CHD risk.

References

1. Mosca L: C-reactive protein—to screen or not to screen? N Engl J Med 347:1615–1617, 2002.
2. Cooper GR, Myers GL, Kimberly MM, Waymack AP: The effects of errors in lipid measurement and assessment. Curr Cardiol Rep 4:501–507, 2002.
3. Keys A, Menotti A, Aravanis C: The Seven Countries Study: 2,289 deaths in 15 years. Prev Med 13:141–154 1984.
4. Stamler J, Wentworth DN, Neaton JD: Is the relationship between serum cholesterol and risk of death from coronary heart disease continuous and graded? Findings on the 356,222 primary screenees of the Multiple Risk Factor Interventional Trial (MR-FIT). JAMA 256:2823–2828, 1986.
5. Wilson PWF, D'Agostino RB, Levy D, et al: Prediction of coronary heart disease using risk factor categories. Circulation 97:1837–1847, 1998.
6. Sharrett AR, Ballantyne CM, Coady SA, et al: Coronary heart disease prediction from lipoprotein cholesterol levels, triglycerides, lipoprotein(a), apolipoproteins A-I and B, and HDL density subfractions: The Atherosclerosis Risk in Communities (ARIC) Study. Circulation 104:1108–1113, 2001.
7. Gardner CD, Fortmann SP, Krauss RM: Association of small low-density lipoprotein particles with the incidence of coronary artery disease in men and women. JAMA 276:875–881, 1996.
8. Campos H, Genest JJ Jr, Blijlevens E, et al: Low density lipoprotein particle size and coronary artery disease. Arterioscler Thromb 12:187–195, 1992.
9. Bostom AG, Cupples LA, Jenner JL, et al: Elevated plasma lipoprotein (a) and coronary heart disease in men aged 55 years and younger: A prospective study. JAMA 276:544–548, 1996.
10. Cantin B, Gagnon F, Moorjani S, et al: Is lipoprotein(a) an independent risk factor for ischemic heart disease in men? The Quebec Cardiovascular Study. J Am Coll Cardiol 31:519–525, 1998.
11. Ridker PM, Hennekens CH, Stampfer MJ: A prospective study of lipoprotein(a) and the risk of myocardial infarction. JAMA 270:2195–2199, 1993.
12. Seed M, Ayres KL, Humphries SE, Miller GJ: Lipoprotein (a) as a predictor of myocardial infarction in middle-aged men. Am J Med 110:22–27, 2001.
13. Gidding SS, Liu K, Bild DE, et al: Prevalence and identification of abnormal lipoprotein levels in a biracial population aged 23 to 35 years (the CARDIA Study). The Coronary Artery Risk Development in Young Adults Study. Am J Cardiol 78:304–308, 1996.
14. Sacks FM, Gerhard M, Walsh BW: Sex hormones, lipoproteins, and vascular reactivity. Curr Opin Lipidol 6:161–166, 1995.
15. Wilson PWF, Anderson KM, Castelli WP: The impact of triglycerides on coronary heart disease: The Framingham Study. Athero Rev 22:59–63, 1991.
16. Wilson PWF, Larson MG, Castelli WP: Triglycerides, HDL-cholesterol and coronary artery disese: A Framingham update on their interrelations. Can J Cardiol 10:5B-9B, 1994.

17. Hokanson JE, Austin MA: Plasma triglyceride level is a risk factor for cardiovascular disease independent of high-density lipoprotein cholesterol level: A meta-analysis of population-based prospective studies. J Cardiov Risk 3:213–219, 1996.

18. Criqui MH, Heiss G, Cohn R, et al: Plasma triglyceride level and mortality from coronary heart disease. N Engl J Med 328:1220–1225, 1993.

19. Manninen V, Tenkanen L, Koskinen P, et al: Joint effects of serum triglycerides and LDL cholesterol and HDL cholesterol concentrations on coronary heart disease risk in the Helsinki Heart Study—implications for treatment. Circulation 85:37–45, 1992.

20. Steinberg D: A critical look at the evidence for the oxidation of LDL in atherogenesis. Atherosclerosis 131 (suppl):5–7, 1997.

21. Rimm EB, Stampfer MJ, Ascherio A, et al: Vitamin E consumption and the risk of coronary heart disease in men. N Engl J Med 328:1450–1456, 1993.

22. Stampfer MJ, Hennekens CH, Manson JE, et al: Vitamin E consumption and risk of coronary heart disease in women. N Engl J Med 328:1444–1449, 1993.

23. MRC/BHF Heart Protection Study of antioxidant vitamin supplementation in 20,536 high-risk individuals: A randomised placebo-controlled trial. Lancet 360:23–33, 2002.

24. Brown BG, Zhao XQ, Chait A, et al: Simvastatin and niacin, antioxidant vitamins, or the combination for the prevention of coronary disease. N Engl J Med 345:1583–1592, 2001.

25. Witztum JL: The oxidation hypothesis of atherosclerosis. Lancet 344:793–795, 1994.

26. Danesh J, Collins R, Appleby P, Peto R: Association of fibrinogen, C-reactive protein, albumin, or leukocyte count with coronary heart disease: Meta-analyses of prospective studies. JAMA 279:1477–1482, 1998.

27. Visser M, Bouter LM, McQuillan GM, et al: Elevated C-reactive protein levels in overweight and obese adults. JAMA 282:2131–2135, 1999.

28. Cushman M, Legault C, Barrett-Connor E, et al: Effect of postmenopausal hormones on inflammation-sensitive proteins: The Postmenopausal Estrogen/Progestin Interventions (PEPI) Study. Circulation 100:717–722, 1999.

29. Ridker PM, Hennekens CH, Buring JE, Rifai N: C-reactive protein and other markers of inflammation in the prediction of cardiovascular disease in women. N Engl J Med 342:836–843, 2000.

30. Danesh J, Whincup P, Walker M, et al: Low grade inflammation and coronary heart disease: Prospective study and updated meta-analyses. Br Med J 321:199–204, 2000.

31. Pearson TA, Mensah GA, Alexander RW, et al: Markers of inflammation and cardiovascular disease: Application to clinical and public health practice: A statement for healthcare professionals from the Centers for Disease Control and Prevention and the American Heart Association. Circulation 107:499–511, 2003.

32. Homocysteine Studies Collaboration: Homocysteine and risk of ischemic heart disease and stroke: 6000 events in 30 observational studies. JAMA 288:2015–2022, 2002.

33. Christen WG, Ajani UA, Glynn RJ, Hennekens CH: Blood levels of homocysteine and increased risks of cardiovascular disease: Causal or casual? Arch Intern Med 160: 422–434, 2000.

34. Selhub J, Jacques PF, Wilson PWF, et al: Vitamin status and intake as primary determinants of homocysteinemia in the elderly. JAMA 270:2693–2698, 1993.

35. Jacques PF, Selhub J, Bostom AG, et al: The effect of folic acid fortification on plasma folate and total homocysteine concentrations. N Engl J Med 340:1449–1454, 1999.

36. Diamond GA, Hirsch M, Forrester JS, et al: Application of information theory to clinical diagnostic testing. The electrocardiographic stress test. Circulation 63:915–921, 1981.

chapter
35

Hypertension in Pregnancy

Sandra J. Taler, M.D.

This chapter addresses basic considerations in the evaluation and management of hypertension in pregnancy. The key to management begins with an accurate disease classification to distinguish preeclampsia, a pregnancy-specific syndrome of reduced organ perfusion, from preexisting chronic hypertension. Although the cause of preeclampsia remains unknown, the pathophysiologic mechanisms and associated risks differ from chronic hypertension, as does management. Hypertension during pregnancy is classified into one of five categories (Table 1).[1]

Prevalence

Hypertensive disorders are estimated to occur in 6% to 8% of pregnancies in the United States. Chronic hypertension occurs in up to 5% of pregnant women, although rates may vary by the population studied. Preeclampsia is more common in nulliparous women, occurring in up to 10% of first-time pregnancies. Risk factors for preeclampsia are listed in Table 2. The prevalence increases to 25% in women with chronic hypertension and is even higher in the setting of renal or other systemic diseases. With recent societal trends to delay childbearing to older maternal ages and the increasing use of fertility drugs resulting in multiple gestation pregnancies, the incidence of preeclampsia is expected to increase.

Hypertensive disorders have a high rate of recurrence (20% to 50%) in subsequent pregnancies.[2] Risk factors for recurrence are shown in Table 3. Although gestational hypertension predicts subsequent essential hypertension, recent studies suggest women with preeclampsia also have a greater tendency to develop sustained hypertension than women with normotensive pregnancies.[2,3]

TABLE 1.	Classification of Hypertension in Pregnancy
Chronic hypertension	• BP ≥ 140 mm Hg systolic or 90 mm Hg diastolic before pregnancy or before 20 weeks' gestation • Persists > 12 weeks postpartum
Preeclampsia	• BP ≥ 140 mm Hg systolic or 90 mm Hg diastolic with proteinuria (> 300 mg/24 hours) after 20 weeks' gestation • Can progress to eclampsia (seizures) • More common in nulliparous women, multiple gestation, women with hypertension for ≥ 4 years, family history of preeclampsia, hypertension in previous pregnancy, renal disease
Chronic hypertension with superimposed preeclampsia	• New-onset proteinuria after 20 weeks; in a woman with hypertension • In a woman with hypertension and proteinuria before 20 weeks' gestation Sudden two- to three-fold increase in proteinuria Sudden increase in BP Thrombocytopenia Elevated AST or ALT
Gestational hypertension	• Hypertension without proteinuria occurring after 20 weeks' gestation • Temporary diagnosis • May represent pre-proteinuric phase of preeclampsia or recurrence of chronic hypertension abated in midpregnancy • May evolve to preeclampsia • If severe, may result in higher rates of premature delivery and growth retardation than mild preeclampsia
Transient hypertension	• Retrospective diagnosis • BP normal by 12 weeks' postpartum • May recur in subsequent pregnancies • Predictive of future essential hypertension

ALT = alanine aminotransferase; AST = aspartate aminotransferase.

TABLE 2.	Maternal Risk Factors for Preeclampsia
	Primigravida
	Family history (maternal or paternal)
	Multiple gestations
	Diabetes mellitus
	Chronic hypertension
	Preexisting renal disease
	Extremes of reproductive age
	Obesity
	Hydatidiform disease
	History of severe early preeclampsia in a prior pregnancy

TABLE 3.	Risk Factors for Recurrent Hypertension in Pregnancy
	Early onset of hypertension in a prior pregnancy
	Chronic hypertension
	Persistent hypertension beyond 5 weeks' postpartum
	High baseline BP early in pregnancy

Preeclampsia

Preeclampsia is a pregnancy-specific syndrome of reduced organ perfusion caused by vasospasm and activation of the coagulation cascade. Although the pathologic changes are primarily ischemic, the cause of preeclampsia remains unknown. In this syndrome, reduced placental perfusion results from the failure to develop the normal low resistance, high-flow vascular connections between endovascular trophoblasts, and the maternal spiral arteries. Postulated causes include inadequate immune tolerance, activation of inflammatory cytokines, and genetic mechanisms. Research efforts have been restricted by the lack of a de novo animal model and the difficulties inherent in predicting which women will develop preeclampsia before it presents.

Clinically, preeclampsia is manifest by hypertension and proteinuria. The degree of blood pressure (BP) elevation may be mild, not reflective of the severity of the disease in other vascular beds. Proteinuria is defined as the urinary excretion of 300 mg protein or greater in a 24-hour urine collection (usually equivalent to a dipstick measure of 30 mg/dL, "1+ dipstick" or more). A random urine protein-to-creatinine ratio correlates closely with 24-hour urine protein measurements in pregnancy.[4] Preeclampsia should be suspected, even in the absence of proteinuria, when other symptoms are present (Table 4).

TABLE 4.	Discriminating Preeclampsia from Chronic Hypertension.	
	Preeclampsia	Chronic Hypertension
Time of diagnosis of hypertension	After 20 weeks	Before 20 weeks
Maternal risk factors for preeclampsia	Yes	No
Hypertension/preeclampsia in prior pregnancies	Yes	Yes
Proteinuria (> 300 mg/24 hours)	Yes	No
Elevated liver enzymes	Yes	No
Thrombocytopenia	Yes	No
Headache, blurred vision, epigastric abdominal pain	Yes	No
Persistent hypertension > 12 weeks' postpartum	No	Yes

Prevention

Prevention of preeclampsia has been frustrated by lack of knowledge of its underlying cause. Current strategies focus on identifying high-risk women for more frequent monitoring to facilitate early detection of preeclampsia and delivery when indicated. Although early small trials suggested benefit, several large multicenter trials of low-dose aspirin failed to demonstrate a benefit over placebo.[5-7] Selective use of aspirin for certain women at higher risk (specifically women with the antiphospholipid syndrome) may be reasonable. Calcium supplementation has effectively reduced the incidence of preeclampsia in women in developing countries who have low calcium intake, but it offers no benefit for low risk women in the United States.[8,9]

Treatment

Treatment for preeclampsia is palliative, as it does not alter the underlying pathophysiology of the disease. Delivery is always appropriate therapy for the mother but may not be so for the fetus, particularly when the fetus is very premature (< 32 weeks' gestation). For a preterm fetus without evidence of fetal compromise in a woman with mild disease, valuable time may be gained by postponing delivery under close monitoring. Regardless of gestational age, delivery should be strongly considered when there are signs of fetal distress or intrauterine growth retardation, or signs of maternal risk, including severe hypertension, hemolysis, elevated liver enzymes, and low platelet count (i.e., the HELLP syndrome), deteriorating renal function, visual disturbance, headache, or epigastric pain (see Table 4). Vaginal delivery is preferable to cesarean delivery to avoid the added stress of surgery.

Antihypertensive therapy is prescribed only for maternal protection. It does not improve perinatal outcomes and may reduce uteroplacental blood flow. The choice of agent and route of administration depends on anticipated timing of delivery. If it is likely to be more than 48 hours until delivery, an oral agent is selected (Table 5). Methyldopa is preferred based on its safety record, with labetalol increasingly used as an alternative based on its efficacy and low side effect profile. If delivery is imminent, parenteral agents are used. Appropriate agents and initial dosages are listed in Table 6. Treatment is initiated for persistent diastolic levels of 105 to 110 mm Hg or higher before induction, aiming for a diastolic BP of 95 to 105 mm Hg.

Chronic Hypertension in Pregnancy

Chronic hypertension complicates pregnancy by increasing the risk of adverse outcomes, including premature birth, intrauterine growth re-

TABLE 5. Oral Treatment of Hypertension in Pregnancy

Agent	Comments
Methyldopa	Preferred based on stable uteroplacental blood flow and long-term child development studies[17]
Beta-blockers	Reports of intrauterine growth retardation (atenolol)[23,24]
	Generally safe
Labetalol	Increasingly preferred to methyldopa because of reduced side effects
Clonidine	Limited data
Calcium antagonists	Limited data
	No increase in major teratogenicity with exposure[25]
Diuretics	Not first-line agents
	Probably safe
ACE inhibitors, ARBs	Contraindicated[26,27]
	Reports of fetal toxicity and death

tardation, fetal death, placental abruption, and need for cesarean delivery. The incidence of these conditions is related to the severity and duration of the hypertension preconception, the presence of target organ damage or coexistent renal disease, and the higher risk for superimposed preeclampsia (25%). Conversely, pregnancy may present additional risks to women with chronic hypertension because of the added stress of volume expansion on compromised cardiac function or increases in proteinuria accelerating renal decline. Women with chronic hypertension may be at higher risk for adverse neonatal outcomes independent of the development of preeclampsia.[10,11] The risks of fetal loss and acceleration of maternal renal disease increase at serum creatinine levels above 1.4 mg/dL at conception, although it may be difficult to delineate the effects of pregnancy from progression of underlying renal disease.[12,13]

TABLE 6. Acute and Parenteral Treatment of Hypertension in Preeclampsia

Hydralazine	5 mg IV bolus, then 10 mg every 20 to 30 minutes to a maximum of 25 mg, repeat in several hours as necessary
Labetalol (second-line)	20 mg IV bolus, then 40 mg 10 minutes later, 80 mg every 10 minutes for 2 additional doses to a maximum of 220 mg
Nifedipine (controversial)	10 mg PO; repeat every 20 minutes to a maximum of 30 mg
	Caution when using nifedipine with magnesium sulfate; can see precipitous BP decrease
	Short-acting nifedipine is not approved by the FDA for managing hypertension
Sodium nitroprusside (rarely when others fail)	0.25 ug/kg/min to a maximum of 5 ug/kg/min
	Fetal cyanide poisoning may occur if used for more than 4 hours

Pre-pregnancy Evaluation

Ideally, women with chronic hypertension should seek evaluation before becoming pregnant to define the severity of their hypertension, review medications, and plan for potential lifestyle changes (Table 7). If the systolic BP is 180 mm Hg or greater, the diastolic BP is 110 mm Hg or

TABLE 7. Management of Chronic Hypertension in Pregnancy	
Before Conception	
Evaluation for secondary hypertension	Pheochromocytoma; Other causes if severe
Evaluation for target organ damage	Cardiac function, LVH Renal disease (serum creatinine, proteinuria)
Change to medications safe for pregnancy	Taper early Titrate later
Lifestyle planning	Restrict aerobic exercise Avoid weight reduction Moderate sodium intake Avoid all alcohol and tobacco
Baseline laboratory testing	Hematocrit, hemoglobin, platelet count, serum creatinine, uric acid, urinalysis
During Pregnancy	
Selection of medications safe for pregnancy	See Table 5
Thresholds for treatment	150 to 160 mm Hg systolic 100 to 110 mm Hg diastolic
Laboratory monitoring	Hematocrit, hemoglobin, platelet count, serum creatinine, uric acid, AST, ALT, quantification of urine protein, serum albumin, LDH, peripheral blood smear, coagulation studies
Delivery	
Maternal indications	Gestational age $\geq$ 38 weeks Platelet count < 100,000 cells/mm^3 Deterioration in hepatic or renal function Suspected placental abruption Severe headache or visual changes Severe epigastric pain, nausea, or vomiting
Fetal indications	Severe fetal growth restriction Concerning fetal testing results Oligohydramnios
Acute or parenteral therapy	See Table 6
Postpartum	
Lactation	Withhold antihypertensive medication Taper medication dosage Select safe medications Monitor closely for adverse effects
ALT = alanine aminotransferase; AST = aspartate aminotransferase; LDH = lactate dehydrogenase; LVH = left ventricle hypertrophy.	

more, or if treatment requires multiple antihypertensive agents, it is particularly important to search for a potentially reversible cause. Some practitioners change to antihypertensive medications known to be safe during pregnancy even before conception. Angiotensin-converting enzyme (ACE) inhibitors and angiotensin receptor blockers (ARBs) should be discontinued before conception or as soon as pregnancy is confirmed.

Planning for pregnancy may require lifestyle changes. Hypertensive women are advised to restrict aerobic exercise during pregnancy based on theoretical concerns that reduced placental blood flow may increase the risk of preeclampsia. Weight reduction is not recommended during pregnancy, even in obese women. Sodium restriction may be continued for those women who have been successfully treated by this approach before pregnancy. As in all pregnancies, alcohol and tobacco use is strongly discouraged.

Treatment

Most women with chronic hypertension in pregnancy have stage 1 to 2 hypertension (i.e., systolic BP of 140 to 179; diastolic BP of 90 to 109 mm Hg, or both). In the short time frame of pregnancy, the risk of cardiovascular complications during pregnancy is low in this setting. Because there is no evidence of pharmacologic treatment leads to improved neonatal outcomes and BP usually decreases during the first half of pregnancy, these women can be monitored with no or reduced drug therapy.[14] Some centers manage patients with chronic hypertension by stopping antihypertensive medications under close observation. For women with evidence of target organ damage or taking multiple agents, medications may be tapered based on BP readings. Medications should be continued if needed to maintain BP control. Evidence suggests that antihypertensive treatment prevents progression of chronic hypertension to severe levels during pregnancy. Treatment should be reinstituted if BP reaches levels of 150 to 160 mm Hg systolic or 100 to 110 mm Hg diastolic.

Secondary hypertension evaluation is usually postponed during pregnancy, with one important exception: all hypertensive women should be screened for pheochromocytoma at the time of hypertension diagnosis because of the high morbidity and mortality associated with this condition if not diagnosed before delivery. When hypertension is severe, further evaluation for secondary causes may be indicated, and treatment may save the life of the fetus. Ultrasound and magnetic resonance scanning techniques offer safe modalities for diagnostic imaging. Laparoscopic adrenalectomy has been successfully performed during the second trimester in settings of primary aldosteronism, resulting in excellent fetal survival.[15,16]

Antihypertensive Drug Selection

The goal of treating pregnant patients with chronic hypertension is to reduce maternal risk, using agents that are safe for the fetus. Methyldopa is preferred by many as first-line therapy, based on reports of stable uteroplacental blood flow and child development studies out to 7.5 years showing no long term adverse effects.[17] Other treatment options are listed in Table 5. For all medication choices, there are still concerns regarding safety in pregnancy. In a recent meta-analysis of 45 randomized, controlled trials of treatment of mild to moderate hypertension in pregnancy using methyldopa, beta-blockers, thiazide diuretics, hydralazine, calcium antagonists, and clonidine, there was a direct linear relationship between a treatment-induced decrease in mean arterial pressure and the proportion of infants who were small for their gestational age.[18] The type of hypertension, type of agent, or duration of therapy did not explain this relationship.

There have been no placebo-controlled trials on treating severe hypertension in pregnancy, and none are likely to be done given ethical concerns. Historical experience with severe chronic hypertension in the first trimester describes fetal loss rates of 50% and significant maternal mortality, primarily occurring in pregnancies complicated by superimposed preeclampsia.[19]

Pregnancy in Women with Renal Disease

Women with renal diseases likely to progress should be encouraged to complete their childbearing while their renal function is well preserved. For women with mild renal disease (serum creatinine < 1.4 mg/dL), fetal survival is moderately reduced, and the underlying disease does not generally worsen. In moderate or severe renal insufficiency, pregnancy may accelerate the hypertension and the renal disease.[12,20,21] A decrease in birth weight correlates directly with increasing maternal serum creatinine concentration.[21] As renal failure progresses, hypertension may worsen because of volume overload, requiring treatment with diuretics or dialysis. Conception should be discouraged in chronic dialysis patients, because pregnancy is associated with significant maternal morbidity. Renal transplant recipients are advised to wait 1.5 to 2.0 years after successful transplantation and undertake pregnancy only if renal function is stable with creatinine of 2.0 mg/dL or less. All pregnancies in transplant recipients are considered high risk with high rates of prematurity.

Treating Hypertension During Lactation

Although all studied antihypertensive agents are excreted into human breast milk, differences in lipid solubility and extent of ionization of the drug at physiologic pH affect the milk-to-plasma ratio.[22] Breastfeeding can usually be done safely with attention to antihypertensive drug choices. For mildly hypertensive mothers who wish to breastfeed for a few months, medication may be withheld with close monitoring of BP. After discontinuation of nursing, therapy can be restarted. For patients with more severe BP elevation, the clinician may consider reducing drug dosages while monitoring the mother and infant. No short-term adverse effects have been reported from exposure to methyldopa or hydralazine. If a beta-blocker is indicated, propanolol and labetalol are preferred. Diuretics may reduce milk volume and thereby suppress lactation. ACE inhibitors and ARBs should be avoided based on reports of adverse fetal and neonatal renal effects. Given the scarcity of data, it is important to monitor all breastfed infants of mothers taking antihypertensive agents for potential adverse effects.

References

1. National High Blood Pressure Education Program Working Group on High Blood Pressure in Pregnancy: Report of the national high blood pressure education program working group on high blood pressure in pregnancy. Am J Obstet Gynecol 2000, 183(suppl):1–22.
2. Zhang J, Troendle JF, Levine RJ: Risks of hypertensive disorders in the second pregnancy. Paediatr Perinat Epidemiol 2001, 15:226–231.
3. Hannaford P, Ferry S, Hirsch S: Cardiovascular sequelae of toxemia of pregnancy. Heart 1997, 77:154–158.
4. Robert M, Sepandj F, Liston RM, et al: Random protein-creatinine ratio for the quantification of proteinuria in pregnancy. Obstet Gynecol 1997, 90:893–895.
5. Caritis S, Sibai B, Hauth J, et al: Low-dose aspirin to prevent preeclampsia in women at high risk. National Institute of Child Health and Human Development Network of Maternal-Fetal Medicine Units [see comments]. N Engl J Med 1998, 338:701–705.
6. ECPPA (Estudo Colaborativo para Prevencao da Pre-eclampsia com Aspirina) Collaborative Group: ECPPA: randomised trial of low dose aspirin for the prevention of maternal and fetal complications in high risk pregnant women. Br J Obstet Gynaecol 1996, 103:39–47.
7. CLASP (Collaborative Low-dose Aspirin Study in Pregnancy) Collaborative Group: CLASP: a randomised trial of low-dose aspirin for the prevention and treatment of pre-eclampsia among 9364 pregnant women. Lancet 1994, 343:619–629.
8. Carroli G, Duley L, Belizan JM, et al: Calcium supplementation during pregnancy: a systematic review of randomised controlled trials. Br J Obstet Gynaecol 1994, 101:753–758.
9. Levine RJ, Hauth JC, Curet LB, et al: Trial of calcium to prevent preeclampsia [see comments]. N Engl J Med 1997, 337:69–76.

10. Rey E, Couturier A: The prognosis of pregnancy in women with chronic hypertension. Am J Obstet Gynecol 1994, 171:410–416.

11. Buchbinder A, Sibai BM, Caritis S, et al: Adverse perinatal outcomes are significantly higher in severe gestational hypertension than in mild preeclampsia. Am J Obstet Gynecol 2002, 186:66–71.

12. Jones DC, Hayslett JP: Outcome of pregnancy in women with moderate or severe renal insufficiency. N Engl J Med 1996, 335:226–232.

13. Jungers P, Chauveau D, Choukroun G, et al: Pregnancy in women with impaired renal function. Clin Nephrol 1997, 47:281–288.

14. Sibai BM, Mabie WC, Shamsa F, et al: A comparison of no medication versus methyldopa or labetalol in chronic hypertension during pregnancy. Am J Obstet Gynecol 1998, 162:960–967.

15. Solomon CG, Thiet M, Moore F. Jr, et al: Primary hyperaldosteronism in pregnancy: a case report. J Reproduct Med 1996, 41:255–258.

16. Aboud E, de Swiet M, Gordon H: Primary aldosteronism in pregnancy—should it be treated surgically? Irish J Med Sci 1995, 164:279–280.

17. Cockburn J, Moar VA, Ounsted M, et al: Final report of study on hypertension during pregnancy: the effects of specific treatment on the growth and development of the children. Lancet 1982, 1:647–649.

18. von Dadelszen P, Ornstein MP, Bull SB, et al: Fall in mean arterial pressure and fetal growth restriction in pregnancy hypertension: a meta-analysis. Lancet 2000, 355:87–92.

19. Sibai BM, Anderson GD: Pregnancy outcome of intensive therapy in severe hypertension in first trimester. Obstet Gynecol 1986, 67:517–522.

20. Hou SH, Grossman SD, Madias NE: Pregnancy in women with renal disease and moderate renal insufficiency. Am J Med 1985, 78:185–194.

21. Cunningham FG, Cox SM, Harstad TW, et al: Chronic renal disease and pregnancy outcome. American Journal of Obstetrics and Gynecology 1990, 163:453–459.

22. White WB: Management of hypertension during lactation. Hypertension 1984, 6:297–300.

23. Rubin PC, Clark DM, Sumner DJ, et al: Placebo-controlled trial of atenolol in treatment of pregnancy-associated hypertension. Lancet 1983, 1:431–434.

24. Butters L, Kennedy S, Rubin PC: Atenolol in essential hypertension during pregnancy. Br Med J 1990, 301:587–589.

25. Magee LA, Schick B, Donnenfeld AE, et al: The safety of calcium channel blockers in human pregnancy: a prospective, multicenter cohort study. Am J Obstet Gynecol 1996, 174:823–828.

26. Hulton SA, Thomson PD, Cooper PA, et al: Angiotensin-converting enzyme inhibitors in pregnancy may result in neonatal renal failure. S Afr Med J 1990, 78:673–676.

27. Schubiger G, Flury G, Nussberger J. Enalapril for pregnancy-induced hypertension: acute renal failure in a neonate. Ann Int Med 1988, 108:215–216.

Preventing Cardiovascular Disease in Women

chapter
36

Andrew P. Miller, M.D.,
Philippe Bouchard, and
Suzanne Oparil, M.D.

More than 61 million Americans suffer from cardiovascular disease (CVD), and women comprise 52% of this group.[1] CVD is the number one killer of women, accounting for one in 2.4 deaths, markedly eclipsing breast cancer at one in 30.[1] Trends in women's mortality have shown a worrisome plateau and a recent increase in deaths attributable to CVD, despite improving diagnostic and therapeutic tools[1] (Fig. 1). This trend may be related to increases in obesity and type-2 diabetes mellitus, coupled with stagnation of improvements in smoking prevention and cessation, dyslipidemia treatment, and hypertension control since 1990.[2]

Although strategies to reduce CVD are effective in both men and women, some gender-specific issues arise in regard to implementation and effectiveness in preventing CVD. This chapter examines strategies for reducing cardiovascular risk factors in women, including *hypertension, dyslipidemia, diabetes mellitus, tobacco abuse, obesity, physical inactivity, and dietary indiscretion.* Menopausal hormone therapy is discussed in relation to its impact on cardiovascular health.

Hypertension

Hypertension is the most common modifiable risk factor for CVD in women. According to the National Health and Nutrition Examination Survey (NHANES III), the prevalence of hypertension and CVD in the U.S. population tracks very closely.[1] There is a striking age-dependent sexual dimorphism in the prevalence of hypertension and CVD. Hypertension and CVD are approximately three times more common in young men (< 35 years old) than in young women. The gender disparity in hypertension prevalence disappears at age 55 years, only to reappear after age 65 years with a reversal in male–female predominance. More than

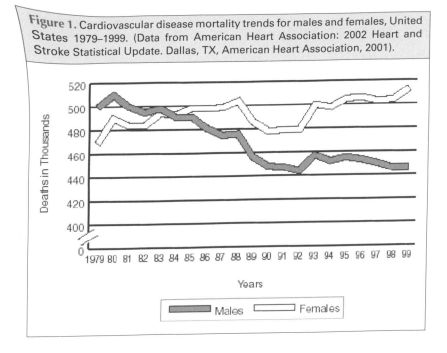

Figure 1. Cardiovascular disease mortality trends for males and females, United States 1979–1999. (Data from American Heart Association: 2002 Heart and Stroke Statistical Update. Dallas, TX, American Heart Association, 2001).

75% of elderly (> 75 years old) U.S. women are hypertensive, but less than two thirds of elderly men have elevated blood pressure (BP). CVD prevalence is equal in both genders at age 65 years with an excess of CVD in elderly (> 75 years old) women.

In absolute numbers, the greatest burden of hypertension in the United States falls on the elderly: an estimated 18.5 million persons older than age 65 years are hypertensive compared with only 7.5 million aged 25 to 44 years.[3] The numbers of hypertensives who are unaware of their condition or are treated but have inadequate BP control are disproportionately greater in the elderly than in the middle-aged and younger age groups. Systolic hypertension is highly prevalent in elderly individuals. Framingham Heart Study data indicate the residual lifetime risk of hypertension was similar for normotensive men and women age 55 to 65 years at 90%, indicating a huge public health burden.[4] More than 50% of 55-year-old participants and two thirds of 65-year-old participants developed hypertension within 10 years.

The Women's Health Initiative (WHI) data underscore the gravity of the hypertension problem in postmenopausal women.[5] WHI enrolled 98,705 women age 50 to 79 years and collected data on risk factors for

CVD, including BP. Baseline characteristics of the cohort are shown in Figure 2. WHI asked three major questions about BP in the cohort:

- What is the prevalence of hypertension among different subgroups (e.g., age, race or ethnicity, concomitant CVD risk factors) of post-menopausal women?
- How is hypertension treated in older women, and is it treated using Joint National Committee (JNC) VI guidelines?
- How adequate is BP control in postmenopausal women?

The overall prevalence of hypertension in women enrolled in WHI was 38% (34,339 women). Another 4% had normal screening BPs while not taking medication but reported a history of hypertension. Among the hypertensives, 64% (22,096) were on treatment but only 36% (12,383) were controlled. Elevated systolic BP with normal diastolic BP was found in 17% (15,821) at the baseline clinical examination. Prevalence rates were directly related to age; hypertension was twice as common in the eighth decade of life as in the sixth decade and varied markedly with race or ethnicity and socioeconomic status. Other major determinants of hypertension prevalence included body weight (48% with body mass index [BMI] > 27.3 vs. 29% with BMI < 27.3), physical activity (45% with no moderate or strenuous activity vs. 31% with ≥ 4 sessions/week), and alcohol consumption (46% in nondrinkers, 32% in moderate drinkers, 36% in heavier drinkers). Concomitant CVD risk factors and history of CVD were associated with marked increases in preva-

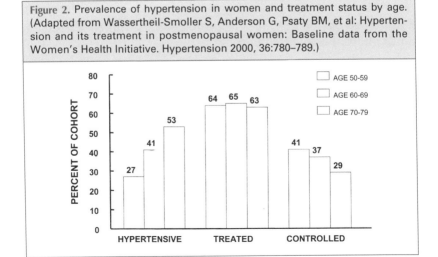

Figure 2. Prevalence of hypertension in women and treatment status by age. (Adapted from Wassertheil-Smoller S, Anderson G, Psaty BM, et al: Hypertension and its treatment in postmenopausal women: Baseline data from the Women's Health Initiative. Hypertension 2000, 36:780–789.)

lence of hypertension. Although current HRT use was associated with a lower prevalence of hypertension than no past use, current HRT use was associated with a 25% greater likelihood of hypertension than past use or never use after adjustment for confounders.

Treatment rates did not vary with age but did vary with race or ethnicity and were highest among black women in this self-selected cohort. Current users of HRT were more likely to be taking antihypertensive medications (OR 1.26, 95% confidence interval [CI] 1.2–1.3) than never users, supporting the concept that HRT users are more health conscious than nonusers. BP control rates were inversely related to age, despite comparable treatment rates in the three decades (see Fig. 2).

The majority of treated hypertensive women received a single drug. Control rates were highest (63%) with monotherapy with diuretics, intermediate with beta-blockers (57%) or angiotensin-converting enzyme (ACE) inhibitors (56%), and lowest with calcium channel blockers (CCBs) (50%). For unclear reasons, adding drugs from different classes did not improve control.

CCBs were used as monotherapy in 16% of participants. Despite the guidelines, diuretics and beta-blockers were used as monotherapy less often (diuretics, 14%; beta-blockers, 9%). Diuretics were used in combination more often than any other drug class. The presence of comorbid conditions influenced drug choice (e.g., beta-blockers were used more often in women with a history of myocardial infarction [MI]; combination therapy was more common in women with a history of CVD; and CCBs were used more frequently in combination with other drugs in diabetics than in nondiabetics).

Pharmacologic Treatment of Hypertension in Women: Effects on Cardiovascular Outcomes

A meta-analysis by gender of seven randomized controlled trials from the Individual Data Analysis of Antihypertensive (INDANA) intervention database showed significant treatment benefits for women (Fig. 3).[6] Significantly lower rates of stroke (total and fatal) and major cardiovascular events were seen in women randomized to thiazide diuretic or beta-blocker than to placebo. Expressed as relative risk, treatment benefits did not differ between the genders.

The Heart Outcomes Prevention Evaluation (HOPE) study evaluated the effects on CVD outcomes of ramipril use in women and men older than age 54 years with documented vascular disease or with diabetes and an additional cardiovascular risk factor.[7] Approximately half of the participants had controlled hypertension at the time of enrollment. Ramipril treatment of the 2480 women reduced the composite endpoint of MI, stroke, or cardiovascular death by 23% with a number needed to

Figure 3. Effects of antihypertensive treatment by gender. Data from the Individual Data Analysis of Antihypertensive (INDANA) intervention database showing significant treatment benefits for women. (Adapted from Gueyffier F, Boutitie F, Boissel J-P, et al: Effect of antihypertensive drug treatment on cardiovascular outcomes in women and men: A meta-analysis of individual patient data from randomized, controlled trials. Ann Intern Med 1997, 126:761–767.)

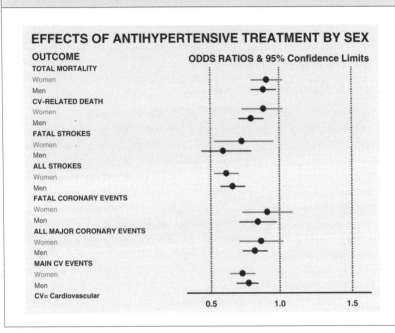

treat (NNT) to prevent one event of 27.[8] Relative risk reduction for CVD death alone was 38 percent in women, a benefit similar to that in men.

The Losartan Intervention For Endpoint reduction in hypertension (LIFE) study randomized 9193 patients, including 4963 women, with hypertension and left ventricular hypertrophy (LVH) by electrocardiogram (ECG) to an antihypertensive treatment regimen based on either the angiotensin receptor blocker (ARB) losartan or the beta-blocker atenolol.[9] Participants randomized to losartan had a 13% reduction in the composite endpoint of MI, stroke or cardiovascular death and 25% reductions in stroke and new-onset diabetes. Benefits of losartan were greater in women than men and in older (> 70 years) than younger persons.

The Antihypertensive and Lipid Lowering to Prevent Heart Attack Trial (ALLHAT) enrolled 42,448 high-risk hypertensive persons, including 19,865 women.[10] The alpha-blocker arm was stopped early because of an excess of heart failure and major CVD.[11,12] ALLHAT found no difference between treatments in the primary (coronary) endpoint or all-cause mortality.[13] Treatment effects were similar in women and men. Because the diuretic was superior to the newer classes of antihypertensive drugs in preventing a variety of CVD outcomes and because diuretics are less costly than the newer agents, ALLHAT investigators concluded that thiazide-type diuretics should be preferred for first-step antihypertensive therapy. They further recommended that a diuretic be included in all multidrug antihypertensive regimens, if possible. These observations, coupled with the additional benefits of thiazide diuretics discussed later, provide a strong rationale for using these agents in high-risk older women with hypertension.

Treatment Recommendations

Thresholds for instituting antihypertensive treatment, BP goals, and choices of antihypertensive drugs are the same for women as for men (Table 1). Current guidelines suggest lifestyle modification and specific drug therapy for the treatment of hypertension, including utilization of specific classes of antihypertensive drugs for compelling indications.[14]

Lifestyle modification is clearly indicated in all persons with clinical hypertension or with BP in the "high normal" range because of its potential for preventing the progression to higher BPs and CVD outcomes and for increasing the efficacy of pharmacologic treatment. Of the lifestyle interventions, weight loss and aerobic exercise are the most efficacious in reducing BP and related CVD risk factors such as dyslipidemia.[15–17]

Important determinants of the intensity of antihypertensive treatment are the severity of hypertension and the presence of other comorbid conditions, including multiple CVD risk factors and established CVD—all of which determine an individual's risk of sustaining CV events. Persons with multiple risk factors or target organ damage should be treated to a lower goal and often require combination therapy, including newer agents with proven benefits beyond BP lowering.

There are no age- or gender-specific recommendations for BP management, with the exception that older persons are generally at higher risk and merit particularly aggressive treatment. The BP-lowering effect of antihypertensive drugs is generally similar in both genders, but some special considerations may dictate treatment choices for women. Beta-blockers tend to be less effective in women than men,[18] and diuretics have added value in older women because their use is associated with decreased bone loss and reduced risk of hip fracture.[19]

Women tend to report more symptoms than men. In the Treatment Of Mild Hypertension Study (TOMHS), women reported twice as many side effects as men.[20] The incidence of side effects in women was similar in placebo- and drug-treated individuals.

TABLE 1. Classification and Management of Blood Pressure for Adults Aged 18 Years or Older

BP Classification	Systolic BP, mmHg*	Diastolic BP, mmHg*	Lifestyle Modification	Initial Drug Therapy Without Compelling Indication	Initial Drug Therapy With Compelling Indications†
Normal	<120	And	<80	Encourage		
Prehypertension	120–139	Or	80–89	Yes	No antihypertensive drug indicated	Drugs for compelling indications‡
Stage 1 hypertension	140–159	Or	90–99	Yes	Thiazide-type diuretics for most; may consider ACE inhibitor, ARB, β-blocker, CCB, or combination	Drug(s) for compelling indications; other antihypertensive drugs (diuretic, ACE inhibitor, ARB, β-blocker, CCB) as needed
Stage 2 hypertension	≥160	Or	≥100	Yes	Two-drug combination for most (usually thiazide-type diuretic and ACE inhibitor, ARB, β-blocker, or CCB)#	Drug(s) for compelling indications; other antihypertensive drugs (diuretics, ACE inhibitor, ARB, β-blocker, CCB) as needed

ACE, angiotensin-converting enzyme; ARB, angiotensin-receptor blocker; BP, blood pressure, CCB, calcium channel blocker.
* Treatment determined by highest BP category.
† Heart failure: diuretic, β-blocker, ACE inhibitor, ARB, aldosterone antagonist. Post-myocardial infarction: β-blocker, ACE inhibitor, aldosterone antagonist. High coronary disease risk: diuretic, β-blocker, ACE inhibitor, CCB. Diabetes: diuretic, β-blocker, ACE inhibitor, ARB, CCB. Chronic kidney disease: ACE inhibitor, ARB. Recurrent stroke prevention: diuretic, ACE inhibitor.
‡ Treat patients with chronic kidney disease or diabetes to BP goal of <130/80 mmHg.
# Initial combined therapy should be used cautiously in those at risk for orthostatic hypotension.

Other adverse responses to drugs may also be gender dependent: whereas women are more likely to develop hyponatremia associated with diuretic therapy, men are more likely to develop gout.[21] Hypokalemia is more common in women taking diuretics, and cough related to ACE inhibitor therapy is three times as common in women as in men[22]; bothersome lower extremity edema induced by CCBs is much more common in women than in men, as is unacceptable minoxidil-induced hirsutism. ACE inhibitors and ARBs are contraindicated in women who are or intend to become pregnant because of the risk of fetal abnormalities.

Dyslipidemia

Lipid levels are strong predictors of risk for CHD in women and men.[23] Women display an age-dependent unfavorable trend in lipid levels. Although high-density lipoprotein (HDL) cholesterol levels are higher in women than in men throughout life, low-density lipoprotein (LDL) and non-HDL cholesterol levels are lower in women than men before menopause and then they increase to exceed levels in men by the end of the sixth decade of life.[24] The biological basis for this "crossover" is not clearly understood, but it may relate to the withdrawal of ovarian estrogen. As the Adult Treatment Panel indicated, postmenopausal women should be targeted for aggressive lipid evaluation and early intervention.

Menopausal Hormone Therapy Effects

The unfavorable changes in total, LDL, and non-HDL cholesterol levels seen during menopause are probably related to the loss of endogenous estrogen.[25] Conversely, favorable effects on lipids occur with estrogen replacement in postmenopausal women. Estrogen (particularly conjugated estrogen) therapy decreases total and LDL cholesterol, increases HDL cholesterol and triglycerides, and decreases serum lipoprotein(a) levels.[25–27] These effects are mediated by estrogen-receptor dependent actions on hepatic expression of apoproteins.[28] Addition of a progestin blunts but does not abolish the favorable effects of estrogen on lipid profiles.[25] The positive effect of estrogen replacement on circulating lipoproteins does not prevent CVD endpoints in women.

Pharmacologic Treatment of Dyslipidemia in Women: Effects on Cardiovascular Outcomes.

Several clinical trials have demonstrated the benefit of 3-hydroxy-3-methylglutaryl coenzyme A reductase inhibitors (statins) in high-risk women (Fig. 4). The Scandinavian Simvastatin Survival Study (4S) was a secondary prevention trial in 4444 participants (~20% women).[29] Subgroup analysis demonstrated a significant reduction in the combined endpoint—CHD death and MI—in women randomized to simvastatin. Likewise, the Cholesterol and Recurrent Events (CARE) trial, a secondary prevention study with 14% women participants, demonstrated a significant reduction in a combined endpoint of CHD death, nonfatal MI or revascularization in women given to pravastatin.[30] Benefits from pravastatin were seen earlier and were twofold greater in women than in men.

The Heart Protection Study (HPS), a randomized, placebo-controlled trial of simvastatin treatment in 20,536 (5082 women) high-risk participants, extended the benefits of statin therapy to women at CVD risk but without a previous event and with "normal" lipid levels.[31] Participants were 40 to 80 years old with either diabetes or known coronary, cerebrovascular, or peripheral vascular disease and were referred by their primary caregiver without an absolute indication for statin therapy. Participants assigned to simvastatin showed significant reductions in mortality, major coronary events, stroke, and a combined endpoint of major vascular events compared with those given placebo. Results were similar for women and men, with a relative risk reduction in the combined endpoint of 23% for women. Participants who entered the trial

Figure 4. Effects of statins on major coronary events in women of large clinical trials. Data from the Scandinavian Simvastatin Survival Study (4S), the Long-term Intervention with Pravastatin in Ischemic Disease Study (LIPID), the Cholesterol and Recurrent Events Trial (CARE), the Airforce/Texas Coronary Atherosclerosis Prevention Study (AFCAPS/TexCAPS), and the Heart Protection Study (HPS). (From Bittner V: Lipoprotein abnormalities related to women's health. Am J Cardiol 2002, 90(8):77-84; with permission.)

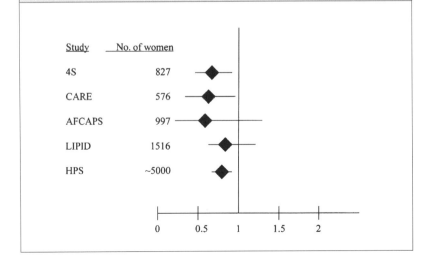

with LDL cholesterol levels less than 111 mg/dL showed marked reductions in the combined endpoint, similar to those in participants who entered the trial with LDL 130 mg/dL or greater. Hepatic dysfunction (alanine aminotransferase > 4XULN) and myopathy (creatine kinase > 10XULN) occurred with equal frequency in active treatment and placebo groups and were exceedingly rare (0.42% and 0.11%, respectively) in the simvastatin group. These results indicate that adding simvastatin to existing treatments in high-risk women and men produces large reductions in MI, stroke, and revascularization rates without introducing important safety issues.

Treatment Recommendations

The foundations for lipid management are published in the Third Report of the Expert Panel on Detection, Evaluation, and Treatment of High Blood Cholesterol in Adults (Adult Treatment Panel III or ATP III) (Table 2).[32] Following ATP III guidelines, a fasting lipid profile should be assessed every 5 years in all persons who are 20 years old or older. Physicians should address lipid levels, calculate a Framingham risk score, and consider instituting pharmacologic therapy in all women at menopause. Specific instructions to patients on lifestyle modification can improve triglyceride, HDL cholesterol, and LDL cholesterol levels.[33] Statin therapy should be initiated in all women with diabetes or known vascular disease and in those with ATP III criteria for pharmacologic treatment. In patients who develop myalgias, liver function test abnormalities, or other symptoms of statin intolerance, consideration should be given to

TABLE 2. LDL Cholesterol Goals and Cutpoints for Therapeutic Lifestyle Changes & Drug Therapy in Different Risk Categories

Risk Category	LDL Goal	Initiate TLC	Consider Drug Therapy
CHD or CHD risk equivalents (10-y risk > 20%)	<100 (mg/dL)	LDL ≥ 100 (mg/dL)	LDL ≥ 130 mg/dL (100–129 mg/dL)
2+ risk factors* (10-y risk ≤ 20%)	< 130 (mg/dL)	LDL ≥ (130 mg/dL)	10-y risk 10–20%: LDL ≥ 130 mg/dL 10-y risk, 10%: LDL ≥ 160 mg/dL
0–1 risk factor*	< 160 (mg/dL)	LDL ≥ (160 mg/dL)	LDL ≥ 190 mg/dL (160–189 mg/dL: LDL-lowering drug optional)

* Risk factors: cigarette smoking; BP ≥ 140 mm Hg or on antihypertensive medications. HDL cholesterol < 40 mg/dL; family history of premature CHD; age (men ≥ 45 years; women ≥ 55 years). Note that the presence of HDL cholesterol ≥ 60 mg/dL removes one risk factor from the total count. Diabetes is a CHD risk equivalent.
CHD = coronary heart disease, LDL = low-density lipoprotein, TLC = therapeutic lifestyle changes

use of niacin or a bile-acid binder (or both) in addition to lifestyle changes. Finally, fasting triglyceride levels above 200 mg/dL should be addressed, first with lifestyle modification and then with a fibrate, recognizing that patients receiving fibrates and a statin require closer monitoring for adverse events.[34–36]

ATP III identifies treatment targets as an LDL cholesterol level of 100 mg/dL or less, HDL cholesterol level of 40 mg/dL or greater, and triglyceride level less than 150 mg/dL. The panel suggests consideration of drug therapy for patients with coronary artery disease or equivalent risk (defined as persons with other vascular disease [peripheral vascular disease, abdominal aortic aneurysm, and symptomatic cerebrovascular disease], diabetes, or a combination of risk factors that confer a 10-year risk for CHD >20% by Framingham risk assessment) at LDL greater than 100 mg/dL, for patients with two risk factors at LDL cholesterol above 130 mg/dL, and for patients with no or one risk factor at LDL above 160 mg/dL. The ATP III guidelines use a Framingham risk assessment to identify patients for more intensive treatment. Gender-specific issues play a role in the evaluation and management of dyslipidemia in women. For example, triglyceride levels are more powerful predictors of CHD risk in women than men.[37]

Goals

- Low risk (≤ 1 risk factor): LDL < 160, HDL > 40, triglycerides < 150
- High risk (≥ 2 risk factors and 10-year risk ≤ 20%): LDL < 130, HDL > 40, triglycerides < 150
- CHD or CHD equivalent: LDL < 100, HDL > 40, triglycerides < 150

Diabetes Mellitus

Diabetes mellitus is a powerful cardiovascular risk factor in women equivalent to a history of MI in predicting future coronary events. The Nurses' Health Study identified a three- to sevenfold increase in cardiovascular events in women with type 2 diabetes compared with nondiabetic women.[38] Diabetes is generally considered to be a more powerful risk factor in women than in men.[39] However, a meta-analysis that corrected for age, hypertension, hypercholesterolemia, and smoking found cardiovascular risk attributable to diabetes similar in men and women (OR 2.3 [95% CI 1.9–2.8] and 2.9 [95% CI 2.2–3.8], respectively).[40] The authors suggested that diabetic versus nondiabetic women may have a less favorable overall CVD risk factor profile than diabetic versus nondiabetic men.

Treatment Recommendations

Prevention of CHD requires a multidisciplinary approach with a comprehensive risk assessment and aggressive risk factor modification in diabetic women. Aggressive lifestyle modification emphasizing weight control and physical activity should be coupled with pharmacologic therapy. Diabetes is associated with low HDL cholesterol levels and elevated triglycerides that couple with hyperinsulinemia to promote atherosclerosis. The metabolic syndrome is defined by three or more of the following in women: impaired glucose tolerance (fasting glucose $\geq$ 110 mg/dL), abdominal obesity (waist circumference > 35 inches), hypertension (BP $\geq$ 130/$\geq$ 85), low HDL cholesterol (< 50 mg/dL), and elevated triglycerides (> 150 mg/dL).[32] This syndrome enhances CVD risk approximately threefold.

Beyond glucose control, the clinical approach to diabetic patients requires treating to three targets. First, BP goals are lowered to systolic BP lower than 130 mm Hg and diastolic BP lower than 80 mm Hg. Two large clinical trials have shown that even within the normal range, BP lowering reduces cardiovascular events in diabetics.[41,42] Furthermore, there is a gender preference in this rigid goal, with diabetic women achieving a more marked reduction in cardiovascular events when diastolic BP is treated to lower than 80 mm Hg.[41] Second, because diabetes carries equivalent risk to known CHD, patients should be treated to an LDL cholesterol goal of less than 100 mg/dL. Triglyceride control is especially important in the diabetic woman because triglycerides become a more prominent secondary endpoint and help to define the metabolic syndrome. Women with triglycerides above 200 mg/dL should be treated to a non-HDL cholesterol goal of less than 130 mg/dL.[32]

Goals

- Reasonable glucose control with HbA1C < 7%
- Systolic BP < 130 mm Hg; diastolic BP < 80 mm Hg
- LDL cholesterol < 100 mg/dL; non-HDL cholesterol < 130 mg/dL

Tobacco Abuse

Smoking is a strong independent and modifiable risk factor for CHD in both women and men. Smoking is synergistic with other risk factors, including oral contraceptive use, in elevating cardiovascular risk. Even passive smoke is a risk factor for CVD and induces endothelial dysfunction in the coronary vasculature.[43] Smoking cessation can be restorative because it leads to gradual elimination of excess risk in women.[44,45]

Treatment Recommendations

The complete cessation of smoking should be stressed, and passive cigarette smoke should be avoided. At every visit, physicians should encourage patients and their families to stop smoking. Pregnancy is an especially critical time to intervene because consideration for the child's welfare may create the stimulus for permanent lifestyle change.[46] If smoking cessation is not possible, a reduction in cigarette use is important both as a means towards future cessation and because the CVD risk of tobacco use is dose related.

Goals

- Complete cessation of cigarette use
- Avoidance of passive smoke

Obesity, Physical Inactivity, and Dietary Indiscretion

Although obesity per se has only a modest impact on CHD risk, the metabolic syndrome is amplified by being overweight or obese.[47] The prevalence of being obese or overweight is increasing at an alarming rate in the United States.[48,49] One major contributor to this trend is physical inactivity. One study that followed 1213 African-American girls and 1166 white girls from age 9 to 19 years demonstrated dramatic declines in physical activity, with nearly half of the 16 and 17 year-old young women reporting no regular leisure-time activity.[50]

Increasing physical activity has a significant positive impact on CVD outcomes. Observations from the WHI show that even small amounts of activity (4.2 metabolic equivalents [MET] h/wk or the equivalent of pleasure walking for 70 min/wk) are associated with nearly a 30% reduction in cardiovascular events.[51] These associations hold irrespective of age, BMI, or race. Similarly, the Nurses' Health Study revealed a 30% to 40% risk reduction for women who participated in regular vigorous exercise ($\geq$ 6 MET).[52] Sedentary women in this study who became active had lower risk than those who remained sedentary.

Combining exercise and diet interventions prevents CHD events in women. A review of 19 intervention trials for physical activity and eight trials of nutritional intervention showed that most behavioral interventions reduce risk, at least in the short term.[46] This review recommended tailoring exercise advice to the individual's age, ethnicity, and physical condition and that a home-based exercise program with self-monitoring, caregiver contracts, and incentives may be effective. Comprehensive nutritional programs including cognitive behavioral therapy, dietitian education, and self-monitoring can reduce weight and improve metabolism. Generalizability is limited because most studies enrolled women of high socioeconomic status. Nevertheless, these clinical trials provide proof that lifestyle modification reduces CVD risk in women.

Treatment Recommendations

Increased physical activity and dietary modification are recommended for all women, particularly those who are overweight, physically inactive, or at high cardiovascular risk.

Goals

Weight:
- Achieve BMI between 18.5 to 24.9 kg/m^2

Physical activity:
- Accumulate $\geq$ 30 minutes of moderate physical activity on most, and preferably all, days.
- Enroll women with recent cardiovascular events in cardiac rehabilitation, a physician-guided home exercise program, or a comprehensive secondary prevention program

Diet:
- Build a diet including fruits, vegetables, and low-fat dairy products.
- Choose foods low in saturated fats and cholesterol; choose and prepare foods with less salt.
- If alcohol is consumed, drink it in moderation.

Menopause and Hormone Replacement Therapy

Rates of cardiovascular events are lower in premenopausal women than age-matched men. With menopause, however, cardiovascular risk and event rates increase markedly for women. Based on evidence from multiple sources, it was predicted that postmenopausal hormone therapy would protect women from CVD. Randomized controlled trials have not supported this prediction.[53–55]

The Heart and Estrogen/progestin Replacement Study (HERS) enrolled 2763 postmenopausal women with coronary disease and an intact uterus and randomized them to 0.625 mg of conjugated equine estrogens (CEE) plus 2.5 mg of medroxyprogesterone acetate (MPA) versus placebo.[53] No significant difference in cardiovascular outcomes between the two groups was seen after an average follow-up of 4.1 years. There was a time trend with more cardiovascular events occurring in the hormone-treated group during year 1 and fewer events in this group during years 4 and 5. This finding led to a "don't start, don't stop" conclusion; because the event curve seemed to diverge with time, the HERS study was continued in an unblinded fashion and published as HERS

II.[54] After 6.8 years average follow-up, HERS II was stopped because the placebo and active treatment groups had similar cardiovascular event rates with hazard ratios of essentially 1.0. The recommendation of the HERS investigators was that menopausal hormone therapy not be used to reduce the risk of CHD events in women with established CHD.

The WHI was designed to address primary prevention of CHD with menopausal hormone therapy.[55] The active treatment limb, which included 16,608 women randomized to placebo or CEE and MPA, was stopped early at 5.2 years of follow-up because of a significant increase in invasive breast cancer. The active treatment group had more CHD events, strokes, and venous thromboembolism but fewer colorectal cancers and hip fractures (Fig. 5).

Current evidence does not support combination therapy in the form of CEE plus MPA for primary or secondary prevention of CVD. The use of unopposed estrogen or combination menopausal hormone therapy in other forms or routes—transcutaneous or intrauterine—remains controversial because of a paucity of outcome data. A tendency to overinterpret the results of HERS and WHI has led to a recent unpopularity of all menopausal hormone therapy. This view seems unjustified given the the positive effects of estrogen on perimenopausal symptoms and bone ar-

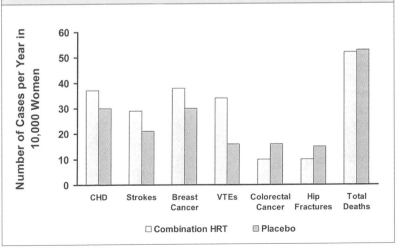

Figure 5. Disease rates for women on combination HRT or placebo. (Adapted from Rossouw JE, Anderson GL, Prentice RL, et al for the writing group for the Women's Health Initiative investigators: Risks and benefits of estrogen plus progestin in healthy postmenopausal women: Principal results from the Women's Health Initiative randomized controlled trial. JAMA 2002, 288:321–333.)

chitecture. Further investigation of other forms of menopausal hormone therapy and the results from the ongoing large clinical trials, including the CEE-alone arm of WHI in more than 12,000 women with hysterectomy, is needed before a definitive stance should be assumed on this topic.

Treatment Recommendations

Menopausal hormone therapy should not be initiated for primary or secondary prevention of cardiovascular disease, but it is beneficial for prevention of osteoporosis and the vasomotor symptoms of ovarian failure. Women taking hormones for the latter indications should continue to receive therapy with counseling that risks of breast cancer, thromboembolic events, and CHD may be increased. Women taking unopposed estrogen after hysterectomy for CVD prevention should continue on therapy pending results of randomized, controlled trials.

References

1. American Heart Association: 2002 Heart and Stroke Statistical Update. Dallas, TX, American Heart Association, 2001.
2. Cooper R, Cutler J, Desvigne-Nickens P, et al: Trends and disparities in coronary heart disease, stroke, and other cardiovascular diseases in the United States: findings of the national conference on cardiovascular disease prevention. Circulation 2000, 102:3137–3147.
3. Hyman DJ, Pavlik VN: Characteristics of patients with uncontrolled hypertension in the United States. N Engl J Med 2001, 345:479–486.
4. Vasan RS, Beiser A, Seshadri S, et al. Residual lifetime risk for developing hypertension in middle-aged women and men: the Framingham Heart Study. JAMA 2002, 287:1003–1010.
5. Wassertheil-Smoller S, Anderson G, Psaty BM, et al: Hypertension and its treatment in postmenopausal women: baseline data from the Women's Health Initiative. Hypertension 2000, 36:780–789.
6. Gueyffier F, Boutitie F, Boissel J-P, et al: Effect of antihypertensive drug treatment on cardiovascular outcomes in women and men: a meta-analysis of individual patient data from randomized, controlled trials. The INDANA Investigators. Ann Intern Med 1997, 126:761–767.
7. Yusuf S, Sleight P, Dagenais G, et al: Effects of an angiotensin-converting-enzyme inhibitor, ramipril, on cardiovascular events in high-risk patients. N Engl J Med 2000, 342:145–153.
8. Lonn E, Roccaforte R, Yi Q, et al: Effect of long-term therapy with ramipril in high-risk women. J Am Coll Cardiol 2002, 40:693–702.
9. Dahlöf B, Devereux RB, Kjeldsen SE, et al: Cardiovascular morbidity and mortality in the Losartan Intervention For Endpoint reduction in hypertension study (LIFE): a randomised trial against atenolol. Lancet 2002, 359:995–1003.
10. Davis BR, Cuttler JA, Gordon DJ, et al: Rationale and design for the Antihypertensive and Lipid-Lowering Treatment to Prevent Heart Attack Trial (ALLHAT): ALLHAT Research Group. Am J Hypertens 1996, 9:342–360.
11. The ALLHAT Collaborative Research Group: Major cardiovascular events in hypertensive patients randomized to doxazosin vs chlorthalidone: the Antihypertensive

and Lipid-Lowering Treatment to Prevent Heart Attack Trial (ALLHAT). JAMA 2000, 283:1967–1975.

12. Davis BR, Cutler JA, Furberg CD, et al: Relationship of antihypertensive treatment regimens and change in blood pressure to risk for heart failure in hypertensive patients randomly assigned to doxazosin or cholthalidone: further analyses from the Antihypertensive and Lipid-Lowering Treatment to Prevent Heart Attack Trial. Ann Intern Med 2002, 137:313–320.

13. The ALLHAT Officers and Coordinators for the ALLHAT Collaborative Research Group: Major outcomes in high-risk hypertensive patients randomized to angiotensin-converting enzyme inhibitor or calcium channel blocker versus diuretic: the Antihypertensive and Lipid-Lowering Treatment to Prevent Heart Attack Trial (ALLHAT). JAMA 2002, 288:2981–2997.

14. Chobanian AV, Bakris GL, Black HR, et al: The seventh report of the Joint National Committee on prevention, detection, evaluation, and treatment of high blood pressure: The JNC 7 report. JAMA 2003, 289:2560–2572.

15. Whelton PK, He J, Appel LJ, et al: Primary prevention of hypertension: clinical and public health advisory from The National High Blood Pressure Education Program. JAMA 2002, 288:1882–1888.

16. Stevens VJ, Obarzanek E, Cook NR, et al: Long-term weight loss and changes in blood pressure: Results of the Trials of Hypertension Prevention, phase II. Ann Intern Med 2001, 134:1–11.

17. Whelton SP, Chin A, Xin X, He J: Effect of aerobic exercise on blood pressure: a meta-analysis of randomized, controlled trials. Ann Intern Med 2002, 136: 493–503.

18. Lewis CE: Characteristics and treatment of hypertension in women: a review of the literature. Am J Med Sci 1996, 11:193–199.

19. Cauley JA, Cummings Sr, Seeley DG, et al: Effects of thiazide diuretic therapy on bone mass, fractures, and falls: the Study of Osteoporotic Fractures Research Group. Ann Intern Med 1993, 118:666–673.

20. Lewis CE, Grandits GA, Flack J, et al: Efficacy and tolerance of antihypertensive treatment in men and women with stage 1 diastolic hypertension. Arch Intern Med 1996, 156:377–385.

21. August P, Oparil S: Hypertension in women. In Oparil S, Weber M, eds. Hypertension. Philadelphia W.B. Saunders, 1999.

22. Os I, Bratland B, Dahlof B, et al: Female sex as an important determinant of lisinopril induced cough. Lancet 1992, 339:372.

23. Manolio TA, Pearson TA, Wenger NK, et al: Cholesterol and heart disease in older persons and women: review of an NHLBI workshop. Ann Epidemiol 1992, 2: 161–176.

24. Bittner V: Lipoprotein abnormalities related to women's health. Am J Cardiol 2002, 90(suppl):77i–84i.

25. The Writing Group for the PEPI Trial: Effects of estrogen or estrogen/progestin regimens on heart disease risk factors in postmenopausal women. JAMA 1995, 273: 199–208.

26. Espeland MA, Marcovina SM, Miller V, et al: Effect of postmenopausal hormone therapy on lipoprotein(a) concentration. Circulation 1998, 97:979–986.

27. Shlipak MG, Simon JA, Vittinghoff E, et al: Estrogen and progestin, lipoprotein(a), and the risk of recurrent coronary heart events after menopause. JAMA 2000, 283: 1845–1852.

28. Mendelsohn ME, Karas RH: The protective effects of estrogen on the cardiovascular system. N Engl J Med 1999, 340:1801–1811.

29. Pedersen TR, Kjekshus J, Berg K, et al on behalf of the Scandinavian Simvastatin Survival Study Group: Randomised trial of cholesterol lowering in 4444 patients with

coronary heart disease: the Scandinavian Simvastatin Survival Study (4S). Lancet 1994, 344:1383–1389.

30. Lewis SJ, Sacks FM, Mitchell JS, et al. Effect of pravastatin on cardiovascular events in women after myocardial infarction. J Am Coll Cardiol 1998, 32:140–146.

31. Collins R, Armitage J, Parish S, et al for the Heart Protection Study Collaborative Group: MRC/BHF Heart Protection Study of cholesterol lowering with simvastatin in 20536 high-risk individuals: a randomized placebo-controlled trial. Lancet 2002, 360:7–22.

32. Grundy SM, Becker D, Clark LT, et al: Executive summary of the third report of the National Cholesterol Education Program (NCEP) expert panel on detection, evaluation, and treatment of high blood cholesterol in adults (Adult Treatment Panel III). JAMA 2001, 285:2486–2497.

33. Kraus WE, Houmard JA, Duscha BD, et al: Effects of the amount and intensity of exercise on plasma lipoproteins. N Engl J Med 2002, 347:1483–1492.

34. Rubins HB, Robins SJ, Collins D, at al: Gemfibrozil for the secondary prevention of coronary heart disease in men with low levels of high-density lipoprotein cholesterol. N Engl J Med 1999, 341:410–417.

35. BIP Study Group. Secondary prevention by raising HDL cholesterol and reducing triglycerides in patients with coronary artery disease. Circulation 2000, 102:21–27.

36. Shek A, Ferrill MJ: Statin-fibrate combination therapy. Ann Pharmacother 2001, 35: 908–917.

37. Hokanson JE, Austin MA: Plasma triglyceride level is a risk factor for cardiovascular disease independent of high-density lipoprotein cholesterol level: a meta-analysis of population-based prospective studies. J Cardiovascular Risk 1996, 3:213–219.

38. Manson JE, Colditz GA, Stampfer MJ, et al: A prospective study of maturity-onset diabetes mellitus and risk of coronary heart disease and stroke in women. Arch Intern Med 1991, 151:1141–1147.

39. Oparil S: Cardiovascular risk reduction in women. J Women's Health 1996, 5: 23–31.

40. Kanaya AM, Grady D, Barrett-Connor E: Explaining the sex difference in coronary heart disease mortality among patients with type 2 diabetes mellitus. Arch Intern Med 2002, 162:1737–1745.

41. Kjeldsen SE, Kolloch RE, Leonetti G, et al: Influence of gender and age on preventing cardiovascular disease by antihypertensive treatment and acetylsalicylic acid: the HOT study. J Hyperten 2000,18:629–642.

42. UK Prospective Diabetes Study Group: Tight blood pressure control and risk of macrovascular and microvascular complications in type 2 diabetes: UKPDS 38. Br Med J 1998, 317:703–713.

43. Otsuka R, Watanabe H, Hirata K, et al: Acute effects of passive smoking on the coronary circulation in young adults. JAMA 2001, 286:436–441.

44. Hermanson B, Omenn GS, Kronmal RA, Gersh BJ: Beneficial six-year outcome of smoking cessation in older men and women with coronary artery disease: results from the CASS registry. N Engl J Med 1988, 319:1365–1369.

45. Kawachi I, Colditz GA, Stampfer MJ, et al: Smoking cessation in relation to total mortality rates in women: a prospective cohort study. Ann Intern Med 1993, 119:992–1000.

46. Krummel DA, Koffman DM, Bronner Y, et al: Cardiovascular health interventions in women: what works? J Womens Health Gend Based Med 2001, 10:117–136.

47. Kannel WB, Wilson PWF, Nam B-H, D'Agostino RB: Risk stratification of obesity as a coronary risk factor. Am J Cardiol 2002, 90:697–701.

48. Flegal KM, Carroll MD, Ogden CL, Johnson CL: Prevalence and trends in obesity among US adults, 1999–2000. JAMA 2002, 288:1723–1727.

49. Mokdad AH, Ford ES, Bowman BA, et al: Prevalence of obesity, diabetes, and obesity-related health risk factors, 2001. JAMA 2003, 289:76–79.

50. Kimm SYS, Glynn NW, Kriska AM, at al: Decline in physical activity in black girls and white girls during adolescence. N Engl J Med 2002, 347:709–715.

51. Manson JE, Greenland P, LaCroix AZ, et al: Walking compared with vigorous exercise for the prevention of cardiovascular events in women. N Engl J Med 2002, 347: 716–725.

52. Manson JE, Hu FB, Rich-Edwards JW, et al: A prospective study of walking as compared with vigorous exercise in the prevention of coronary heart disease in women. N Engl J Med 1999, 341:650–658.

53. Hulley S, Grady D, Bush T, et al for the Heart and Estrogen/progestin Replacement Study (HERS) Research Group: Randomized trial of estrogen plus progestin for secondary prevention of coronary heart disease in postmenopausal women. JAMA 1998, 280:605–613.

54. Grady D, Herrington D, Bittner V, et al for the HERS Research Group: Cardiovascular disease outcomes during 6.8 years of hormone therapy: Heart and Estrogen/progestin Replacement Study Follow-up (HERS II). JAMA 2002, 288:49–57.

55. Rossouw JE, Anderson GL, Prentice RL, et al for the writing group for the Women's Health Initiative investigators: Risks and benefits of estrogen plus progestin in healthy postmenopausal women: principal results from the Women's Health Initiative randomized controlled trial. JAMA 2002, 288:321–333.

Hypertension in African Americans

chapter
37

Elijah Saunders, M.D.,
Wallace Johnson, M.D.,
and Charlotte Jones-Burton, M.D.

Epidemiology

Based on the Third National Health and Nutrition and Examination Survey (NHANES III), the prevalence of hypertension in the United States in people aged 18 to 74 years is approximately 25%, with significantly higher rates in African Americans at 32.4% compared with 23.3% in non-Hispanic whites. This difference begins after puberty and persists into adult life. In fact, by age 65 years, approximately 75% of African American women are hypertensive compared with approximately 50% of white women. African Americans have an earlier onset of hypertension, which is more severe and results in more target organ damage. Hypertension in African Americans leads to an 80% higher stroke mortality rate, a 50% higher heart disease mortality rate, and a 320% higher rate of hypertension-related end-stage renal disease (ESRD) than the general population.[1]

Several hypotheses have been generated to explain higher rates of hypertension in African-Americans. One explanation is based on the voyage from Africa to America on slave ships (i.e., the Middle Passage). Grim and others have speculated that during these arduous trips, slaves were placed in a Darwinian "survival of the fittest" situation in which survival depended on "high-sodium–retaining" genes.[1] After individuals with these genes assumed lifestyles in environments where sodium was plentiful, the hypothesis suggests, the risk of hypertension escalated. This theory remains controversial.

Another related explanation espouses significant differences in sodium handling between blacks and whites. African Americans have increased sodium sensitivity, retaining more sodium than whites and exhibiting a greater increase in blood pressure (BP).[2] Yet another hypothesis involves plasma renin activity. Low renin forms of hypertension are found in black and white hypertensives. There is no ethnic difference in the pathophysiology of this subset of hypertension, a frequent misconception. Although many African American hypertensives have normal to high circulating renin activity, as a group, they are more likely than white hypertensives to manifest suppressed circulating renin activity. The authors speculate that there may be upregulation of the tissue angiotensin II system in blacks, which may be dissociated from the circulating renin angiotensin system.

Although various "physiological" explanations exist for the disparity in rates of hypertension between African Americans and white Americans, socioeconomic factors (including access to health care), mistrust of white physicians, and delay in diagnosis must be taken into account. Despite the dismal statistics regarding the high prevalence of hypertension in African Americans, African Americans can achieve overall declines in BP similar to those in European Americans. Blacks do experience fewer cardiovascular complications when their access to health care and treatment equals that given to whites (Figs. 1 and 2).

Comorbidity Associated with Hypertension in African Americans

Hypertension is a major risk factor for atherosclerotic cardiovascular diseases (CVDs) including stroke, heart failure, coronary heart disease, peripheral artery disease, and renal disease. Hypertension also clusters

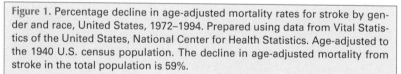

Figure 1. Percentage decline in age-adjusted mortality rates for stroke by gender and race, United States, 1972–1994. Prepared using data from Vital Statistics of the United States, National Center for Health Statistics. Age-adjusted to the 1940 U.S. census population. The decline in age-adjusted mortality from stroke in the total population is 59%.

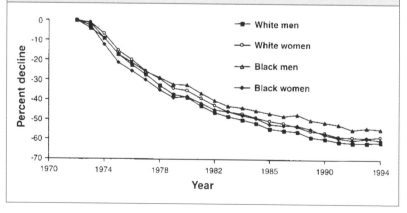

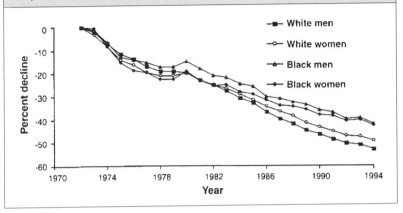

Figure 2. Percentage decline in age-adjusted mortality rates by gender and race for coronary heart disease, United States, 1972–1994. Prepared using data from Vital Statistics of the United States, National Center for Health Statistics. Age-adjusted to the 1940 U.S. census population. The decline in age-adjusted mortality for coronary heart disease in the total population is 53.2%.

with a number of other risk factors, including obesity, insulin resistance or glucose intolerance, and dyslipidemia.[2] African Americans have higher rates of stage 2 (> 160/> 100 mmHg) hypertension, other cardiovascular risk factors, and delays in diagnosis and treatment. It is not surprising that African Americans have greater hypertension-related morbidity and mortality than white Americans.

Obesity

Although the incidence of obesity continues to increase in all racial and ethnic, age, and gender groups, more African Americans, especially women, are affected. Strikingly, 65.9% of African American women and 56.7% of African American men are classified as overweight (body mass index [BMI] $\geq$ 25 kg/m^2) or obese (BMI $\geq$ 30 kg/m^2) compared with 47.0% and 60.6% of white women and men, respectively.[3,4] The Framingham Heart Study demonstrated a positive relationship between body weight and BP. In this population, 70% of new hypertensive patients were obese.[3] Even if individuals do not meet the BMI criteria for obesity, the presence of central or visceral obesity is strongly associated with a cluster of risk factors, including insulin resistance, impaired glucose tolerance and diabetes, atherogenic dyslipidemia, obesity, and hypertension.[4] Clustering of risk factors, known as the **metabolic syndrome,** confers an increased risk of cardiovascular morbidity and mortality. The American Heart Association has classified obesity as a modifiable risk factor for coronary artery disease.[5] Furthermore, modest long-term weight loss decreases BP.[6]

Insulin Resistance

Growing data support hyperinsulinemia as a significant factor in the genesis of hypertension.[7] Elevated insulin levels and insulin resistance associated with hypertension may be more common in African Americans. Insulin resistance is an impaired response to insulin of tissues, particularly skeletal muscle, adipose tissue or liver, or whole body.[8] Initially, the body compensates for insulin resistance by increasing insulin production to maintain a normal glucose level. Eventually, the beta cells fail to overcome the insulin resistance through hypersecretion. In one study, individuals who were most sensitive to insulin did not develop hypertension or cardiovascular disease (CVD) over a 4-year follow-up period, but one in five individuals with the greatest degree of insulin resistance developed CVD or hypertension.[9]

Diabetes Mellitus

Approximately 2.8 million African Americans have diabetes mellitus, making it one of the most serious diseases affecting this population.[10] Moreover, an estimated 700,000 African Americans have diabetes and do not know it. Diabetes is more prevalent among African Americans than whites, and African Americans are more likely to develop diabetic complications. African Americans have a frequency of diabetic retinopathy that is 40% higher than in whites. Similarly, diabetic ESRD is four times higher in blacks than in whites.[11] Often, diabetes and hypertension occur concomitantly, significantly increasing an individual's risk for developing CVD.

Cardiovascular Disease

Cardiovascular disease is the leading cause of death in the United States. Coronary heart disease (CHD) accounts for 54% of deaths from all CVDs. Although the prevalence of CHD is lower in black men than in white men, the mortality associated with CHD is higher in blacks.[12] There is no clear explanation about the pathogenesis and clinical manifestations of coronary artery disease in African Americans. However, some data indicate that African Americans are often underdiagnosed and untreated, both procedurally and surgically, for CHD.[13]

Congestive heart failure is increasing in the general population, but particularly in African Americans. A likely reason for this is that African Americans are more prone to concomitant diseases such as diabetes, hypertension, obesity, and CHD. Among African Americans, hypertension is the most common cause of heart failure.

Cerebrovascular Disease

Stroke is the third leading cause of death in the U.S. population, accounting for one of every 14 deaths. The age-adjusted prevalence of stroke for Americans age 20 years and older is higher in African American men and women than white American men and women, 2.5% and 3.2% vs. 2.2% and 1.5%, respectively. Young African Americans have a two- to threefold greater risk of ischemic stroke than their white counterparts and are more likely to die as a result of stroke.[14] In the black community, stroke is a common complication of hypertension. Two mechanisms explain the effect of hypertension on the development of cerebrovascular disease. Namely, hypertension increases the risk of atherothrombotic cerebral infarction by accelerating atherosclerosis, and hypertension increases the risk of cerebral hemorrhage by promoting the development of cerebral vascular microaneurysms.[15] Tight BP pressure control could prevent more than 50% of strokes in African Americans.[16]

Kidney Disease

In the United States, kidney disease affects approximately 20 million people. African Americans have four times the risk of developing ESRD, representing 32% of patients with ESRD. Furthermore, African American men ages 25 to 44 years are 20 times more likely to develop ESRD as a result of elevated BP than white men in the same age group.[17] Hypertension and diabetes mellitus are the major causes of ESRD. Recently, type 2 diabetes mellitus replaced hypertension as the primary cause of ESRD among African Americans.[18]

Resistent Hypertension in African Americans

Up to 95% of hypertensive African Americans have primary (i.e., essential) hypertension. However, if there are compelling circumstances (e.g., resistant hypertension despite multiple antihypertensive medications), further workup should be done to rule out secondary causes and aggravating causes of hypertension.

Sleep apnea and sleep-disordered breathing have been associated with hypertension.[19,20] Untreated sleep apnea induces sustained arterial hypertension. Because African Americans have a higher incidence of resistant hypertension, this diagnosis should be explored in patients with risk factors and symptoms consistent with sleep apnea (i.e., obesity, loud snoring, witnessed apneic episodes).

Although the prevalence of primary hyperaldosteronism was thought to be very low, it may be as high as 8% to 30% in selected hypertensive populations. In one trial, 20% of patients referred to a university clinic for resistant hypertension were found to have primary hyperaldosteronism.[21] In this study, the prevalence was similar in black and white subjects. Primary hyperaldosteronism is treatable either with an aldosterone antagonist or, in the case of an adrenal adenoma, with an adrenalectomy. In patients with resistant hypertension, hypokalemia, and metabolic alkalosis, this diagnosis should be pursued.

Therapeutic Targets for African Americans

Hypertension is a major modifiable risk factor for CVD. Despite this widely recognized fact, it is estimated that at least 35% of hypertensive patients are unaware of their diagnosis, and only 27% of treated patients have a BP level <140/90 mmHg (NHANES III).[22] However, the treatment of hypertension significantly reduces CVD. It is postulated that this failure to treat patients with hypertension to goal BP highlights the difficulty of maintaining individuals on long-term treatment for an asymptomatic disease.[23]

Because the prevalence of hypertension and sequelae of this disease are so overwhelming in African Americans, treatment of hypertension in this population must be given the highest priority. Identification of individuals in this high-risk population with high normal BP, more recently termed "pre-hypertension," will allow health care practitioners to encourage lifestyle modifications that may prevent or delay the onset of hypertension. The Seventh Report of the Joint National Committee on Prevention, Detection, Evaluation, and Treatment of High Blood Pressure (JNC VII) identifies lifestyle changes as losing weight, limiting daily alcohol intake, increasing daily aerobic activity, stopping smoking, and adjusting one's diet.[24] The Dietary Approaches to Stop Hypertension (DASH) diet lowers BP more in hypertensive African Americans than hypertensive whites.

The debate over racial differences in response to antihypertensive agents has occurred for decades. Undoubtedly, social influences have shaped the interpretation of data and led to the establishment of various opinions. These opinions include blacks responding better to diuretics; poorer to beta-blockers, angiotensin-converting enzyme (ACE) inhibitors, and angiotensin receptor blockers (ARBs); and equally to calcium antagonists than whites. These telescoped opinions have been used to establish race as an important variable in creating an antihypertensive regimen, perhaps to the disadvantage of African American hypertensives.[25] Several trials have documented successful treatment of African Americans to goal BP. However, ample data document the need for the use of multiple agents to achieve BP control. All classes of anti-hypertensive agents lower BP in African Americans.[26]

Factors to consider before prescribing antihypertensive medication include the degree of BP elevation, the presence of target organ damage or dysfunction, and the presence of other risk factors. Recently, the Hypertension in African Americans Working (HAAW) Group of the International Society on Hypertension in Blacks (ISHIB) published an evidence-based consensus statement regarding the management of high BP in African Americans[26] (Fig.3). For the first time, dual therapy is recommended as initial treatment for patients with systolic BP > 15

Figure 3. Clinical algorithm for achieving target BP in African-American patients with high BP. *Asterisk* indicates to initiate monotherapy at the recommended starting dose with an agent form any of the following classes: diuretics, beta-blockers, CCBs, ACE inhibitors, or ARBs. *Dagger* indicates to initiate low-dose combination therapy with any of the following combinations: beta-blocker and diuretic, ACE inhibitor and diuretic, ACE inhibitor and CCB, or ARB and diuretic. (Adapted from Douglas JG, Bakris GL, Epstein M, et al: Management of high blood pressure in African Americans. Consensus statement of the Hypertension in African American Working Group of the International Society on Hypertension in Blacks. Arch Intern Med 163:525–541, 2003.)

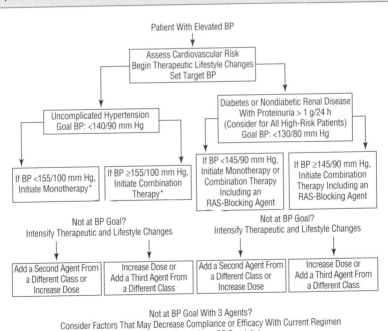

mmHg or diastolic BP 0.10 mmHg above their targets. This evidence-based approach is a marked departure from the traditional "stepwise" approach. Because African American hypertensives usually have higher BP before initiating therapy, monotherapy does not lower BP to the same extent as in white hypertensives. Thiazide diuretics have been the cornerstone of initial treatment of hypertension in African Americans. Additionally, calcium channel blockers (CCBs) have been another class of agents touted as having greater BP-lowering effects in African Americans. However, the studies had limitations in supporting the success of thiazide diuretics and CCBs in treating African American hypertensives. These limitations included monitoring diastolic BP, instead of systolic BP, for response; reporting response rates that reflected an arbitrary endpoint (i.e., diastolic BP 10 mmHg or more below baseline) rather than the target BP; and using study agents as a "proxy for class effect."[28]

The Antihypertensive and Lipid-Lowering Treatment to Prevent Heart Attack Trial (ALLHAT)[27,28] randomized 42,418 patients, including 35% African Americans, to a diuretic (chlorthalidone), an ACE inhibitor (lisinopril), or an alpha-blocker (doxazosin) plus a dihydropyridine CCB (amlodipine). The doxazosin arm of the trial was terminated early after patients in this arm developed more CHF than chlorthalidone-treated patients. There was no significant difference observed in the remaining three drugs in preventing major coronary events, the primary outcome of the trial. Chlorthalidone was superior to lisinopril in lowering BP and in preventing aggregate CVD, including stroke and CHF. Additionally, chlorthalidone was superior to amlodipine in preventing CHF. Based on these results, the authors concluded that thiazide diuretics are superior in preventing one or more major forms of CVD and should be the preferred agent for first-step antihypertensive therapy. However, a majority of patients in ALLHAT required an additional agent to lower BP. Despite the continued evidence in favor of thiazide diuretics, monotherapy is usually insufficient, particularly in African Americans.[28]

Another key component of the HAAW group recommendations is the use of a renin-angiotensin-aldosterone system (RAAS) blocking agent (i.e., ACE inhibitor or ARB) in the treatment of complicated hypertension. Patients with complicated hypertension include those with diabetes, evidence of target organ damage, and a history of a cardiovascular event. The Heart Outcomes Prevention Evaluation (HOPE) trial found that ramipril reduced cardiovascular events in high-risk patients with or without high BP.[29] Even though monotherapy with ACE inhibitors provide a more potent blood pressure reduction in white hypertensives,[30,31] the response in African American hypertensives is clinically significant. Increasing the doses of ACE inhibitor provides better antihypertensive efficacy in African Americans.[38] Adding a low-dose diuretic to the ACE inhibitor enhances BP reduction in African American hypertensives.[32]

JNC VI recommends substituting ARBs when ACE inhibitors are not tolerated.[26] ARBs have less cough associated with their use, and it has been suggested that hyperkalemia is less likely. Recent clinical trials confirmed the benefits of ARBs on the progression of renal disease in patients with type 2 diabetes.[33–36] ARBs are effective in reducing albumin excretion, ESRD, doubling of baseline serum creatinine level, and heart failure. These benefits were achieved without significant reduction in BP. Even though African American hypertensives do not experience similar BP reductions as white hypertensives, some evidence supports the use of RAAS-blocking agents in high-risk populations for other reasons (i.e., protection of target organs, reduction of cardiovascular mortality).

Compelling evidence now exists that progression to ESRD can be slowed in African Americans. The African American Study of Kidney Disease and Hypertension (AASK)[37] trial enrolled 1094 African Americans and is the first trial with significant power to evaluate the effects of inhibition of the RAAS in African Americans. The primary outcome evaluated was the rate of change in glomerular filtration rate (GFR) over approximately 36 months. The decline in GFR was 36% slower in the ramipril group compared with the amlodipine group. Furthermore, the risk reduction in secondary outcomes (i.e., a decline in GFR, ESRD, or death) for ramipril versus amlodipine was 38%. BP was considerably lower during the follow-up period than at baseline, but there was no significant difference between the treatment groups. These data supports the initial use of an ACE inhibitor in African Americans with hypertensive kidney disease.

The HAAW group has recommended the following combinations for initial treatment in African American hypertensives with BP > 155/100 mmHg at the onset: beta-blocker and diuretic, ACE inhibitor and diuretic, ARB and diuretic, or ACE inhibitor and CCB. The authors acknowledge that other combinations may be effective, and three drugs are often needed to reach target BP. Regardless of which medical regimen is chosen, a new paradigm is clearly indicated for the management of high-risk hypertensives such as African Americans. Lifestyle modifications can have a major impact on BP reduction, particularly in African American hypertensives. As physicians change their approach to identifying, diagnosing, and treating African Americans with hypertension, this disease and its manifestations will hopefully move from being "not so silent" to being controlled and quiescent.

References

1. Blaustein MP, Grim CE: The pathogenesis of hypertension: Black-white differences. In Saunders E, Davis FA, eds. Cardiovascular Diseases in Blacks. Philadelphia, 1991; pp 97–113.

2. Reaven GM: Role of insulin resistance in human disease. Diabetes 37:1595–1607, 1988.

3. Kannel WB, Brand N, Skinner JJ, et al: The relationship of adiposity to blood pressure and development of hypertension. The Framingham Study. Ann Intern Med 67:48–59, 1967.

4. Lemieux I, Pascot A, Couillard C, et al: Hypertriglyceridemic waist: a marker for atherogenic metabolic triad (hyperinsulinemia;hyperapolipoprotein B; small dense LDL) in men? Circulation 102:179–184, 2000.

5. Eckel RH, Krauss RM: American Heart Association call to action: Obesity as a major risk factor for coronary heart disease. Circulation 97:2099–2100, 1998.

6. Stevens VJ: Long-term weight loss and changes in blood pressure: Results of the Trials of Hypertension Prevention, phase II. Ann Intern Med 134:1–11, 2001.

7. MacFalane SI, Banjeri M, Sowers JR: Insulin resistance and cardiovascular disease. J Clin Endocrin Metab 86:713–718, 2001.

8. Hansen BC: The metabolic syndrome X. Ann NY Acad Sci 18:1–24, 1999.

9. Yip Y, Facchini FS, Reaven GM: Resistance to insulin-mediated glucose disposal as a predictor of cardiovascular disease. J Clin Endocrinol Metab 83:2773–2776, 1998.

10. National Institute of Diabetes and Digestive and Kidney Diseases: National Diabetes Statistics fact sheet: General information and national estimates on diabetes in the United States, 2000. Bethesda, MD, U.S. Department of Health and Human Services, National Institutes of Health, 2002.

11. Available at URL: http://www.diabetes.org/main/info/facts/facts_nephropathy.jsp.

12. Available at URL: http://www.americanheart.org/downloadable/heart/10461207852142003HDSStatsBook.pdf.

13. Peterson ED, Shaw LK, DeLong ER, et al: Racial variation in the use of coronary-revascularization procedures. Are the differences real? Do the matter? N Engl J Med 336:480–486, 1997.

14. Available at URL: www.strokecenter.org/pat/stats.htm.

15. Williams GS: Hypertensive vascular disease. In Fauci AS, et al, eds. Harrison's Principals of Internal Medicine, 14th edition. 1384, 1998.

16. Cooper ES, Caplan LR. Cerebrovascular disease in hypertensive blacks. In Saunders E, Davis FA, eds. Cardiovascular Diseases in Blacks. Philadelphia, 1991, pp 145–155.

17. National Kidney Disease Education Program. (NIH Publication No. 03–5349). Bethesda, MD, National Institutes of Health, 2003.

18. Flack JM, Peters R, Mehra VC, Nasser SA: Hypertension in special populations. Cardiol Clin 20:303–319, 2002.

19. Kales A, Bixler EO, Cadieux RJ, et al: Sleep apnea in a hypertensive population. Lancet 2:1005–1008, 1984.

20. Nieto FJ, Young TB, Lind BK, et al: Association of sleep disordered breathing, sleep apnea, and hypertension in a large community-based study. Sleep Heart Study. JAMA 283:1829–1836, 2000.

21. Calhoun DA, Nishizaka MK, Zaman MA, et al: Hyperaldosteronism among black and white subjects with resistant hypertension. Hypertension 40:892–896, 2002.

22. Burt VL, Cutler JA, Higgins M, et al: Trends in the prevalence, awareness, treatment and control of hypertension in the adult US population. Data from the health examination surveys, 1960 to 1991. Hypertension 26:60–69, 1995.

23. Kaplan NM: Treatment of hypertension: Insights from the JNC VI report. Am Fam Physician 58:1323–1330, 1998.

24. Joint National Committee on Prevention, Detection, Evaluation, and Treatment of High Blood Pressure: The sixth report of the Joint National Committee on Prevention, Detection, Evaluation, and Treatment of High Blood Pressure. Arch Intern Med 157:2413–2446, 1997.

25. Jamerson K, DeQuattro V: The impact of ethnicity on response to antihypertensive therapy. Am J Med 101(suppl 3A):22S-32S, 1996.

26. Douglas JG, Bakris GL, Epstein M, et al: Management of high blood pressure in African Americans. Consensus statement of the Hypertension in African American Working Group of the International Society on Hypertension in Blacks. Arch Intern Med 163:525–541, 2003.

27. ALLHAT Collaborative Research Group: Major cardiovascular events in hypertensive patients randomized to doxazosin vs chlorthalidone: The Antihypertensive and Lipid-Lowering Treatment to Prevent Heart Attack Trial (ALLHAT). JAMA 283:1967–1975, 2000.

28. The ALLHAT Officers and Coordinators, for the ALLHAT Collaborative Research Group: Major outcomes in high-risk hypertensive patients randomized to angiotensin-converting inhibitor or calcium channel blocker vs diuretic: The Antihypertensive and Lipid-Lowering Treatment to Prevent Heart Attack Trial (ALLHAT). JAMA 288:2981–2197, 2002.

29. Yusef S, Sleight P, Pogue J, et al. for the Heart Outcomes Prevention Evaluation Study Investigators: Effects of an angiotensin-converting enzyme inhibitor, ramipril, on cardiovascular events in high-risk patients. N Engl J Med 342:145–153, 2000.

30. Hanes DS, Weir MW: Gender considerations in hypertension pathophysiology and treatment. Am J Med 101(suppl 3A):10S-21S, 1996.

31. Hall WD: A rational approach to the treatment of hypertension in special populations. Am Fam Physician 60:156–162, 1999.

32. Saunders E. Blockade of the renin-angiotensin system in African Americans with hypertension and cardiovascular disease. J Clin Hypertens (Greenwich) 5(1 suppl 1):12–17, 2003.

33. Parving HH, Lehnert H, Brochner-Mortensen J, et al: Irbesartan in Patients with Type 2 Diabetes and Microalbuminuria Study Group: The effect of irbesartan on the development of diabetic nephropathy in patients with type 2 diabetes. N Engl J Med 345: 870–878, 2001.

34. Lewis EJ, Hunsicker LG, Clarke WR, et al: Renoprotective effect of the angiotensin-receptor antagonist irbesartan in patients with nephropathy due to type 2 diabetes. N Engl J Med 345:851–860, 2001.

35. Brenner BM, Cooper ME, de Zeeuw D, et al: for the RENAAL Study Investigators: Effects of losartan on renal and cardiovascular outcomes in patients with type 2 diabetes and nephropathy. N Engl J Med 345:861–869, 2001.

36. Viberti G: Microalbuminuria reduction with valsartan in patients with type 2 diabetes mellitus: A blood pressure-independent effect. Circulation 106:672–678, 2002.

37. Agodoa LY, Appel L, Bakris GL, et al: Effect of ramipril vs amlodipine on renal outcomes in hypertensive nephrosclerosis: A randomized controlled trial. JAMA 285:2719–2728, 2001.

38. Saunders E, Weir MR, Kong BWW, et al: A comparison of the efficacy and safety of a beta-blocker, a calcium-channel blocker, and a converting enzyme inhibitor in hypertensive blacks. Arch Intern Med 150:1707, 1990.

.

Hypertension in Adolescents

Bonita Falkner, M.D.

chapter

38

Hypertension is a clinical problem that occurs in children and adolescents, as well as adults. Although hypertension does not occur as frequently in adolescents as it does in adults, hypertension is not uncommon in adolescents. In adults, hypertension is defined according to the level of blood pressure (BP) that is linked with a substantial increase in the risk for cardiovascular events such as stroke or ischemic heart disease. Although it is now known that the relationship of BP level to cardiovascular disease (CVD) risk is continuous across the range of BP, BP $\geq$ 140/90 mmHg is diagnostic of hypertension in adults. Hypertension is defined somewhat differently in young individuals: because (1) there is a normal upward trend in BP throughout childhood that is related to growth and (2) the occurrence of the typical hypertension-related cardiovascular events is rare in adolescents. Therefore, hypertension in young people, up through age 17 years, is defined as systolic or diastolic BP that is equal to or greater than the 95th percentile of the normal BP range for age, gender, and height.[1]

In adolescents, the BP level that is indicative of hypertension is < 140/90 mmHg. Charts are available that provide the precise BP levels for age, gender, and height. Table 1 provides a simplified approximation of the 95th percentile for adolescent boys and girls. As shown in the table, the BP level that defines hypertension in adolescents is between 120/80 and 135/85 mmHg, depending on age and gender. The systolic BP level that designates hypertension is somewhat lower in girls than in boys. The diagnosis of hypertension in adolescents also requires that the systolic or diastolic BP must be consistently elevated on at least three separate measurement sessions. With these definition guidelines, it is estimated that the occurrence of hypertension in adolescents is between 1% and 3%, with variation in adolescent hypertension rates related somewhat to race and the prevalence of obesity.

Secondary hypertension, or hypertension caused by some underlying condition such as renal, cardiovascular, or endocrine abnormality, had,

TABLE 1. Values for Hypertension in Adolescents* Blood Pressure (mmHg)		
Age (years)	Boys	Girls
12–14	120/80	120/80
14–15	130/82	125/82
16–18	135/85	130/85
* 95th percentile		

in the past, been considered to be the most likely explanation for hypertension in young individuals. But with the development of a large body of data on BP in the young and an improved understanding of the normal range of BP levels in healthy children and adolescents, this thinking has changed. In adolescents, primary or essential hypertension appears to be the most frequent type of hypertension and probably accounts for > 50% of hypertension in adolescents. However, hypertension that is secondary to another disorder occurs more frequently in young than in older patients. Therefore, after the presence of hypertension is established in an adolescent, clinical decisions must be made regarding how extensive the evaluation for possible underlying causes of hypertension should be. The other clinical decision in the management of hypertensive adolescents involves how to treat the hypertension. Typical types of adolescent hypertension are used here to discuss these issues.

Hypertension in Athletes

A common source for the detection of hypertension in adolescents, especially boys, is the physical examinations required for sports participation. These athletes appear to be very healthy and are without symptoms. The typical story is that the adolescent athlete has had no health problems, and the elevated BP measurement was an unexpected finding. Most of the time, these children are not permitted to participate in competitive sports until they have obtained medical clearance from a physician, which, for boys in particular, makes the solution to this problem urgent. The steps to be taken in resolving the BP problems for adolescent athletes are to (1) verify the BP elevation, (2) conduct the necessary diagnostic evaluation, and (3) determine what treatment is most appropriate.

Confirming the presence of hypertension requires repeated BP measurements that are at or above the 95th percentile for age and gender (see Table 1). In performing repeat measurements in the office, attention should be given to the body size of the child and the size of the BP cuff to be used. Adolescent boys who are engaged in some competitive sports, such as football, can be very large, with muscular upper arms. For these large boys, the standard size BP cuff is too small. Use of a BP cuff that is too small can result in an inappropriately elevated BP measurement. A larger BP cuff that is appropriate for the size of the upper arm is necessary to obtain accurate blood pressure measurements. When an elevated BP measurement has been obtained with a cuff that was too small, sometimes simply using an appropriate size BP cuff can resolve the problem.

If the repeated BP measurements continue to be marginal or only slightly elevated and the presence of hypertension continues to be uncertain, obtaining ambulatory BP measurements over a 24-hour period can be very helpful. Again, the correct cuff size should be used with the 24-hour monitor. The cutpoint for elevated BP measurement should be programed in the analysis of the measurements over 24 hours. The standard programs for adults uses 140/90 mmHg as the cutpoint for elevated readings, but the appropriate BP cutpoint for adolescents should be used in interpretation of the results. In general, < 25% of the 24-hour BP measurements are elevated and if there is a normal nighttime dip in the BP, the adolescent may have "white coat hypertension." If this is the case, no further evaluation is necessary, and routine health care is recommended.

When hypertension in an adolescent is verified by repeated BP measurements that are equal to or greater than the 95th percentile, an appropriate evaluation is necessary. The purposes of the evaluation are to determine if there is a secondary cause for the hypertension and to determine if there is evidence of target organ injury. The degree of BP elevation and information obtained from a medical history and physical examination are used to decide how extensive the diagnostic evaluation should be. Adolescents with more severe hypertension and absence of the typical risk factors for essential hypertension are more likely to have a secondary cause. Alternatively, adolescents who have only slight BP elevation along with a family history of hypertension or excess body weight are more likely to have essential hypertension. When taking a history from an adolescent athlete, include questions about bodybuilding such as use of diet supplements and other drugs and weight-training regimens that include power weightlifting. These behaviors can have an adverse effect on BP in young individuals.

Blood pressure measurements that are 15 to 20 mmHg above the 95th percentile in an adolescent should be considered significantly elevated, and a careful diagnostic evaluation is appropriate. Depending on other findings from the history and physical examination, testing should be performed to determine if there is a renal, renal vascular, cardiac, or endocrine cause for the hypertension. More frequently, however, the athlete has BP measurements that are closer to the 95th percentile, which can make it more difficult to determine the extent of the workup. Many of these adolescents are very serious about their participation in sports, and sometimes an athletic scholarship for college is an issue. In these situations, a thorough evaluation can be the most appropriate course to follow. The basic evaluation includes blood chemistries, complete blood count, urinalysis, and a renal ultrasound. An echocardiogram is helpful in determining if the hypertension is of sufficient length and degree to effect left ventricular hypertrophy (LVH). When requesting an echocardiogram in an adolescent, it is important to specify that the echocardiogram is being obtained to determine cardiac structure and determine if LVH is present.

Strategies for treatment of hypertensive adolescents include lifestyle changes and antihypertensive pharmacologic therapy. Adolescents who take athletic performance seriously are generally physically active and have appropriate body weight. These adolescents should not be restricted from participation in sports. Exceptions include patients in whom potentially serious cardiac valvular abnormalities or significant asymmetric septal hypertrophy are detected, in which physical activity should be limited until the child has been evaluated by a pediatric cardiologist. Otherwise, these adolescents should be encouraged to continue physical activity, although little BP benefit can be expected from further increasing physical activity and weight reduction. However, even athletic adolescents can benefit from dietary changes to reduce sodium intake and change from processed and fast foods to fresh fruits and vegetables in the style of the Dietary Approaches to Stop Hypertension (DASH) diet.

If the BP is consistently above the 95th percentile or if there is evidence of target organ damage such as proteinuria or LVH by echocardiogram, then pharmacologic therapy is appropriate. When drugs are indicated to improve BP control, it is best to select medications that are unlikely to have an effect on physical performance. For this reason, it is preferred to use drugs in the classes of angiotensin-converting enzyme (ACE) inhibitors, angiotensin receptor blockers (ARBs), or calcium channel blockers (CCBs) as first-choice medications. Athletes begun on ACE inhibitors and ARBs should be instructed on the importance of adequate fluid and electrolyte replacement during training and competition because excessive hypotension can occur. Beta-blockers and diuretics are not preferred first-choice medications because of possible adverse effects on physical performance. During the course of controlling BP, it is important to educate the adolescent about high BP and the importance of achieving a satisfactory level of BP control for now and into the future.

Adolescent Couch Potatoes

Among adolescents, as well as adults, more common lifestyles involve physical inactivity, dietary patterns that include disproportional amounts of processed foods with frequent snacks, and use of leisure time with sedentary activities such as television viewing. These lifestyles are contributing substantially to the obesity epidemic. A consequence of obesity in adolescence is hypertension. The hypertension is not necessarily caused directly by the obesity, but the obesity tends to permit earlier expression of essential hypertension. Most of the time, adolescents with high BP and obesity also have other characteristic risk factors for essential hypertension, including a family history of hypertension and cardiovascular disease. In these individuals, the hypertension is typically mild, with the degree of BP elevation near or just above the 95th percentile. The management of adolescent "couch potatoes" with elevated BP entails a process similar to management of adolescent athletes with hypertension. It includes verification of the hypertension, appropriate evaluation, and treatment.

Hypertension in overweight, sedentary adolescents is verified by repeated BP measurements that are at or above the 95th percentile (see Table 1). As with large, muscular athletes, the use of a BP cuff that is appropriate for the size of the adolescent is important. When the diagnosis of hypertension is in question, 24-hour ambulatory BP monitoring can also provide useful information on the level of BP elevation throughout the day and determine if the normal nighttime BP dipping occurs.

After it is established that an obese adolescent has hypertension, the issues to be addressed in the evaluation are somewhat different. Obesity and hypertension are two components of the **metabolic syndrome,** also known as the **syndrome of insulin resistance.** Therefore, the diagnostic evaluation should include an assessment for undetected comorbidities associated with obesity and high BP. A medical history and physical examination are the first steps in an evaluation. Then, as with athletes, the basic evaluation should include blood chemistries, complete blood count, and urinalysis. Unless some clues pertaining to possible underlying renal disease are detected, a renal ultrasound may not be necessary. However, additional metabolic studies should be done, including a fasting blood sample for measurement of lipids, glucose, and insulin. If there is a family history for diabetes, it would be appropriate to also do a HbA1c or an oral glucose tolerance test. When evidence of the metabolic syndrome is present,[3] it is appropriate to determine if evidence of cardiovascular injury is also present. At the present time, the best clinical measures to examine this possibility are echocardiography to determine if LVH is present and a urine sample for microalbuminuria.

Initial treatment for adolescent couch potatoes should strongly emphasize lifestyle changes, including increasing physical activity, making diet changes, and decreasing excess body weight. If the adolescent smokes, this behavior should also be changed. Strong motivation on the part of the adolescent is essential to successfully achieve changes in lifestyles. All possible strategies should be considered for these adolescents, including joining fitness clubs, engaging in after-school activities, and consulting with nutritionists. It can be helpful to set realistic goals in achieving change and to begin with small but attainable changes in physical activity and diet. For example, simply eliminating sodas and walking a few extra blocks a day would have substantial long-range benefit if sustained.

It is obvious that the primary treatment should be to effect positive changes in health-related behaviors that promote the obesity and adverse lifestyles. It is also important to treat related medical problems. If the efforts to achieve lifestyle changes are not successful or if the BP does not decrease to a satisfactory level despite some changes, additional medical treatment is indicated. When an adolescent continues to have BP measurements that are at or above the 95th percentile, pharmacologic treatment is appropriate. In selecting antihypertensive drug treatments for overweight, sedentary adolescents, comorbidities associated with the metabolic syndrome should be considered. The first-choice medications are those that do not have an adverse effect on metabolic parameters. If there is evidence of cardiovascular injury such as LVH or microalbuminuria, drugs that are angiotensin inhibitors are appropriate for initial pharmacologic treatment. If the adolescent has a strong family history of diabetes or has impaired glucose tolerance, continued monitoring of glucose metabolism is important. Alterations in plasma lipid levels, if present, also require monitoring and possible treatment. Overweight adolescents with hypertension are demonstrating chronic cardiovascular disease in its early phase. Without any intervention, many of these individuals will likely experience cardiovascular events prematurely in their adult years.

Adolescent Girls with Hypertension

The normal distribution for BP tends to be lower in adolescent girls compared with adolescent boys. The lower normal range of BP for girls is most likely because girls are shorter than boys. As seen in Table 1, the level of BP that designates hypertension in adolescent girls is somewhat lower than in adolescent boys. There are some special considerations in adolescent girls regarding elevated BP. A common clinical occurrence is an adolescent girl who is noted to have elevated BP while taking oral contraceptives. Some young women do experience an increase in BP when taking oral contraceptives. The newer oral contraceptives that are currently in use have lower amounts of exogenous hormones in the tablets. However, some young women and adolescent girls still experience an increase in BP when taking these drugs.

In evaluating an adolescent girl who is noted to have high BP while taking birth control pills, it is important to determine what her BP level was before taking the oral contraceptives. In other words, determine if the patient had unrecognized hypertension. For example, a 15-year-old girl who had a BP of 136/84 mmHg recorded before she began taking the birth control pills could have been hypertensive, and the birth control pills were not necessarily causative of her high BP. If the adolescent girl was clearly normotensive or even if it is unknown if she was normotensive before taking the oral contraceptives, it would be appropriate to discontinue the birth control pills and monitor her BP to determine if readings decrease to a normotensive range. This would be the most logical and reasonable management course to follow. However, it is also important to consider the reason that the adolescent girl is taking the birth control pills. Although oral contraceptives can be prescribed for reasons other than preventing pregnancy in sexually active women, pregnancy prevention is by far the most common indication, especially when prescribed for adolescent girls. Before discontinuing the oral contraceptives in a sexually active adolescent girl, careful discussion of alternative birth control methods should be considered, along with consideration about how effective the alternatives would be for pregnancy prevention.

As noted, the level of BP that indicates hypertension is lower in adolescent girls than in boys. Adolescent girls with marked hypertension may require special consideration. For example, a BP level of 145/90 mmHg in a 14-year-old girl is severe hypertension. Although the absolute number for BP level is not that high, it is more than 20 mmHg above the cutpoint for hypertension for a 14-year-old girl. This level of BP in an adolescent girl would be comparable to stage 2 hypertension in an adult. Girls with severe hypertension, particularly girls who do not have the typical risk factors for essential hypertension, are the adolescents who are most likely to have secondary hypertension. A slender white girl who has a negative or minimal family history of hypertension and has a BP of 145/90 mmHg on repeated measurement is unlikely to have essential hypertension. Adolescent girls who have BP measurements that are 15 to 20 mmHg above the designated cutpoint for hypertension and also have none of the typical risk factors for essential hypertension should be evaluated thoroughly for a secondary cause. Adolescent boys with similar severity of BP elevation and absence of risk factors should be managed similarly. Underlying causes of hypertension that are identified in adolescents with hypertension are most frequently renal or renal-vascular causes. Unless substantial clinical clues exist that indicate a different direction for the evaluation (e.g., signs and symptoms of hyperthyroidism), the most productive focus of the clinical evaluation is on underlying renal disease.

High-Risk Adolescents

Some adolescents with known chronic medical problems are also at risk for hypertension. Two clinical problems in particular require careful attention to monitoring BP and early intervention for BP control, even with mild elevations in BP. Adolescents with diabetes mellitus are at risk for developing diabetic nephropathy. Most diabetic adolescents have type 1 diabetes. However, as a consequence of the obesity epidemic, type 2 diabetes is progressively more commonplace in adolescents, especially ethnic minorities. Even in the absence of proteinuria or micro-albuminuria, BP levels in both type 1 and type 2 diabetic adolescents should be controlled to avoid renal injury. Medications used for treatment of hypertension in diabetic adolescents are similar to those used in the treatment of hypertension in adults with diabetics. Drugs that interfere with angiotensin action such as ACE inhibitors or ARBs are preferred first-choice medications for BP control.

Hypertension is associated with many types of chronic renal diseases that can occur in adolescence, including chronic glomerulonephritis, chronic pyelonephritis, and various types of renal dysplasia. Elevated BP in adolescents with chronic renal disease is secondary to the renal disease. The elevated BP can also augment progression of the renal disease. To preserve renal function, medications should be used to ensure optimal BP control in adolescents with known renal disease.

Summary

Hypertension is a common problem that can be detected in adolescents. Because hypertension in children and adolescents is currently defined as BP that exceeds the 95th percentile, the level of BP that designates hypertension in adolescents is lower than 140/90 mmHg. Hypertension in adolescents is often essential hypertension. When the hypertension is only slightly above the 95th percentile and the adolescent is overweight and has a strong family history hypertension, essential hypertension is the most likely diagnosis. However, adolescents who have marked elevation in BP and a paucity of risk factors should be evaluated for secondary causes of the hypertension. Whether the adolescent has essential or secondary hypertension, BP should be controlled using both pharmacologic and nonpharmacologic treatment strategies.

References

1. National High Blood Pressure Education Program Working Group on Hypertension Control in Children and Adolescents: Update on the 1987 Task Force Report on High Blood Pressure in Children and Adolescents: a working group report from the National High Blood Pressure Education Program. Pediatrics 98:649–658, 1996.
2. Appel LJ, Moore TJ, Obarzanek E, et al. for the DASH Collaborative Research Group: A clinical trial of the effects of dietary patterns on blood pressure. N Engl J Med 336:1117–1124, 1997.
3. Ford ES, Giles WH, Dietz WH: Prevalence of the metabolic syndrome among US adults. JAMA 287:356–359, 2002.

Hypertension in Surgical Patients

chapter

39

Randa K. Noseir, M.D., and
Thomas J. Ebert, M.D., Ph.D.

Definition and Risk Assessment

Postponing elective surgery has psychological, social, political, and economic consequences and preoperative hypertension is the most common avoidable medical condition that results in postponing surgery. Yet it is still unclear what level of arterial pressure should be used as a guideline for postponing surgery because prospective outcome studies have not been performed. Three decades ago, Prys-Roberts et al.[1] demonstrated that poorly controlled preoperative blood pressure (BP) (i.e., untreated hypertensive patients) was associated with an increased frequency of arrhythmia, intraoperative BP instability, and myocardial ischemia. More recently, preoperative chronic hypertension has been associated with both pre- and postoperative silent ischemia and clearly ischemia is a predictor for adverse cardiac outcome.[2–5] Moreover, a patient history of hypertension has been associated with perioperative cardiovascular death in noncardiac surgical procedures.[6] Nowadays, with more consistent treatment of hypertension and improved medical therapy for controlling hypertension, focus has been shifted to determine if admission or immediate preoperative BP has a predictive role in adverse cardiac outcome.[3,7,8] Patients with elevated BP readings on admission to the hospital have exaggerated pressor responses to laryngoscopy and intubation, are more likely to develop perioperative myocardial ischemia and are more likely to require vasodilator therapy.[7] One retrospective study[8] indicated that whereas increased BP on admission to the hospital was not associated with cardiovascular death, a diagnosis of hypertension was associated with perioperative cardiovascular death.[10] This leads to two important points: 1) long-standing, not "white coat," hypertension is likely to result in vascular injury and end-organ damage to cardiac, renal, and cerebral tissue, thereby placing patients at risk of adverse outcome and 2) preoperative elevations in BP are generally treated rather than ignored by anesthesia caregivers. Patients with acute hypertension are commonly treated before anesthetic induction with rapidly acting

421

intravenous antihypertensive agents that likely improve patient outcomes (although this has not been prospectively studied).

Postoperative Hypertension: Risk Factors and Outcomes

Regardless of preoperative BP and adequate treatment of hypertension before initiating anesthesia, it is quite clear that hypertension can develop in the intra- and postoperative period and put multiple organs at risk, leading to myocardial infarction, congestive heart failure, stroke, and renal failure. Factors promoting perioperative hypertension include increases in sympathetic activity secondary to preoperative anxiety, tracheal intubation, surgical stimulation, rapid intravascular fluid shifts, and postoperative pain. These factors may induce hypertensive states in otherwise normotensive patients. In addition, patients with preexisting hypertension have exaggerated postoperative BP increases, likely caused by pain, anxiety, and catecholamine surges adding to an already noncompliant vasculature. Risk factors for postoperative hypertension are listed in (Table 1). Hypertension and tachycardia in the post-anesthesia care unit (PACU) are associated with long-term morbidity and mortality, including unplanned admission to intensive care units and hospital mortality.[9] However, anesthetic factors provide only a small contribution toward predicting risk for postoperative hypertension; patient and surgical factors have greater influence (Fig. 1).[9] In the postoperative period,

TABLE 1. Risk Factors for Hypertension in the Postanesthesia Care Unit for Patients Having General Anesthesia

Characteristic	Patients with Hypertension, %	Adjusted Relative Odds*
Patient Factors		
Age		1.05
Smoker	2.8	1.54
Renal disease	10.0	4.83
Intraoperative Factors		
Case duration		
2 to 4 hours	3.5	2.16
> 4 hours	7.4	3.30
Cases finishing after 6 PM	4.0	1.41
Intracranial surgery	8.5	2.09
Intraoperative hypertension	17.4	4.60
Intraoperative tachycardia	3.8	1.79
PACU Factors		
Hypoventilation	6.7	2.54
Substantial pain	3.6	1.79
Nausea or vomiting	2.6	1.45

* Adjusted relative odds ratio < 1.0 have been omitted. (Adapted from Rofe et al.[9])

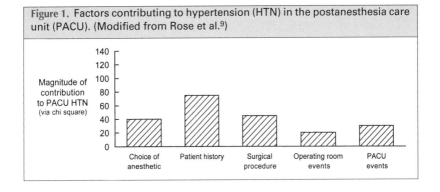

Figure 1. Factors contributing to hypertension (HTN) in the postanesthesia care unit (PACU). (Modified from Rose et al.[9])

the increased afterload imposed by hypertension can lead to increased myocardial work and predisposes patients to ischemia, impaired left ventricular ejection leading to pulmonary edema, wound hematoma, arrhythmia, intracerebral hemorrhage, acute renal failure, cerebral edema, and encephalopathy.

Practical Implications for the Perioperative Management of Hypertensive Patients

There has been controversy about when to treat and how rapidly to decrease BP in the perioperative period. Management goals to maintain hemodynamic stability depend on many factors, especially preoperative BP (i.e., the patient's "normal" BP). General indication for intraoperative intervention are a systolic or diastolic pressure change 20% to 30% above resting BP, signs of organ dysfunction (e.g., ST segment depression), or a patient disease state (e.g., increased intracranial pressure, CAD) that mandates tight BP control to avoid morbidity.

Recent guidelines have been offered for the perioperative management of hypertensive patients (Table 2),[8] using the Joint National Committee on the Detection, Evaluation, and Treatment of High Blood Pressure (JNC-VI) classification of arterial BP. They are consistent with the American College of Cardiology/American Heart Association (ACC/AHA) guidelines that recommend deferring anesthesia if the diastolic BP is above 110 mm Hg.[10] However, both systolic and diastolic BP should be taken into account because there is now evidence that systolic BP is independently associated with target organ damage[11] and increased risk of postoperative silent myocardial ischemia.[2] Substantial benefit has also been shown for treatment of isolated systolic hypertension in elderly individuals.[12] The justification for postponing surgery is to provide the opportunity to improve the patient's medical condition to an extent

TABLE 2.   Guidelines for Care when Hypertensive Patients Present for Anesthesia and Surgery

Stages of Hypertension	Guidelines and Justification
Stages 1, 2 (systolic BP 140–179 mm Hg, diastolic BP 90–109 mm Hg)	Anesthesia and surgery may proceed Studies were unable to demonstrate association between poorly controlled HTN in stages 1 and 2 and cardiac complications[8,17]
Stage 3 (systolic BP > 180 mm Hg, diastolic BP > 110 mm Hg)	Anesthesia and surgery should be deferred to allow arterial blood pressure to be treated and end-organ function to be optimized Studies demonstrated an association between poorly controlled HTN (stage 3) and the occurrence of intraoperative[1] and postoperative[3] myocardial ischemia and arrhythmia

Stages as described by Sixth Joint National Committee on the Detection, Evaluation and Treatment of High Blood Pressure (JNC VI Classification).[18]

TABLE 3.   Management of Anesthesia for Hypertensive Patients

Preoperative Evaluation
- Continue most antihypertensive agents, including beta and calcium channel blockers, orally with sip of water
- Withhold morning angiotensin-converting enzyme (ACE) inhibitor or angiotensin receptor agonists (ARAs)[19,20]
- Consider case cancellation to improve medical therapy if systolic BP > 180 or diastolic BP > 110 mm Hg
- Review routine laboratory analysis to assess renal, cerebral, and cardiac function
- Consider invasive BP monitoring
- Premedication with benzodiazepines for anxiolysis
- Consider beginning beta-blocker therapy with atenolol, metoprolol, or esmolol infusion

Induction of Anesthesia
- Expect exaggerated BP decreases with propofol or sodium thiopental induction
- Expect exaggerated BP increases to intubation, especially if etomidate is used for induction
- Pretreat generously with opioid and consider topical or systemic lidocaine before laryngoscopy
- Perform short-duration laryngoscopy

Maintenance of Anesthesia (to minimize fluctuations in intraoperative BP)
- Titrate rapid acting volatile anesthetic to control BP
- Avoid desflurane because of sympathetic stimulation properties[21]
- Consider opioids or alpha$_2$ agonists to prevent sympathetic surges with surgical stimulation
- Monitor for and aggressively treat myocardial ischemia or arrhythmia

Postoperative Management
- Anticipate hypertension on emergence from anesthesia, especially if patient has preexisting hypertension, pretreat with esmolol or labetalol before emergence and extubation
- For high-risk patients, consider intravenous sodium nitroprusside or nitroglycerine for rapid BP control; also continue chronic beta-blocker therapy and reinstitute ACE inhibitor or ARAs
- Continue invasive monitoring until BP is controlled

that would reasonably be expected to decrease risk factors substantially.[13] Unfortunately, no definitive data have established whether perioperative (i.e., pre-, intra-, and postoperative) treatment of hypertension reduces intra- or postoperative risk for major adverse cardiac, renal, or cerebral outcomes. Some insight can be gleaned from patient studies in which a moderately elevated BP was treated with a single oral dose of a β-blocking agent. This reduced the incidence of myocardial ischemia and cardiovascular morbidity, suggesting more intense medical therapy directed at controlling heart rate (and presumably BP) may improve outcome.[14,15] Perioperative management of patients with essential hypertension who are scheduled for surgery is outlined in Table 3. Prys-Roberts[16] has offered a flow diagram for the management of hypertensive patients presenting for anesthesia and surgery. It was modified recently to include the management of isolated systolic hypertension (15) (Fig. 2). It is important that when deferring anesthesia and surgery for elevated BP, appropriate antihypertensive therapy is started and follow up is arranged.

Figure 2. Flow diagram for the management of hypertensive patients for surgery. (Adapted from Prys-Roberts.[13])

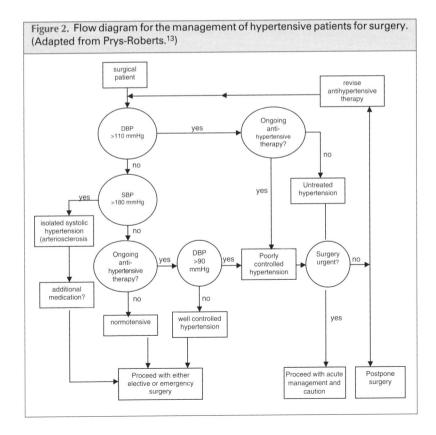

References

1. Prys-Roberts C, Meloche R, Foëx P: Studies of anaesthesia in relation to hypertension. I: cardiovascular responses of treated and untreated patients. Br J Anaesth 1971, 43:122–1371.
2. Hollenberg M, Mangano DT, Browner WS, et al: Predictors of postoperative myocardial ischemia in patients undergoing noncardiac surgery: the Study of Perioperative Ischemia Research Group. JAMA 1992, 268:205–209.
3. Howell J, Hemming AE, Allman KG, et al: Predictors of postoperative myocardial ischemia: the role of intercurrent arterial hypertension and other cardiovascular risk factors. Anaesthesia 1997, 52:107–111.
4. Mangano DT, Browner WS, Hollenberg M, et al: Long-term cardiac prognosis following noncardiac surgery. JAMA 1992, 268:233–239.
5. Raby KE, Goldman L, Creager MA, et al: Correlation between preoperative ischemia and major cardiac events after peripheral vascular surgery. N Engl J Med 1989, 321:1296–1300.
6. Howell SJ, Sear YM, Yeates D, et al: Risk factors for cardiovascular death after elective surgery under general anesthesia. Br J Anaesth 1998, 80:14–19.
7. Bedford RF, Feinstein B: Hospital admission blood pressure: a predictor for hypertension following endotracheal intubation. Anesth Analg 1980, 59:367–370.
8. Howell SJ, Sear YM, Yeates D, et al: Hypertension, admission blood pressure and perioperative cardiovascular risk. Br J Anaesth 1996, 51:1000–1004.
9. Rose DK, Cohen MM, DeBoer DP: Cardiovascular events in the postanesthesia care unit. Contribution of risk factors. Anesthesiology 1996, 84:772–781.
10. Eagle KA, Brundage BH, Chaitman BR, et al: Guidelines for perioperative cardiovascular evaluation for noncardiac surgery: report of the American College of Cardiology/American Heart Association Task Force on Practice Guidelines: Committee on Perioperative Cardiovascular Evaluation for Noncardiac Surgery. Circulation 1996, 93:1278–1317.
11. Stamler J, Stamler R, Neaton JD: Blood pressure, systolic and diastolic, and cardiovascular risks. US population data. Arch Intern Med 1993, 153:598–615.
12. SHEP Cooperative Study Group: Prevention of stroke by antihypertensive drug treatment in older persons with isolated systolic hypertension: final results of the systolic hypertension in the elderly program (SHEP). JAMA 1991, 265:32–55.
13. Prys-Roberts C. Isolated systolic hypertension: pressure on the anesthetist? Anaesthesia 2001, 56:505–510.
14. Pasternack PF, Grossi EA, Baumann G, et al: Beta blockade to decrease silent myocardial ischemia during peripheral vascular surgery. Am J Surg 1989, 158:113–116.
15. Stone JG, Foëx P, Sear JW, et al: Myocardial ischemia in untreated hypertensive patients: effect of a single small oral dose of a β-adrenergic blocking agent. Anesthesiology 1988, 68:495–500.
16. Prys-Roberts C: Chronic antihypertensive therapy. In Cardiac Anesthesia. New York: Grune and Stratton, 1983, pp 345–62.
17. Goldman L, Caldera DL: Risks of general anesthesia and elective operation in the hypertensive patient. Anesthesiology 1979, 50:285–292.
18. The Sixth Report of the Joint National Committee on Detection, Evaluation and Treatment of High Blood Pressure: NIH Publication No. 98–4080, November 1997.
19. Brabant SM, Bertrand M, Eyraud D, et al: The hemodynamic effects of anesthetic induction in vascular surgical patients chronically treated with angiotensin II receptor antagonists. Anesth Analg 1999, 88:1388–1392.
20. Colson P, Ryckwaert F, Coriat P: Renin angiotensin system antagonists and anesthesia. Anesth Analg 1999, 89:1143–1155.
21. Ebert TJ, Muzi M, Lopatka CW: Neurocirculatory responses to sevoflurane in humans: a comparison to desflurane. Anesthesiology 1995, 83:88–95.

HOT TOPICS

SECTION IX

SECTION IX
Pharmacotherapeutic Considerations:
Maximizing Opportunities and
Minimizing Threats

chapter
40

Use of Nonsteroidal Anti-inflammatory Drugs in Hypertensive Patients

Perry V. Halushka, Ph.D., M.D.*

Because hypertensive patients tend to be older, heavier, and more likely to have degenerative joint disease than the general population, concomitant use of nonsteroidal anti-inflammatory drugs (NSAIDs) is especially common. Moreover, these patients are at high risk for coronary heart disease, and many are likely to benefit from low-dose aspirin. This chapter addresses commonly encountered and clinically important questions concerning aspirin, other nonselective NSAIDs, and cyclooxygenase (COX)-2 selective inhibitor (coxibs), including:

- Are nonselective NSAIDs cardioprotective, and are there differences between them?
- Are coxibs cardioprotective; if not, why?
- If low-dose aspirin is required for cardioprotection in patients on coxibs, is the gastrointestinal (GI) benefit lost?

When definitive answers are missing, the current practice is defined and trials in progress are noted, so that providers can make informed therapeutic decisions.

Physiologic Effects of Prostaglandins and Thromboxane A_2

Both the beneficial and unwanted effects of aspirin and the nonselective NSAIDS reflect inhibition of fatty acid COX, the proximate enzymes responsible for the synthesis of prostaglandins and thromboxane A_2 (Fig. 1).

*The author is a paid consultant to the Pharmacia Corporation, St. Louis, Missouri.

Figure 1. Metabolism of arachidonic acid via the enzyme fatty acid cyclooxygenase-1. The final major products (eicosanoids) of this pathway for each cell or organ are depicted in the *boxed area*. All classical nonselective NSAIDs inhibit the enzyme. The eicosanoids contribute to the physiologic functions of the various organs and cells. Aspirin is an irreversible inhibitor of fatty acid COX.

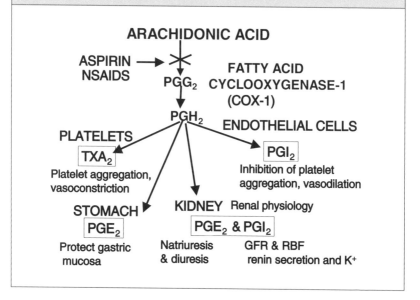

There are two fatty acid COX enzymes, named COX-1 and COX-2. COX-1 was discovered first.[1] COX-1 is constitutively present in most cells in the body. Metabolism of arachidonic acid via COX-1 and the subsequent formation of prostaglandins and thromboxane A_2 modulate cellular physiology locally in an autocrine/paracrine manner (see Fig. 1).

Human platelets contain only COX-1. The intermediate endoperoxide (PGH_2) is rapidly converted to thromboxane A_2 via the enzyme thromboxane synthase.[2] Thromboxane A_2 is a potent, labile and effective proaggregatory and vasoconstrictor substance.[3] The bleeding diathesis that occurs with aspirin and NSAIDs is caused by the inhibition of platelet thromboxane A_2 synthesis. The cardiovascular benefits of aspirin result from the irreversible inhibition of COX-1 in the platelet.[4–6] Because the platelet is anucleate, it cannot synthesize new COX-1; thus, the effect of aspirin lasts for the lifespan of the platelet. For a recent discussion of aspirin use for cardiovascular prophylaxis see Lauer.[7]

Endothelial cells synthesize predominately prostacyclin (PGI_2), which is anti-aggregatory and vasodilator. Endothelial cells posses both COX-1 and COX-2. All of the classic nonselective NSAIDS and aspirin inhibit endothelial cell PGI_2 synthesis. In addition, the selective COX-2 inhibitors significantly inhibit endothelial cell PGI_2 synthesis.[8]

In the stomach, the major prostaglandin formed is PGE_2, which has cytoprotective properties and decreases gastric acid secretion. Inhibition of COX-1 in the stomach contributes to NSAID-induced ulcers.

The kidneys possess both COX-1 and COX-2. The cellular distribution of the two enzymes are different (see Harris for review.[9]) Both enzymes catalyze the formation of PGE_2 and PGI_2, which participates in maintaining renal blood flow, glomerular filtration, and sodium excretion. Thus, inhibition of their synthesis can lead to salt and water retention, edema, elevation of blood pressure (BP), and interference with some antihypertensive drugs[10] (see Frishman for review[11]).

Metabolism of arachidonic acid via COX-1 leads to the formation of products that are involved in normal physiologic processes. Thus, inhibition of COX-1 is associated with some unwanted side effects, especially GI actions, of the nonselective NSAIDs.[12]

Fatty Acid Cyclooxygenase-2 (COX-2)

In 1990, a second COX was discovered and named COX-2[13] (see Smith et al. for review[1]). COX-2 was originally believed to be expressed only after being induced by a variety of stimuli, most notably those of a pro-inflammatory nature, but also growth factors, to name just a few. In contrast, glucocorticoids inhibited its expression.[14] Most cells and tissues in which it was found are involved in inflammation (Table 1). Thus, the hypothesis was advanced that selective COX-2 inhibition would have anti-inflammatory effects without untoward effects. In fact, the lower incidence of adverse GI effects was demonstrated in two large clinical trials (CLASS and VIGOR).

Subsequent studies found COX-2 was constitutively present in endothelial cells and the kidney and brain (see previous discussion). Because it is constitutively present in the kidneys, the precautions concerning the use of nonselective NSAIDs in hypertensive patients apply to the selective COX-2 inhibitors (coxibs).[9,11]

TABLE 1. Distribution of Fatty Acid COX-2	
Regulation:	Inducible
Tissues:	Activated macrophages and monocytes, osteoblasts, synoviocytes, fibroblasts, lung and colon carcinoma, vascular smooth muscle, amnion and decidua, ovarian follicles
Regulation:	Constitutive
Tissues:	Kidney, endothelial cells, and brain

Coxibs and Cardiovascular Diseases

Because the coxibs do not inhibit COX-1, the platelet can still synthesize thromboxane A_2 and contribute to the pathogenesis of acute coronary and cerebrovascular syndromes.[15] The potential that coxibs may contribute to these syndromes was first raised in the Vioxx Gastrointestinal Outcomes Research (VIGOR) trial,[16] a large-scale outcomes trial, designed primarily to demonstrate GI safety (rofecoxib, Vioxx) (Table 2). In this study, there was a significant increase (0.4% vs. 0.1%) in coronary events compared with the active comparator, naproxen. In the Celecoxib Long-term Arthritis Safety Study (CLASS), published about the same time, there was no increased incidence of cardiovascular events compared with celecoxib with ibuprofen or diclofenac.[17] The design of the two trials deserves careful analysis and has lead to several possible explanations for the increased incidence in cardiovascular events in the VIGOR trial but not in the CLASS trial.

Whereas in the VIGOR trial were not allowed to take low-dose aspirin, they were allowed aspirin in the CLASS trial. This raises the possible conclusion that the excessive number of events was attributable to the patients who were candidates for low-dose aspirin therapy and did not receive it. This possibility remains tenable. A second explanation is that naproxen is cardioprotective. As a result of this notion, a series of retrospective analyses of large databases were conducted to test this possibility. These studies have generated a confusing picture, which is summarized in Table 3. Some studies showed a potential cardioprotective effect of naproxen, but others have not. The notion that naproxen may have some cardioprotective effect results from its long half-life compared with the other active comparators (Table 4) and thus its prolonged antiplatelet effect. Based on the studies to date, the notion that naproxen is cardioprotective remains an open issue. Naproxen should not be considered as a substitute for the cardioprotective effects of aspirin.

TABLE 2. Design and Enrollment Criteria of the CLASS and VIGOR Trials*	
CLASS	**VIGOR**
OA and RA	RA
Allowed aspirin use	No aspirin allowed
Allowed low-dose antacids	Allowed low dose (OTC) H_2RA and antacids
Minimum duration: 6 months	Min duration: 6 months
Four times the OA dose/2× RA dose (800 mg)	Two times the OA dose (at pain dose 50 mg)
Comparators: ibuprofen 800 mg TID and diclofenac 75 mg BID	Comparator: Naproxen 500 mg BID

BID = twice a day; OA = osteoarthritis; OTC = over the counter; RA = rheumatoid arthritis; TID = three times a day.
*Patients with OA, RA, or both were enrolled in the trials.

TABLE 3. Retrospective Studies of the Potential Cardioprotective Effects of Naproxen

Relative Risk, %	Confidence Interval	Data Base	Protective
1.18	(95% CI$_2$, 0.61–2.29)	UK-GPRD[19]	No
0.95	(95% CI, 0.82–10.9)	US-Medicaid[20]	No
0.84	(95% CI, 0.72–0.98)	US-Medicaid[21]	Yes
0.57	(95% CI, 0.31–1.06)	UK-GPRD[22]	Yes
0.79	(95% CI, 0.63–0.99)	Quebec database[23]	Yes

This column indicates whether a cardioprotective effect of naproxen was found.

The possibility that a coxib could lead to a prothrombotic state has been considered, given the combination of uninhibited platelet COX-1 and thus thromboxane A_2 formation and inhibition of endothelial cell COX-2 and decreased prostacyclin formation. In this regard, the recent examination of one large database provides some potential insight into the differences between the CLASS and VIGOR trials and whether the coxibs have potential to produce a prothrombotic diathesis. In the CLASS trial, the dose of celecoxib was two times the rheumatoid arthritis dose or four times the osteoarthritis (OA) dose (800 mg) (see Table 2). In the VIGOR trial, the dose for rofecoxib was also two times the RA dose or 50 mg (see Table 2). In that retrospective analysis, there was no increased risk for a cardiovascular event in patients taking celecoxib up to 800 mg. Similarly, there was no increased risk for a cardiovascular event with rofecoxib for doses up to and including 25 mg. However, there was an increased relative risk for the 50-mg dose. The 50-mg daily dose used in the VIGOR trial is approved for only 5 days for pain. Thus, one possible explanation for the increase in cardiovascular events may be a thrombotic diathesis at the higher dose of rofecoxib but not at the lower dose approved for chronic treatment.

At this time, it appears that any patient who is a candidate for low-dose aspirin therapy should not discontinue it when taking a coxib.[5] The question arises concerning treating elderly patients with arthritis. Do you use a nonselective NSAID and low-dose aspirin or a coxib and low-dose aspirin? The CLASS trial showed that the incidence of GI events

TABLE 4. Half-Life Values for Nonselective NSAIDs Used in the CLASS and VIOXX Clinical Trials

Nonselective NSAID	Half-Life, Hours
Diclofenac	2
Ibuprofen	3
Indomethacin*	2
Naproxen	~ 14

* Indomethacin is included for comparison purposes.

was not significantly different for aspirin plus celecoxib versus a nonselective NSAID. Thus, the advantage of a coxib is potentially lost in patients requiring low-dose aspirin therapy. The question that remains is; Is the combination of low-dose aspirin plus a coxib safer for the GI tract than a nonselective NSAID and aspirin? From a strictly intuitive approach, the former would appear to be safer, but there is no data to support this. However, the incidence of GI events with the combination of aspirin and celecoxib is less compared with nonselective NSAIDS with aspirin.[18]

Summary

The coxibs have similar efficacy in the treatment of arthritis as the nonselective NSAIDS. Although devoid of the GI side effects, they have the same renal precautions as the nonselective NSAIDs. Thus, they can lead to edema, increase BP, and interfere with the antihypertensive effects, particularly beta-blockers and angiotensin-enzyme converting inhibitors. Whether they lead to a thrombotic diathesis or simply do not provide cardiovascular prophylaxis remains an unresolved question.

Acknowledgements

The author gratefully acknowledges the helpful discussions with Ms. Deanna S. Jackson, Pharm.D.

References

1. Smith W, DeWitt D, Garavito R: Cyclooxgenases: structural, cellular, and molecular biology. Ann Rev Biochem 2000, 69:145–182.
2. Hamberg M, Svensson J, Samuelsson B: Thromboxanes: a new group of biologically active compounds derived from prostaglandin endoperoxides. Proc Natl Acad Sci USA 1975, 72:2994–2998.
3. Davis-Bruno KL, Halushka PV: Molecular pharmacology and therapeutic potential of thromboxane A_2 receptor antagonists. Adv Drug Res 1994, 25:173–202.
4. Catella-Lawson F, Reilly MP, Kapoor SC, et al: Cyclooxygenase Inhibitors and the Antiplatelet Effects of Aspirin. N Engl J Med 2001, 345:1809–1817, 2001.
5. Patrono C, Coller B, Dalen JE, et al: Patelet-active drugs: the relationships among dose, effectiveness, and side effects. Chest 1998, 114:(suppl S)470–488.
6. Roth GJ, Stanford N, Majerus PW: Acetylation of prostaglandin synthase by aspirin. Proc Natl Acad Sci 1979, 72:3073–3076.
7. Lauer MS: Aspirin for the primary prevention of coronary events. N Eng J Med 2002, 346:1468–1473.
8. McAdam BF, Catella-Lawson F, Mardini I, et al: Systemic biosynthesis of prostacyclin by cyclooxygenase (COX)-2: the human pharmacology of a selective inhibitor of COX-2. Proc Natl Acad Sci 1999, 96:272–277.

9. Harris RC: Cyclooxygenase-2 inhibition and renal physiology. Am J Cardiol 2002, 89(suppl D):10–17.

10. Schwartz JI, Vandormael K, Malice MP, et al: Comparison of rofecoxib, celecoxib, and naproxen on renal function in elderly subjects receiving a normal salt diet. Clin Pharmacol Ther 2002, 72:50–61.

11. Frishman WH: Effects of nonsteroidal anti-inflammatory drug therapy on blood pressure and peripheral edema. Am J Cardiol 2002, 89(suppl D):18–25.

12. Warner TD, Giuliano F, Vojnovic I, et al: Nonsteroid drug selectivities for cyclo-oxygenase-1 rather than cyclo-oxygenase-2 are associated with human gastrointestinal toxicity: a full in vitro analysis. Proc Natl Acad Sci 1999, 96:7563–7568.

13. O'Banion MK, Winn VD, Young DA: cDNA cloning and functional activity of a glucocorticoid-regulated inflammatory cyclooxygenase-1. Proc Natl Acad Sci 1992, 89:4888–4892.

14. Masferrer JL, Zweifel BS, Seibert K, et al: Selective regulation of cellular cyclooxygenase by dexamethasone and endotoxin in mice. J Clin Invest 1990, 86:1375–1379.

15. Halushka PV, Pawate S, Martin ML: Thromboxane A_2 and other eicosanoids. In Von Bruchhusen F, Walter U (eds). Handbook of Experimental Pharmacology, Platelets and Their Factors. Berlin, Germany: Springer-Verlag, 1997. p 459–482.

16. Bombardier C, Laine L, Reicin A, et al: Comparison of upper gastrointestinal toxicity of rofecoxib and naproxen in patients with rheumatoid arthritis. N Eng J Med 2000, 343:1520–1528.

17. Silverstein F, Faich G, Goldstein J, et al: Gastrointestinal toxicity with celecoxib vs. nonsteroidal anti-inflammatory drugs for osteoarthritis and rheumatoid arthritis: the CLASS study: randomized controlled trial. JAMA 2000, 284:1247–1255.

18. Deeks JJ, Smith LA, Bradley MD. Efficacy, tolerability, and upper gastrointestinal safey of celecoxib for treatment of osteoarthritis and rheumatoid arthritis: systematic review of randomised controlled trials. Br Med J 2002, 325:619–626.

19. Garcia-Rodriguez LA, Varas D, Patrono C: Differential effects of aspirin and non aspirin nonsteroidal antiinflammatory drugs in the primary prevention of myocardial infarction in postmenopausal women. Epidemiology 2000, 11:382–387.

20. Ray WA, Stein CM, Hall K, et al: Non-steroidal anti-inflammatory drugs and risk of serious coronary heart disease: an observational cohort study. Lancet 2002, 359:118–123.

21. Solomon DH, Glynn RJ, R. I, et al: Nonsteroidal anti-inflammatory drug use and acute myocardial infarction. Arch Intern Med 2002, 162:1099–1104.

22. Watson DJ, Rhodes T, Cai B, et al: Lower risk of thromboembolic cardiovascular events with naproxen among patients with theumatoid arthritis. Arch Intern Med 2002, 162:1105–1110.

23. Rahme E, Pilote L, LeLorier J: Association between naproxen use and protection against acute myocardial infarction. Arch Intern Med 2002, 162:1111–1115.

Amiloride-sensitive Hypertension

David A. Calhoun, M.D.

chapter
41

Low-renin, volume-dependent hypertension is common, particularly among patients with resistant hypertension. The cause of such hypertension is most often multifactorial, and the most important contributing factors are age, dietary salt intake, and renal insufficiency. In rare cases, the underlying cause of the low-renin hypertension is a single gene mutation resulting in inappropriate sodium and fluid retention, with a consequential increase in blood pressure (BP). Such monogenic hypertensive syndromes, although they are uncommon, provide important mechanistic insight into the cause of low-renin, resistant hypertension; when these syndromes are recognized, targeted antihypertensive therapy may be used.

Liddle's disease is a rare, autosomal dominant disorder that phenotypically resembles primary hyperaldosteronism even though aldosterone excretion is suppressed. The syndrome is caused by a mutation in the epithelial sodium channel (ENaC) that results in inappropriate sodium retention and potassium wasting at the level of the distal nephron, with subsequent volume expansion-related suppression of renin activity and development of severe hypertension. Treatment of patients with Liddle's disease is best accomplished with use of amiloride or triamterene, both K^+-sparing diuretics, in conjunction with low dietary salt ingestion. Concomitant use of other classes of antihypertensive agents may be necessary, particularly in older patients.

Historical Background

In 1963, Grant Liddle described a 16-year-old girl who had been referred to Vanderbilt University for evaluation of resistant hypertension.[1] She was suspected of having hyperaldosteronism, based on the development of severe hypertension, hypokalemia (serum potassium 2.6 mEq/L), and a metabolic alkalosis (serum CO_2 30 mEq/L). Two siblings were similarly affected. Primary hyperaldosteronism was excluded and, suppressed urinary aldosterone excretion was documented. Evaluation of other urinary steroids, likewise, did not indicate mineralocorticoid excess. Administration of spironolactone, an aldosterone antagonist, had no effect. In contrast, triamterene, administered in conjunction with low-dietary salt ingestion, effectively lowered the BP and corrected the hypokalemia. Based on these observations, Liddle correctly deduced that this disorder ". . .stems from an unusual tendency of the kidneys to conserve sodium and excrete potassium even in the virtual absence of mineralocorticoids."[1]

Within the original Liddle pedigree, resistant hypertension was common, as was premature cardiovascular disease, such as stroke and congestive heart failure.[2] Evaluation of the extended family clearly established the autosomal dominant inheritance of the disorder, with early but variable penetrance. Although hypokalemia was characteristic of presenting family members, subsequent evaluation of the family identified affected individuals with normal or minimally reduced serum potassium.[3]

Liddle's original index case subsequently developed renal insufficiency, progressing to end-stage renal disease in 1989. She underwent cadaveric kidney transplantation,[3] which effectively cured her Liddle's disease, normalizing renin activity, aldosterone excretion, and serum potassium. Postoperatively, her BP was more easily controlled. Similar benefit was reported for a young French woman with Liddle's disease who also underwent kidney transplantation.[4] Although development of severe renal insufficiency is uncommon among patients with Liddle's disease, these cases clearly verify the renal cause of the disorder.

Epithelial Sodium Channel

The ENaC complex consists of three homologous subunits, α, β, and γ, each of which has two membrane-spanning regions and a large extracellular domain. The ENaC is expressed in the apical membranes of many Na^+-absorptive epithelia, such as renal tubules, the distal colon, and the lungs. Activation of ENaC in the luminal plasma membrane of the connecting segment and cortical collecting duct contributes importantly to sodium and fluid balance (Fig. 1). Although regulation of ENaC activity is poorly understood, aldosterone, through stimulation of the cytosolic mineralocorticoid receptor, results in genomic effects that increase transcription of genes encoding ENaC subunits.[5] Possible direct or nongenomic stimulation of ENaC by aldosterone has also been described.[6]

Genetic linkage analysis of the original Liddle's family identified a causal mutation in the β subunit of ENaC.[7] Since then, additional polymorphisms in the β or γ subunit that have been identified as causing Liddle's disease.[8] The effect of each of the mutations is to cause a gain of

Figure 1. Liddle's disease is caused by inappropriate constitutive activation of the epithelial Na^+ channel on the apical membrane of renal tubular cells (*left side*), which is normally upregulated by aldosterone. However, in Liddle's disease, the ENaC is highly active despite suppression of aldosterone. Amiloride and triamterene block the sodium channel (*right side*). Spironolactone, which inhibits sodium absorption by binding to the cytoplasmic aldosterone receptor, is not effective in patients with Liddle's disease (*right panel*). (Reproduced with permission from Warnock et al.[2])

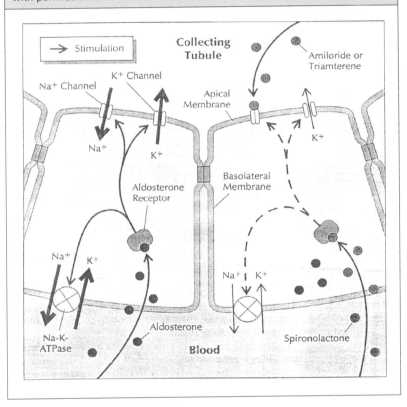

function or constitutive activation of ENaC, resulting in inappropriate sodium and fluid retention. The exact mechanism by which subunit mutations result in constitutive ENaC activation remains unknown but may be related to increased channel longevity or a direct kinetic effect.[9,10]

Prevalence

The original family with Liddle's disease was white. Since then, Liddle's disease has been observed in many ethnic groups, including African-American, European, Japanese, African, and Hispanic. Genetic analysis of selected hypertensive populations has consistently found Liddle's disease to be rare, probably having been identified in less than 50 families worldwide.[11,12] Although polymorphisms of ENaC are common, particularly among persons of African descent, the majority of these mutations have not been shown to cause Liddle's disease. Whether such mutations may contribute to more subtle abnormalities of ENaC dysfunction than observed in Liddle's disease, and, thereby, contribute to the development of hypertension, remains a possibility.

In a recent report, it was found that a small group of subjects in London of African descent with a novel mutation of the ENaC β subunit (T594M), manifested a significant BP response to amiloride.[13] This mutation is reportedly present in approximately 5% of black subjects in London. These results are provocative in that they support the possibility that novel or unrecognized polymorphisms of ENaC, particularly in black populations, may contribute to the development of hypertension much more commonly than currently thought.

Clinical Characteristics

Liddle's disease classically manifests as mineralocorticoid excess (i.e., resistant hypertension, low renin activity, hypokalemia, metabolic alkalosis), but with suppressed aldosterone excretion, hence use of the descriptive term *pseudohyperaldosteronism*. Reports subsequent to Liddle's original description clearly indicate a wide variability in the clinical presentation, with affected individuals being described with mild hypertension or even high to normal BP levels and with only minimally low or even normal serum potassium levels (Table 1).[14]

From a practical standpoint, Liddle's disease might be suspected in young patients with a strong family history of hypertension who present with new onset of hypertension, particularly if it is severe or resistant to pharmacologic therapy. Evidence of potassium wasting in the setting of low aldosterone excretion should increase the level of suspicion.

Diagnosis

Liddle's disease can be suspected in patients with the characteristic phenotype, but definitive confirmation requires direct sequencing of polymerase chain reaction-amplified genonomic DNA for causative ENaC polymorphisms. Although it is done routinely for experimental reasons, such screening is not available commercially. Alternatively, analysis of urinary steroids by mass spectrometry yields an excretion profile characteristic of Liddle's disease, but such analysis, is likewise, currently limited to certain research laboratories.

TABLE 1. Clinical Features of Family Members Affected and Unaffected by Liddle's Disease

	Age, years	BP, mm Hg	pK+, mmol/L	PRA, ng/mL/h	PAC, ng/dL	Ualdo, µg/day)
Affected						
1	16	142/100	3.1	< 0.22	< .99	< 0.67
2	43	126/98	3.4	1.91	3.26	0.99
3	34	160/108	4.6	< 0.22	3.72	0.78
4	46	123/74	4.6	0.61	1.88	0.67
5	27	118/72	5.1	1.51	4.22	1.38
6	63	118/84	3.5	1.51	< .99	ND
Mean	37 ± 7	138 ± 8/89 ± 6	4.1 ± 0.3	1.0 ± 0.29	2.5 ± 0.57	0.90 ± 0.14
Unaffected						
1	20	122/84	4.8	0.68	13.8	7.0
2	44	118/68	4.8	1.91	18.0	13.1
3	36	130/77	4.4	0.90	15.1	14.4
4	68	102/64	5.6	0.40	4.8	7.9
Mean	42 ± 10	118 ± 6/73 ± 5	4.9 ± 0.3	0.97 ± 0.32	12.9 ± 2.8*	10.6 ± 1.8*

BP = blood pressure; ND = not done; PAC = plasma aldosterone concentration; pK+ = plasma potassium; PRA = plasma renin activity; Ualdo = urinary aldosterone; mean values ±SEM.
*Different from affected, $p < 0.001$. (Adapted with permission from Findling et al.)[8]

Because they do not have easy access to confirm the diagnosis of Liddle's disease, most clinicians must rely on a presumptive or tentative diagnosis. In such situations, a therapeutic trial of amiloride seems reasonable, particularly in patients resistant to other classes of antihypertensive agents. Although the range of the different biochemical parameters in Liddle's disease have not been well defined, affected persons should present with low plasma renin activity (< 1.0 mg/mL/h) and suppressed aldosterone excretion (plasma aldosterone concentration < 5 ng/dL or 24-hour urinary aldosterone < 4 µg/day) (see Table 1). A strong family history of hypertension and evidence of potassium wasting increases the likelihood of Liddle's disease.

Treatment

Treatment of patients with Liddle's disease is aimed at blocking the ENaC with use of amiloride (5 to 20 mg/day) or triamterene (50 to 300 mg/day) and concomitant restriction of dietary salt. Some individuals may respond better to amiloride or triamterene, or vice versa, so both agents should be tried individually before deciding K+-sparing diuretics are ineffective. With either drug, dietary salt restriction is necessary to maximize the antihypertensive efficacy. Aldosterone antagonists are ineffective in treating patients with Liddle's disease. Thiazide or loop diuretics can be added for additional BP or volume control. Such agents may exacerbate the potassium wasting that typically occurs in patients with Liddle's disease.

The K^+-sparing diuretics are available in a fixed-dosed combination with hydrochlorothiazide; however, the combination products are dosed to minimize thiazide-induced hypokalemia. Treatment generally requires higher doses of amiloride or triamterene than are provided in the fixed-dosed combination pills. Accordingly, in treating patients with Liddle's disease, it is generally better to dose the K^+-sparing diuretic separately and add other agents as necessary for additional BP control.

If a patient has normal renal function, risk of hyperkalemia or acute renal insufficiency is low with the use of amiloride or triamterene. However, such adverse effects can occur, necessitating the need for careful monitoring of renal function. We initiate therapy at the lowest dose and titrate at no sooner than 6-week intervals. Patients with underlying renal insufficiency or diabetics and patients receiving angiotensin-converting enzyme inhibitors or angiotensin receptor blockers are at increased risk of hyperkalemia and require more aggressive surveillance. In these higher risk patients, electrolytes should be assessed within 2 weeks of initiating therapy with either of the K^+-sparing diuretics.

Perspectives

Although uncommon, Liddle's disease provides important insight into the cause of low-renin hypertension. Notably, of the several monogenic forms of hypertension that have been identified all cause hypertension by inducing inappropriate sodium and fluid retention at the level of the distal nephron. In the case of glucocorticoid-remediable aldosteronism (GRA) and apparent mineralocorticoid excess syndrome (AME), cortisol and aldosterone, respectively, underlie classic mineralocorticoid-induced hypertension. In Liddle's disease, constitutive ENaC activation in the absence of mineralocorticoid excess causes excessive sodium and fluid retention.

The common final pathway of these inherited disorders may be relevant to the cause of hypertension in general. It is hypothesized that these hypertensive syndromes may be more common than suggested by genetic screenings. Perhaps because of unrecognized polymorphisms in known culprit genes or polymorphisms in novel genes that cause similar syndromes, genetic mutations—either singularly or in combination—that result in excessive renal sodium and fluid retention may play a much broader role in causing hypertension than currently thought. If so, genetic screening may allow for identification of persons at high risk of developing hypertension and guide therapy to more effectively counteract underlying causes. Effective and broader genetic screening of hypertensive populations will test this possibility.

References

1. Liddle GW, Bledsoe T, Coppage WS: A familial renal disorder simulating primary aldosteronism but with negligible aldosterone excretion. Trans Am Assoc Physicians 1963, 76:199–213.

2. Warnock DG, Bubien JK: Liddle syndrome: clinical and cellular abnormalities. Hospital Practice 1994, 15:95–105.

3. Botero-Velez M, Curtis JJ, Warnock DG: Liddle's syndrome revisited: a disorder of sodium reabsorption in the distal tuble. N Eng J Med 1994, 300:178–181.

4. Noblins M, Kleinknecht D, Dommergues JP, et al: Syndrome de Liddle (ou pseudo-hyperaldosteronism): evolution à long terme ét etude des flux potassiques érythrocytaires dans 4 observations. Arch Fr Pédiatr 1992, 49:685–692.

5. Asher C, Wald H, Rossier BC, Garty H: Aldosterone-induced increase in abundance of Na^+ subunits. Am J Physiol Cell Physiol 1996, 271(suppl C):605–611.

6. Zhou Z-H, Bubien JK: Nongenomic regulation of ENaC by aldosterone: Am J Physiol Cell Physiol 2001, 281(suppl C):1118–1130.

7. Shimkets RA, Warnock DG, Bositis CM, et al: Liddle's syndrome: heritable human hypertension caused by mutations in the beta subunit of the epithelial sodium channel. Cell 1994, 79:407–414.

8. Oh Y, Warnock DG: Disorders of the epithelial Na^+ channel in Liddle's syndrome and autosomal recessive pseudohypoaldosteronism, type 1. Exp Nephrol 2000, 8:320–325.

9. Snyder PM, Price MP, McDonald FJ, et al: Mechanism by which Liddle's syndrome mutations increase activity of a human epithelial Na^+ channel. Cell 1995, 83:969–978.

10. Firsov D, Schild L, Gautschi I, et al: Cell surface expression of the epithelial Na channel and a mutant causing Liddle syndrome: a quantitative approach. Proc Natl Acad Sci USA 1996, 93:15370–15375.

11. Persu A, Barbry P, Bassilana F, et al: Genetic analysis of the β subunit of the epithelial, Na+ channel in essential hypertension. Hypertension 1998, 32;129–137.

12. Iwai N, Baba S, Mannami T, et al: Association of sodium channel γ-subunit promoter variant with blood pressure. Hypertension 2001, 38:86–89.

13. Baker EH, Duggal Am Dong Y, et al: Amiloride, a specific drug for hypertension in black people with T594M variant? Hypertension 2002, 40;13–17.

14. Findling JW, Raff H, Hansson, et al: Liddle's syndrome: prospective genetic screening and suppressed aldosterone secretion in an extended kindred. J Clin Endocrinol Metab 1997, 82:1071–1074.

Adverse Drug Reactions in Patients with Hypertension

chapter
42

Domenic A. Sica, M.D.

Adverse reactions and drug–drug interactions are common occurrences with many drug classes and, in particular, with antihypertensive medications. These occurrences take many forms, including electrolyte changes, alterations in level of renal function, nonspecific or idiosyncratic side effects, and side effects that specifically relate to systemic drug levels. There is considerable interplay between several antihypertensive compounds and the CYP_{450} system and a keen understanding of this system is needed to avoid what can sometimes be life-threatening drug–drug interactions with antihypertensive medications. This chapter comments on the individual drug classes, noting the pros and cons of their use as well as the hidden "pearls" that maximize the gain and minimize the risk of such drug therapy. In many instances, the reported side effect or drug–drug interaction reflects a class effect and is so stated.

Diuretics

Diuretics are important primary and adjunctive therapy in the treatment of hypertension. They are of particular use when administered—even in doses as low as 6.25 mg of hydrochlorothiazide (HCTZ)—in conjunction with other classes of antihypertensive medications in the form of fixed-dose combination therapy. The acute response to diuretics is volume dependent. The change in plasma volume stimulates both the sympathetic nervous (SNS) and renin-angiotensin-aldosterone (RAA) axes in a patient-specific fashion. The extent to which either or both of these systems is activated determines the efficiency with which diuretics acutely reduce blood pressure (BP). The chronic vasodepressor effect of thiazide-type diuretics is more closely related to a persistent reduction in total peripheral resistance than to an effect of volume reduction. The dose–response relationship for BP reduction with a thiazide-type diuretic such as HCTZ is extremely flat at doses > 25 mg/day. Much of the early negative biochemical and metabolic experience with diuretics was related to the very high doses (100–200 mg/day) that had been in common use. The frequency of metabolically negative side effects such as hypokalemia, hypomagnesemia, glucose intolerance, and hypercholesterolemia is much lower with low-dose diuretic therapy (Table 1).

Beta-blockers

Beta-blockers vary considerably in their pharmacologic features, and their efficacy and side effect profiles vary depending on the specific compound and the drug delivery system. Beta-blockers have a relatively flat dose–response curve for BP reduction. Escalating doses of beta-blockers induce salt and water retention; therefore, diuretics may become a necessary adjunctive form of therapy. Beta$_1$-cardioselective agents have some advantages, particularly at low-end doses. These include a smaller risk of paradoxical pressor effects during major stresses than is seen with nonselective beta-blockade. Nonselective beta-blockade may be preferred though in the treatment of certain concomitant illnesses, such as essential tremor or migraine headache. In addition, beta-blockers reduce BP without decreasing peripheral vascular resistance, which may be one factor behind why these drugs negatively impact intermittent claudication or Raynaud's phenomenon. Abrupt discontinuation of a beta-blocker—particularly when administered in high doses—may be followed by adrenergically mediated withdrawal symptoms. Therefore, a stepwise reduction in dose is advised. Beta-blockers given together with either verapamil or diltiazem can precipitously decrease heart rate. This combination should be given cautiously, if at all (Table 2).

Angiotensin-converting Enzyme Inhibitors

The pharmacologic features of angiotensin-converting enzyme (ACE) inhibitors are uniform except for differences in half-life, pharmacokinetics, and tissue binding. ACE inhibitors have a steep dose–response curve for BP reduction at low doses; thereafter, the dose–response relationship is fairly flat. Multiple dose titrations of an ACE inhibitor are seldom warranted except in patients with congestive heart failure (CHF). The highly tissue bound ACE inhibitors are not more effective in controlling BP, but they may maintain BP control better in the face of a missed medication dose because of their prolonged duration of action. The BP-lowering effect and tissue protection afforded by ACE inhibitor therapy may be attenuated by coadministration of aspirin, although this still remains a con-

TABLE 1. Diuretics	
Generic and Brand Names	**Comments**
Chlorthalidone (Hygroton)	More prolonged effect than HCTZ; greater likelihood of hypomagnesemia; diuretic used in ALLHAT trial with strongly positive cardiovascular outcomes data
Hydrochlorothiazide (Hydrodiuril, Microzide)	Short-acting diuretic; impotence is not uncommon (class effect); decreases urine calcium excretion and is used in nephrolithiasis and adjunctively in osteoporosis management (class effect); decreases lithium clearance in lithium-treated patients with an increased risk of lithium toxicity; diuretic-related hyponatremia more common (class effect) than is the case with loop diuretics
Indapamide (Lozol)	May cause less potassium loss than other thiazide diuretics
Metolazone (Mykrox, Zaroxylyn)	Improved bioavailability with Mykrox compared with Zaroxylyn results in lower dose being given; effective at GFR < 40 cc, unlike other thiazide diuretics; Zaroxylyn is the preferred form of metolazone when used with a loop diuretic in diuretic-resistant states
Loop Diuretics	
Bumetanide (Bumex)	Short-acting loop diuretic; associated with significant hypercalciuria (class effect for loop diuretics)
Furosemide (Lasix)	Shorter duration of action; multiple daily dosing to avoid rebound sodium retention (same for bumetanide)
Torsemide (Demadex)	Long duration of action; independent vasodepressor effect
Ethacrynic acid (Edecrin)	Only nonsulfonamide diuretic; ototoxicity
Potassium Sparing	
Amiloride (Midamor)	Hyperkalemia; decreases urine calcium excretion above and beyond what occurs with HCTZ; magnesium sparing (class effect) and useful in the hypomagnesemia associated with cis-platinum or amphotericin; reduces polyuria associated with lithium
Spironolactone (Aldactone)	Dose-dependent gynecomastia; long half-life; hyperkalemia; increases digoxin levels
Triamterene (Dyrenium)	Hyperkalemia, triamterene stones can occur; increased risk of nephrotoxicity when administered together with NSAIDs; interferes with the tubular secretion of creatinine (similar to creatinine, it is an organic cation) and reduces the reliability of serum creatinine values as a marker of renal function

troversial issue as to the degree of this interaction. ACE inhibitor use is not accompanied by salt and water retention or increased heart rate. Perioperative hypertension may be treated intravenously with the ACE inhibitor enalaprilat.

Side effects associated with ACE inhibitors include cough, angioedema, and a unique form of functional renal insufficiency. Cough and

Generic and Brand Names	Comments
TABLE 2.	**Beta-Adrenergic Blocking Drugs**
Acetbutolol (Sectral)	Cardioselective, intrinsic sympathomimetic activity (ISA); lupuslike reactions reported; immunologic monitoring is indicated during therapy (this is not a class effect for beta-blockers)
Atenolol (Tenormin)	Cardioselective; renally cleared; (may require dose adjustment in advanced renal disease; reduces plasma and urine aldosterone (class effect)
Betaxolol (Kerlone)	Cardioselective; rebound hypertension or withdrawal symptomatology upon abrupt discontinuation (class effect)
Bisoprolol (Zebeta)	Cardioselective; indicated as first-step therapy as combination product
Carteolol (Cartrol)	Abrupt withdrawal of clonidine while receiving a beta-blocker may exaggerate the rebound hypertension because of unopposed alpha-stimulation (class effect)
Esmolol (Brevibloc)	Available as an intravenous form; ultra short-acting
Metoprolol (Lopressor, Toprol XL)	Cardioselective, long-acting preparation available; strong outcomes data in congestive heart failure; diphenhydramine inhibits the metabolism of metoprolol in extensive metabolizers, thereby prolonging the negative chronotropic and inotropic effects of the drug; genetic polymorphism for CYP2D6 expression, with slow metabolizers displaying an exaggerated beta-blocker effect at low doses
Nadolol (Corgard)	Renally cleared; diminishes the effectiveness of epinephrine in the setting of anaphylaxis (class effect)
Penbutolol (Levatol)	Increases serum potassium by blocking $beta_2$-mediated intracellular flux of potassium; most prominent when the presence of renal failure precludes excretion of potassium
Pindolol (Visken)	ISA; does not decrease the risk of a second MI as do other beta-blockers without ISA activity
Propranolol (Inderal, Inderal-LA, Innopran-XL)	Long-acting preparation available, Innopran-XL form indicated for nighttime dosing; strong cardiovascular outcomes data; indicated in post-MI patients; useful for essential tremor; adjunct therapy for anxiety and panic attacks; NSAID therapy may attenuate the antihypertensive effect; cimetidine may increase the blood levels by as much as twofold (because of decreased metabolism); hydralazine increases the oral bioavailability of short-acting forms of propranolol
Timolol (Blocadren)	Available as ophthalmic solution for open-angle glaucoma; as much as ⅔ of administered dose may enter the nasolacrimal duct, only to be swallowed and absorbed with ensuing systemic beta-blockade

angioedema are class effects, and there is no benefit of switching to another ACE inhibitor to escape these problems. The occurrence of functional renal insufficiency with an ACE inhibitor does not preclude a patient from future ACE inhibitor therapy unless bilateral renal artery stenosis is present. There is no level of renal function at which ACE inhibitors cannot be used because these agents are not intrinsically nephrotoxic. ACE inhibitor therapy commonly reduces glomerular filtration rate by 20% when first started. If clinically relevant hyperkalemia occurs in this setting, consideration should be given to temporarily discontinuing the ACE inhibitor and reassessing other factors that may have contributed to the development of hyperkalemia (Table 3).

TABLE 3. ACE Inhibitors	
Generic And Brand Names	**Comments**
Benazepril (Lotensin)	Not FDA approved for CHF; diarrhea occurs with ACE inhibitors, which can be related to angioedema of the gut
Captopril (Capoten)	Neutropenia, skin rash, and dysgeusia occur more frequently than with other ACE inhibitors; increased risk of developing hypoglycemia (not a class effect per se); very high-dose therapy ($\geq$ 1g) associated with development of membranous nephropathy; antacids significantly decrease captopril absorption
Enalapril (Vasotec)	Available as intravenous enalaprilat; suppresses red blood cell production, a property that be used therapeutically in posttransplant erythrocytosis
Fosinopril (Monopril)	Renal and hepatic elimination; aspirin may interfere with the hemodynamic effect of ACE inhibitors in patients with severe CHF and may reduce the antihypertensive effect (class effect)
Lisinopril (Prinivil, Zestril)	Development of hyperkalemia (class effect; suggested to be less with renally or hepatically cleared ACE inhibitors)
Moexipril (Univasc)	Not FDA approved for CHF; ACE inhibitors may cause fetal or neonatal injury or death when used during the second or third trimester of pregnancy; hypotension, neonatal anemia, hyperkalemia, neonatal skull hypoplasia, anuria, and renal failure have occurred in fetuses and neonates (class effect)
Perindopril (Aceon)	Not FDA approved for CHF; concomitant use with lithium may increase lithium levels significantly (class effect): angioedema, which is a potentially life-threatening process, can occur (class effect); rechallenge should never occur with the causal compound or another ACE inhibitor in the class
Quinapril (Accupril)	Pancreatitis reported (class effect); severe hyperkalemia can develop when given together with trimethoprim-sulfamethoxazole (Bactrim) (class effect); reduces the absorption of tetracycline by ~ 35% possibly because of high magnesium content of tablets
Ramipril (Altace)	Indicated in high-risk hypertensives; small changes in serum creatinine (e.g., a 20% increase) can occur as a normal physiologic response in renal failure patients (class effect); therapy need not be stopped
Trandolapril (Mavik)	Renal and hepatic elimination; first-dose hypotension, particularly if volume contracted (class effect)

Angiotensin Receptor Blockers

Pharmacologic features of angiotensin receptor blockers (ARBs), (e.g., absorption, protein binding, and volume of distribution) vary from compound to compound but have less influence on efficacy than receptor affinity, which also varies from compound to compound in this class. All ARBs are indicated for once-daily dosing but may occasionally lose efficacy at the end of their dosing interval, thereby necessitating twice-daily dosing. All ARBs are eliminated by some combination of renal and hepatic clearance. This distinguishes the ARBs from ACE inhibitors, which are predominantly renally cleared. ARBs have a steep dose–response curve for BP reduction at low doses; thereafter, the dose–response relationship is fairly shallow. Side effects are uncommon with ARBs and do not relate to dose; accordingly, higher doses of ARBs are now routinely tried absent the likelihood of dose-dependent side effects. Cough does not occur with ARBs, and angioedema is rare. The occurrence of functional renal insufficiency with an ACE inhibitor does not preclude a patient from future therapy with an ARB, unless bilateral renal artery stenosis is present. ARBs may be used in patients with renal insufficiency. Hyperkalemia appears to be less common with ARBs than with ACE inhibitors (Table 4).

Calcium Channel Blockers

Calcium channel blockers (CCBs) fall into two classes: dihydropyridines and nondihydropyridines; the latter class includes verapamil and diltiazem. Dihydropyridine-type CCBs are generally more potent but, in the process, can activate the sympathetic nervous system. This does not occur with verapamil or diltiazem. Diltiazem and verapamil have modest negative inotropic effects and can inhibit atrioventricular conduction. The availability of sustained-release delivery systems for CCBs has further advanced the use of these drugs, in part, because side effects decrease as the intensity of exposure to drug is lessened. CCBs can have a fairly steep dose–response curve for BP reduction. The amount by which BP is reduced with a CCB is a function of the pretherapy BP; thus, the higher the BP at the start of therapy, the greater the decrease in BP. Dihydropyridine CCBs can be effectively combined with a beta-blocker, an ACE inhibitor, or a peripheral alpha-antagonist such as doxazosin or terazosin.

The side effect profiles of drugs in this class are similar and, in many instances, are dose dependent. Side effects associated with CCBs typically relate to vasodilation and include headaches, flushing, and dependent edema. The latter relates to CCBs being more potent arteriolar than venodilators and is both dose dependent and more common in women. The peripheral edema with CCBs does not occur as a consequence of salt and

TABLE 4.   Angiotensin Receptor Blockers

Generic and Brand Names	Comments
Candesartan (Atacand)	First-dose hypotension, particularly if volume contracted (class effect)
Eprosartan (Teveten)	Small changes in serum creatinine (e.g., a 20% increase) can occur as a normal physiologic response in renal failure patients (class effect); therapy need not be stopped; purported dual mechanism of effect with a decrease in sympathetic nervous system activity
Irbesartan (Avapro)	Metabolized to an inactive metabolite by CYP2C9; genetic polymorphism exists for CYP2C9 with the CYP2C9*2 and CYP2C9*3, exhibiting reduced catalytic activity and therein a greater BP-lowering response to the drug (this represents a small part of the population); indicated in type 2 diabetic nephropathy
Losartan (Cozaar)	Anemia secondary to decrease in erythropoietin amount or effect (class effect); angioedema (rarely); (class effect); metabolized to an active metabolite by CYP2C9 and CYP3A4; although inhibitors and stimulators of these isozymes alter production of the active metabolite, it appears not to translate into any alteration in BP control; indicated in type 2 diabetic nephropathy
Olmesartan (Benicar)	Contraindicated in the second and third trimester of pregnancy (class effect)
Telmisartan (Micardis)	Increase in serum potassium but less than that seen with ACE inhibitors (class effect); interaction with digoxin with increases in digoxin levels; monitoring of digoxin level advised with start or increase in the dose of digoxin
Valsartan (Diovan)	Use with caution in patients with bilateral renal artery stenosis or unilateral stenosis with a solitary kidney (class effect); can be given together with an ACE inhibitor with an improvement in heart failure outcomes

water retention; thus, it is poorly responsive to diuretic therapy. The coadministration of venodilators, such as ACE inhibitors, ARBs, or nitrates, generally reduces or eliminates CCB-induced peripheral edema. Most side effects of CCBs are class specific, with the exception of constipation and atrioventricular block, which occur more commonly with verapamil.

A final consideration with CCBs relates to the issue of drug interactions. Concomitant administration of CCBs (i.e., nifedipine, diltiazem, nicardipine, verapamil) and digitalis glycosides (digoxin) can result in up to a 50% increase in serum digoxin concentrations. The metabolism of a number of CCBs is slowed when they are taken together with grapefruit juice. The effects of grapefruit juice may last several hours, and juice consumed some time before taking felodipine may still affect felodipine levels. Increased felodipine bioavailability with grapefruit juice is chiefly caused by inhibition of primary metabolism in the intestinal wall via the cytochrome P450 enzyme system; alternatively, felodipine half-life is not affected by grapefruit juice. The magnitude of the grapefruit juice and felodipine interaction is highly variable among individuals but is reproducible within individuals. The potential for an interaction is especially relevant for patients with severe hypertension or stable angina because both can have ischemic complications with felodipine, leading to myocardial infarction or unstable angina. This interaction can occur with grapefruit juice, grapefruit segments, tangelos, and Seville orange juice.

In addition, verapamil and diltiazem inhibit the CYP3A4 isozyme, thereby slowing the metabolism of drugs such as cyclosporine, nifedipine, simvastatin, quinidine, and theophylline. These drug–drug interactions present as an exaggeration of the physiologic effect of the interfered with compound (e.g., theophylline toxicity or additive BP reduction when verapamil or diltiazem is given together with nifedipine) or with concentration-related side effects (e.g., the increased risk of rhabdomyolysis when verapamil is coadministered with simvastatin). Such drug–drug interactions may prove financially beneficial (e.g., the reduced dose of cyclosporine required when it is given together with verapamil or diltiazem) (Table 5).

Peripheral Alpa-Antagonists

The effectiveness of alpha$_1$-adrenergic blocking drugs is related, in part, to the degree of sympathetic activation of the patient. This is the only class of antihypertensive drugs that consistently improves plasma lipid profiles and reduces insulin resistance. Alpha$_1$-adrenergic blocking drugs, similar to a number of other antihypertensives, can provoke salt and water retention, a process that tends to limit their antihypertensive effect. These drugs are effective in the treatment of the symptoms of benign prostatic hyperplasia (BPH), so they are commonly used in older hypertensive men. The Antihypertensive and Lipid-Lowering Treatment to Prevent Heart Attack Trial (ALLHAT) has shown a higher rate of new-onset CHF with doxazosin compared with chlorthalidone, each having been used as first-step therapy in older hypertensives with preexisting CVD risk factors; accordingly, as first-step therapy, these drugs do not have a place in treatment. However, in difficult-to-treat hypertensives, these compounds are of proven utility as adjunctive therapy to ACE inhibitors or CCBs. Side effects of alpha$_1$-adrenergic blockers are dose dependent and commonly include dizziness, lethargy, and fatigue (Table 6).

Central Alpha-Agonists

A small dose of clonidine (0.1–0.2 mg bid) augments the effect of most other agents. Dose titration of clonidine beyond 0.4 mg per day is often

TABLE 5. Calcium Channel Blockers	
Generic and brand name	**Comments**
Dihydropyridines	
Amlodipine (Norvasc)	Very long acting; minimal grapefruit juice effect; minimal effect on cyclosporine levels (monitoring recommended); no digoxin interaction of note; gingival hyperplasia can occur (class effect)
Felodipine (Plendil)	Bioavailability of felodipine is two- to threefold greater with grapefruit juice with a doubling of hemodynamic effects and an increase in vasodilator side effects; the interaction is highly variable; this is not a class effect for all CCBs
Isradapine (Dynacirc, Dynacirc SR)	Minimal interaction with cyclosporine; itraconazole (CYP3A4) inhibitor slows metabolism and therein increases the rate of vasodilator side effects
Nicardipine (Cardene-SR)	Coadministration with cimetidine increases blood levels
Nifedipine (Procardia XL, Adalat CC)	Minimal interaction with cyclosporine; minimal interaction with grapefruit juice; dose may need to be reduced when coadministered with cimetidine; coadministration with diltiazem increases concentrations by 100–200% and results in additive BP reduction
Nimodipine	Indicated for subarachnoid bleed
Nisoldipine (Sular)	Significant grapefruit juice effect; consider stopping grapefruit juice before beginning treatment; foods high in fat content increase the release of nisoldipine from the controlled-release core delivery system; peak concentrations may increase $\le$ 300%; because of greater release of the drug proximally and presumably greater presystemic metabolism, total exposure is decreased about 25%
Nondyhydropyridines	
Diltiazem (Cardizem, Cardizem-CD or SR, Cardizem -LA, Tiazac)	Decreases the metabolism off cyclosporine and tacrolimus by inhibition of CYP3A4; decreases metabolism of other CYP3A4 metabolized substances such as theophylline and simvastatin; use carefully with beta-blockers
Verapamil (Calan, Calan-SR, Isoptin-SR, Covera-HS , Verelan-PM)	Decreases the metabolism off cyclosporine by inhibition of CYP3A4; decreases metabolism of other CYP3A4 metabolized substances such as theophylline and simvastatin; use carefully with beta-blockers; aspirinlike effect to decrease platelet aggregability

followed by troubling side effects, such as lethargy and dry mouth, although these side effects can occur at lower doses. In addition, escalating doses of clonidine are prone to induce salt and water retention; thus, when it—or similar compounds—are given, a diuretic is a useful ad-

TABLE 6. Peripheral Alpha-Antagonists	
Generic and Brand Names	**Comments**
Doxazosin (Cardura)	Long acting; urinary incontinence in women; careful use in the setting of systolic dysfunction; improves insulin resistance (class effect); additive effect to ACE inhibitor or CCB treatment (class effect)
Terazosin (Hytrin)	Long acting; dose-dependent fluid retention (class effect); useful for symptomatic relief in benign prostatic hypertrophy (class effect)
Prazosin (Minipres)	Short-acting compound; reflex activation of sympathetic nervous system with tachycardia that is dose dependent; first-dose hypotension, particularly if volume contracted or on a beta-blocker but less so with newer, long-acting compounds

junctive form of therapy. Clonidine is available in a transdermal delivery system, which is particularly useful in the management of labile hypertensives; multiply medicated patient; hospitalized patients who cannot take medications by mouth; and patients prone to early morning surges in BP, which are adrenergically mediated. Its use is limited by the occurrence of skin irritation. The salt and water retention observed with oral clonidine may be less with the transdermal delivery system.

Clonidine has become established as a drug of choice for hypertensive urgencies with the recent demise of sublingual nifedipine. Its hourly administration, in doses of 0.1 to 0.2 mg, successfully reduces BP in a large number of patients. Rebound hypertension occurs in some patients receiving oral clonidine if the drug is suddenly terminated, particularly in patients with excessive adrenergic tone, who require high medication doses, or who are receiving clonidine together with a beta-blocker and inadvertently continue beta-blocker therapy while discontinuing clonidine. Rebound hypertension can be avoided by frequent administration of oral clonidine (three or four times daily) or by use of a transdermal delivery system. Clonidine overdose produces paradoxical hypertension attributable to peripheral alpha$_2$-adrenergic receptor stimulation, which supercedes the BP-lowering effect of central alpha$_2$-adrenergic receptor stimulation (Table 7).

Combined Alpha- and Beta-Adrenergic Blockers

These drugs are nonselective beta-blockers, and their beta-blocking effect typically exceeds their alpha-blocking effect. Their use is generally reserved for complicated hypertensive patients when an antihypertensive effect beyond that of a beta-blocker is sought. Salt and water retention is common at higher doses of drugs in this class. Labetalol, ei-

TABLE 7. Central Alpha-Agonists

Generic and Brand Names	Comments
α-methyldopa (Aldomet)	Autoimmune hemolytic anemia, drug fever, and liver dysfunction can occur; postural hypotension is not uncommon
Clonidine (Catapres)	Bradycardia can occur with all drugs in this class; adjunct therapy for systolic heart failure; has analgesic and anesthesia-sparing effects; available in an intravenous form
Guanabenz (Wytensin)	NSAIDs attenuate the BP-reducing effect of all drugs in this class; pretreatment with drugs in this class increases the pressor response to ephedrine or ephedra-containing herbals such as *ma huang*
Guanfacine (Tenex)	Less withdrawal symptomatology because of a longer half-life

ther orally or intravenously, has been used to treat hypertensive emergencies, particularly associated with cocaine use or in the postoperative setting. Carvedilol is an effective adjunct therapy in the patient with systolic CHF (Table 8).

Direct Vasodilators

Hydralazine is rarely used in the management of hypertension, having been supplanted by safer and generally more effective agents. It is used in pregnancy-induced hypertension and in CHF patients intolerant of ACE inhibitors. Minoxidil is a potent vasodilator that is generally reserved for refractory hypertension. Early use of minoxidil often simplifies the process of establishing BP control in such patients. Minoxidil, if given in doses > 5 mg daily, often causes tachycardia or salt and water

TABLE 8. Combined Alpha- and Beta-Blockers

Generic and brand name	Comments
Labetalol (Normadyne, Trandate)	All beta-blocker–related side effects can occur; orthostatic hypotension is a common and troubling side effect; elevations in transaminases occur in ≤ 8% of treated patients; may prevent rebound hypertension with clonidine, unlike pure beta-blockers, which may increase the risk
Carvedilol (Coreg)	Decreases microalbuminuria in hypertensive patients; subject to genetic polymorphism of the CYP2D6 isozyme, which may contribute to inter-subject variability in its pharmacokinetics; poor metabolizers may exhibit exaggerated response or toxicity such as a significant fall in pulse rate

TABLE 9. Direct Vasodilators	
Generic and Brand names	**Comments**
Hydralazine (Apresoline)	In slow acetylators, women, and HLA-DR 4 phenotypes, there appears to be a correlation with the lupuslike syndrome and high doses (> 200–400 mg/day), although patients receiving smaller doses have also developed systemic lupus erythematosus
Minoxidil (Loniten)	Usually requires a diuretic and beta-blocker; hair growth common; in women, may require depilatories; idiosyncratic pericardial effusions rarely occur

retention, counterregulatory responses that negate the BP-lowering effect of this compound. In these circumstances, dose escalation of minoxidil may actually be accompanied by an increase in BP. Effective minoxidil-based regimens typically include a diuretic and a beta-blocker to combat these counterregulatory events. Salt and water retention with minoxidil may be of sufficient severity to require the use of combination diuretic therapy with a loop diuretic and metolazone. Minoxidil use is frequently accompanied by an increase in left ventricular mass, a process that can be prevented by coadministration of an ACE inhibitor (Table 9).

References

1. Sica DA, Gehr TW: 3-Hydroxy-3-methylglutaryl coenzyme A reductase inhibitors and rhabdomyolysis: Considerations in the renal failure patient. Curr Opin Nephrol Hypertens 11:123–133, 2002.
2. Schoolwerth AC, Sica DA, Ballermann BJ, Wilcox CS; Renal considerations in angiotensin converting enzyme inhibitor therapy: A statement for healthcare professionals from the Council on the Kidney in Cardiovascular Disease and the Council for High Blood Pressure Research of the American Heart Association. Circulation 104:1985–1991, 2001.
3. Flockhart DA, Tanus-Santos JE: Implications of cytochrome P450 interactions when prescribing medication for hypertension. Arch Intern Med 162:405–412, 2002.
4. Kane GC, Lipsky JJ: Drug-grapefruit juice interactions. Mayo Clin Proc 75:933–942, 2000.
5. Shionori H: Pharmacokinetic drug interactions with ACE inhibitors. Clin Pharmacokinet 25:20–58, 1993.
6. Frishman WH, Kowalski M, Nagnur S, Sica D: Cardiovascular considerations in using topical, oral, and intravenous drugs for the treatment of glaucoma and ocular hypertension: Focus on beta-adrenergic blockade. Heart Dis 3:386–397, 2001.
7. Anderson JR, Nawarskas JJ: Cardiovascular drug-drug interactions. Cardiol Clin 19: 215–234, 2001.
8. Opie LH: Adverse cardiovascular drug interactions. Curr Probl Cardiol 25:621–676, 2000.

Index

Page numbers in **boldface** type indicate complete chapters.

A

Abdominal examination, in blood pressure evaluation, 7

Acetbutolol, side effects of, 446

Acidosis, metabolic, diuretics-related, 53

Adenoma, aldosterone-secreting, 238, 280, 418

Adenosine receptor blockers, as orthostatic hypotension treatment, 318

Adolescents
  female, physical inactivity in, 405
  hypertension in, **411–419**
    in athletes, 412–414
    in high-risk individuals, 418
    obesity-related, 411, 415–416
    sedentary lifestyle-related, 415–416
    treatment for, 414

Adrenalectomy, laparoscopic, during pregnancy, 375

Adrenergic blockers. *See also* Alpha-blockers; Alpha$_1$-blockers; Beta-blockers
  combined alpha- and beta, 452–453

Adult Treatment Panel, 386

African Americans
  health crisis among, 147–148, 153
  hypertension in, **399–409**

African Americans (*Cont.*)
  hypertension in (*Cont.*)
    comorbidity associated with, 399, 400–403
    epidemiology of, 399–400
    prevalence of, 264, 399–400
    renal tubular uric acid reabsorption associated with, 53
    resistant, 403–404
    target organ damage associated with, 293
  hypertension treatment in, 404–407
    age factors in, 239
    barriers to, 132–133
    as combination therapy, 255–256, 302
    in isolated systolic hypertension, 271–272
    promotion of, 135
  left ventricular hypertrophy in, 286
  lipoprotein (a) in, 361
  metabolic syndrome in, 25
  microalbuminuria in, 24–25, 33

African American Study on Kidney disease and hypertension (AASK), 109–110, 254, 299, 301, 303, 407

Africans, endothelial sodium channel mutations in, 438

Albumin/creatinine ratio, 28, 33
Albuminuria, 25–26. *See also*
    Macroalbuminuria; Microal-
    buminuria
  blood pressure target goal in, 235
  effect of transforming growth fac-
    tor-β1 on, 29
  measurement of, 26–28
Alcohol use
  as blood pressure increase cause, 5
  comorbidity with depression, 133
  contraindications to
    orthostatic hypotension, 315
    pregnancy, 375
  as hypertension cause
    in elderly patients, 271
    in postmenopausal women, 381
  moderate, 155
    for hypertension control, 231,
      232
  restriction of, as left ventricular
    dysfunction treatment, 290
  as single-dose antihypertensive
    drug therapy failure cause,
    239
Aldactone. *See* Spironolactone
Aldosterone antagonists, use in myo-
    cardial infarction patients,
    234–235
Aldosteronism
  glucocorticoid-remediable, 440
  primary
    diagnosis of, 238
    during pregnancy, 375
    as refractory hypertension cause,
      280–281
Alkalosis, metabolic, bicarbonate
    levels in, 52, 53
Alpha-blockers
  as isolated systolic hypertension
    treatment, 272
  renoprotective effects of, 303, 304
  as sexual dysfunction cause, 353
  use in diabetic hypertensive pa-
    tients, 258
Alpha₁-blockers
  pharmacologic features of, 450
  side effects of, 450, 452

Amaurosis fugax, 68
American College of Sports Medi-
    cine, 207
American Diabetes Association, 111,
    251, 252–253
American Heart Association, 70,
    113, 168
American Indians, diastolic dysfunc-
    tion in, 43
American Medical Association,
    148
American Society of Hypertension,
    241
  Clinical Hypertension Specialist
    certification by, 282
Amiloride
  as Liddle's disease treatment, 435,
    437, 439, 440
  as refractory hypertension treat-
    ment, 281
  as salt-sensitive hypertension treat-
    ment, 281
  side effects of, 445
Aminoglycosides, as hypertension
    cause, in organ transplant re-
    cipients, 336
Amitriptyline, 197
  side effects of, 198
Amlodipine
  cardioprotective effects of,
    232–233
  as isolated systolic hypertension
    treatment, 271–272
  lack of renoprotective effects,
    109–110
  pharmacologic features of, 451
Amphotericin, as hypertension cause,
    in organ transplant recipients,
    336
Amyloid A, as coronary heart disease
    risk factor, 363, 364
Anemia, as orthostatic hypotension
    cause, 314, 318
Anesthesia
  hypertension as contraindication
    to, 423, 424
  in hypertensive surgical patients,
    421, 422, 423, 424, 425

Angioedema, angiotensin-converting enzyme inhibitors-related, 257, 459–460

Angiography
of carotid artery stenosis, 70, 74
computed tomography, 70
magnetic resonance
carotid, 70
for renovascular hypertension diagnosis, 61

Angioplasty, percutaneous
as carotid artery disease treatment, 75–76
as renal artery stenosis treatment, 62–63, 325, 326, 327, 328–330, 331, 332
versus medical therapy, 331

Angiotensin-converting enzyme inhibitors (ACEIs)
aspirin-related attenuation of, 444–445
cardioprotective effects of
in diabetic patients, 258, 292
in microalbuminuria patients, 301
as congestive heart failure prophylaxis/treatment, 291, 294
in diabetic patients, 292
contraindications to
pregnancy, 373, 375, 386
renal artery stenosis, 446–447
cost of, 142
as diastolic dysfunction heart failure treatment, 288
as endothelial dysfunction treatment, 247–248
as hypertension treatment, 300, 444–445
in adolescents, 414, 428
in African Americans, 404, 405, 406–407
in diabetic patients, 234, 255–256
diuretic-related potentiation of, 255–256
efficacy of, 232
in high-normal blood pressure, 126

Angiotensin-converting enzyme inhibitors (ACEIs) (*Cont.*)
as hypertension treatment (*Cont.*)
inefficacy of, for refractory hypertension, 279
in initial combination treatment, 240
as initial treatment, 231
for hypertension treatment
for hypertensive emergencies, 293
in isolated systolic hypertension, 272
in postmenopausal women, 382
for renovascular hypertension, 330
indications for, 385
as left ventricular hypertrophy treatment, 290
as metabolic syndrome treatment, 246
as microalbuminuria treatment, 32, 33
natural, 184, 185, 187
pharmacologic features of, 444–445
post-myocardial infarction administration of, 234–235
renoprotective effects of, 51, 52, 53, 235, 300–301, 304, 305
in combination with angiotensin-receptor blockers, 302
side effects of, 257, 445–447
gender differences in, 386
sexual function effects, 350–351, 352, 353
use in adolescents, 430
use in organ transplant recipients, 340

Angiotensin I, 57

Angiotensin II, 29, 57, 300
in erectile dysfunction, 348–350

Angiotensin II antagonists, lack of sexual function effects, 350–351, 352, 353–354, 355

Angiotensin-receptor blockers
  cardioprotective effects of, in dia-
    betic patients, 257
  as congestive heart failure treat-
    ment, 294
  contraindications to
    pregnancy, 373, 375, 386
    renal artery stenosis, 448
  as diastolic dysfunction heart fail-
    ure treatment, 288
  as high-normal blood pressure
    treatment, 126
  as hypertension treatment
    in adolescents, 414
    in African Americans, 404, 405,
      407
    in diabetics, 234
    efficacy of, 233
    inefficacy of, in refractory hyper-
      tension, 279
    in initial combination treatment,
      240
    in initial treatment, 231
    in isolated systolic hypertension,
      272
    in renovascular hypertension, 330
  indications for, 385
  as left ventricular hypertrophy
    treatment, 290
  as metabolic syndrome treatment,
    246–247
  as microalbuminuria treatment, 32,
    33
  natural, 188
  pharmacologic features of, 448
  renoprotective effects of, 235,
    301–302, 304, 305
    in diabetic patients, 256, 257
  side effects of, 448, 449
  as stroke prophylaxis, 235
Ankle-brachial index (ABI)
  measurement and interpretation of,
    77, 79
  in peripheral arterial disease, 76,
    77, 79, 80, 81, 83
Anticoagulants, as cerebrovascular
    disease prophylaxis, 70, 72

Antidepressants, 195–200
  as orthostatic hypotension cause,
    314
  side effects of, 195, 198, 314
Antihypertensive and Lipid-Lowering
    Treatment to Prevent Heart At-
    tack Trial (ALLHAT), 73, 126,
    232–233, 271–272, 281, 292,
    383–384, 420, 450
Antihypertensive compounds, nat-
    ural, 184–188
Antihypertensive drug therapy. See
    also specific antihypertensive
    drugs
  in adolescents, 414, 416
    with diabetes, 418
  in African Americans, 404–407
  blood pressure target goals in,
    105–118
  cardioprotective effects of, 105
    blood pressure target goals in,
      110–113
  clinical trials of, 105–106,
    107–113, 124
    post-hoc analysis in, 108
  as combination therapy, 142–143,
    231
    in African Americans, 404–407
    blood pressure goal achieve-
      ment in, 299
    indications for, 385
    initial use of, 240–241
    with nonpharmacologic inter-
      ventions, 181
    in organ transplant recipients,
      340
    for refractory hypertension,
      279
  as congestive heart failure prophy-
    laxis/treatment, 290–292, 294
  cost-effectiveness of, 114–115
    in diabetic patients, 259
  cost of, 142
  dosages of
    fixed-dose, 233
    low-dose, 233
    in obese patients, 279

Antihypertensive drug therapy
(*Cont.*)
efficacy of, ambulatory blood pressure measurement assessment of, 4
guided by home blood pressure measurement, 17, 18
for high-normal blood pressure, 125
in high-risk patients, 234–235
for hypertensive emergencies, 293
indications for, 399
initial, evidence-based selection of, **231–236**
initial monotherapy
age by race paradigm in, 239
failure of, **237–242**
intensity of, 106–115
for isolated systolic hypertension, 267–270, 271–273
during lactation, 377
as left ventricular hypertrophy prophylaxis/treatment, 47, 290–291
long-acting, 233
noncompliance with, 129–130, 238–239
as refractory hypertension cause, 278
in organ transplant recipients, 335, 339–341
patient profiling for, 239
in postmenopausal women, 383–384
for preeclampsia, 372
during pregnancy, 372, 373, 375–376
renoprotective effects of, in diabetes mellitus, 252–253
for renovascular hypertension, 330–332
residual microalbuminuria during, 33
side effects of, **444–454**
gender differences in, 384
orthostatic hypotension, 281, 314

Antihypertensive drug therapy (*Cont.*)
side effects of (*Cont.*)
sexual dysfunction, 345, 347, 350–354
as therapy noncompliance cause, 141–142
as stepped care, 240
as stroke prophylaxis, 72–73, 105
in surgical patients, 421–422
for "white coat" hypertension, 227
in women, 382–386
Antioxidants
antihypertensive effects of, 185, 186
as coronary heart disease prophylaxis, 361
as endothelial dysfunction treatment, 247–248
Anti-Parkinson drugs, as orthostatic hypotension cause, 314
Antiplatelet therapy
for carotid disease, 70
as cerebrovascular disease prophylaxis, 70, 72
Antipsychotic drugs, as orthostatic hypotension cause, 314
Anxiety, as hypertension cause, 239
Aortic coarctation, 7, 9
differentiated from intermittent claudication, 78
Aortorenal bypass, 63
Aphasia, 68–69
Apnea-hypopnea index (AHI), 89, 90
Apolipoprotein A, 360, 361
Apolipoprotein B, 360
Apparent mineralocorticoid excess, 440
Appetite suppressants
as orthostatic hypotension cause, 314
as refractory hypertension cause, 280
Appropriate Blood Pressure Control in Diabetes (ABCD) trial, 252, 299
Arachidonic acid, cyclooxygenase-assisted metabolism of, 428, 429

L-Arginine
  antihypertensive effects of, 186
  as endothelial dysfunction treat-
    ment, 247–248
  as peripheral arterial disease treat-
    ment, 82
Arrhythmias, 7
Arterial stiffness
  as coronary heart disease cause,
    267
  as isolated systolic hypertension
    cause, 265–266
Arteriography, for renovascular hy-
    pertension diagnosis, 59
Arteriolar hyperresponsiveness, in
    hypertension, 123–124
Arteriosclerosis
  definition of, 265
  differentiated from atherosclerosis,
    265–266
  of the renal artery, 57, 58, 60,
    62–63. See also Hypertension,
    renovascular
Arthritis, of the hip, differentiated
    from intermittent claudication,
    78
Asians
  barriers to hypertension control in,
    132
  high-sodium diets of, 133
Aspirin
  angiotensin-converting enzyme
    inhibitor-attenuating activity
    of, 444–445
  cardioprotective effects of, 428
  in cyclooxygenase-2 inhibitor
    therapy, 427, 430, 431–432
  in peripheral arterial disease, 81
  gastrointestinal effects of, 427,
    428, 431–432
  interaction with angiotensin-
    converting enzyme inhibitors,
    458–459
  as preeclampsia prophylaxis, 372
  prostaglandin-inhibiting activity of,
    428–429
  as stroke prophylaxis, 70

Association for the Advancement of
    Medical Instrumentation, 3,
    16
Asymptomatic Carotid Artery Study
    (ACAS), 75
Atenolol
  antihypertensive efficacy of, in dia-
    betics, 110
  as isolated systolic hypertension
    treatment, 272
  as left ventricular hypertrophy
    treatment, 290
  pharmacologic features of, 446
  renoprotective effects of, 303
  side effects of, 350, 352, 446
  as stroke prophylaxis, 72–73
Atherosclerosis
  of carotid artery. See Carotid artery
    disease
  differentiated from arteriosclerosis,
    265–266
  of lower extremity vasculature. See
    Carotid artery disease
  oxidized low-density lipoproteins-
    related, 361
  as renovascular hypertension
    cause, 325
  role of nutrients in, 181
  as sexual dysfunction cause, 345,
    346
  as systemic disease, 67
Atherosclerosis Risk in Communities
    (ARIC) study, 174
Athletes, adolescent, hypertension in,
    412–414

B
Baker's cyst, differentiated from inter-
    mittent claudication, 78
Bariatric surgery, for weight loss,
    205, 210, 211, 279
Behavioral strategies, for blood pres-
    sure reduction
  in lifestyle modifications, 157–158
  in stress reduction, **223–229**
  in weight management, 208–209,
    211

Benezapril
  renoprotective effects of, 300, 301
  side effects of, 447
Beta-blockers
  cardioprotective effects of, in dia-
    betic patients, 258
  as congestive heart failure prophy-
    laxis/treatment, 291, 292, 294
  contraindication as high-normal
    blood pressure treatment, 126
  cost of, 142
  dose-response curve of, 444
  drug interactions of, 444
  as hypertension treatment
    in African Americans, 404, 405,
      407
    contraindication in adolescent
      athletes, 414
    efficacy of, 232, 233
    gender differences in, 384
    in initial hypertension, 138
    in isolated systolic hypertension,
      272
    in orthostatic hypotension, 318
    in postmenopausal women,
      382
    in pregnancy, 373, 376
  indications for, 385
  as left ventricular hypertrophy
    treatment, 290
  as metabolic syndrome treatment,
    246
  natural, 187
  pharmacologic features of, 444
  renoprotective effects of, 303, 304
  side effects of, 444, 445
    elevated blood glucose, 126
    impaired lipid metabolism, 126
    sexual dysfunction, 345,
      350–351, 352, 353
  as stroke prophylaxis, 235
  use during lactation, 377
  use in organ transplant recipients,
    340
  withdrawal from, 444
Beta-carotene, as coronary heart disease prophylaxis, 361

Betaxolol, pharmacologic features of,
  445
Bicarbonate levels, in hypertensive
  patients, 52, 53
Bile-acid binders, as statin alternative, 388–389
Biofeedback, as hypertension treatment, 223–224, 226–227
Bipolar disorder, 194–195
Bisoprolol, side effects of, 446
Blood glucose, antihypertensive drug
  therapy -related elevation in,
  126
Blood pressure. *See also* Hypertension; Hypotension
  borderline elevation in, 119
  circadian pattern of, 311
  diastolic
    aging-related increase in, 264,
      265
    excessive therapeutic lowering
      of, 272–273
    as hypertension treatment focus,
      141
    as mortality predictor, 106–107
    normal, 385
    in stage 1 hypertension, 385
    in stage 2 hypertension, 385
    in uncontrolled hypertension,
      140
    in undiagnosed hypertension,
      140
    in untreated hypertension,
      140
  high-normal, 1, 2, **119–128**
    ambulatory blood pressure mea-
      suring in, 4
    clinical importance of, 119–126
    control of, 125–126
    definition of, 119
    progression to hypertension,
      121, 123–124
  initial evaluation of, **1–11**
  normal, 2, 385
  optimal, 2
  stage 1, 385
  stage 2, 385

Blood pressure (*Cont.*)
 systolic. *See also* Hypertension,
  isolated systolic
  aging-related increase in,
   263–265
  high-normal, 2
  as hypertension treatment focus,
   139, 141
  normal, 2, 263, 385
  optimal, 2
  relationship with stroke risk,
   108, 109
  in stage 1 hypertension, 385
  in stage 2 hypertension, 385
  in uncontrolled hypertension,
   107, 137, 140
  in undiagnosed hypertension,
   140
  in untreated hypertension, 140
  water ingestion-related increase in,
   316
Blood Pressure Lowering Treatment
   Trialists' Collaborative, 113
Blood pressure measurement
 in adolescents, 411
  in athletes, 412–413
  in obese adolescents, 415
 ambulatory, 3
  versus home blood pressure
   monitors, 17
  for orthostatic hypotension diagnosis, 312, 314
  for supine hypertension evaluation, 320
  in "white coat" hypertension,
   278–279
 cuff size in, 143
 in diabetic patients, 253
 with home monitors, 3, **13–21,**
   126
  accuracy of, 16
  ambulatory measurement *versus,*
   17
  auscultatory-type, 13, 14
  oscillometric-type, 13–14, 17
  patient instruction in use of,
   17–19

Blood pressure measurement (*Cont.*)
 with home monitors (*Cont.*)
  types of, 13–15
  in "white coat" hypertension,
   278–279
 laboratory evaluation of, 7–10
 in physician's office
  limitations of, 2–3
  in "white coat" hypertension, 3
 for target blood pressure goal
  achievement, 143
 with 24 -hour monitoring
  in adolescent athletes, 413
  in overweight adolescents, 415
 in "white coat" hypertension, 3,
   278–279
Bodybuilders, hypertension in, 413
Body fat
 distribution of, 204
 excessive, 203
Body mass index (BMI), 203–204
 measurement of, 211
 microalbuminuria-related increase
  in, 31
 in obesity, 203–204, 205
  as weight loss surgery indication, 210
Body surface area, use in glomerular
  filtration rate calculation,
   50–51
Breast cancer, estrogen replacement
  therapy-related, 393
Breastfeeding, antihypertensive therapy during, 377
Breathing, controlled, as hypertension treatment, 226, 227
British Hypertension Society, 111, 251
 Working Party on Blood Pressure
  Measurement, 16
Bronchodilators, as orthostatic hypotension cause, 314
Bruits
 abdominal, 7
  renovascular hypertension-
   related, 58
 carotid, 69
Bumetanide, side effects of, 445

Bupropion, 197, 210
  side effects of, 198

C
Caffeine
  as antihypertensive drug therapy
    failure cause, 239
  as orthostatic hypotension treat-
    ment, 318
Calcineurin inhibitors, as hyperten-
    sion cause, in organ transplant
    recipients, 336–337
Calcium
  antihypertensive effects of,
    170–171, 172, 184
  cardioprotective effects of,
    170–172
  as preeclampsia prophylaxis,
    372
Calcium channel blockers. See also
    specific calcium channel
    blockers
  cardioprotective effects of, in dia-
    betic patients, 258
  in combination therapy, 448
  as congestive heart failure prophy-
    laxis, 291
  as diastolic dysfunction heart fail-
    ure treatment, 288
  dihydropyridine
    contraindication in diabetic re-
      nal disease, 258
    drug interactions of, 451
    as isolated systolic hypertension
      treatment, 272
    pharmacologic features of,
      448
    as refractory hypertension treat-
      ment, 279
    renoprotective effects of,
      302–303, 304
    use in organ transplant recipi-
      ents, 339
  drug interactions of, 340, 449,
    450
  grapefruit juice interaction with,
    449–450, 451

Calcium channel blockers. (Cont.)
  as hypertension treatment
    in adolescents, 414
    in African Americans, 404, 405,
      406, 407
    in diabetic patients, 258
    efficacy of, 232, 233
    as initial combination treatment,
      240
    as initial treatment, 231
    for isolated systolic hyperten-
      sion, 272
    in postmenopausal women, 382
    in pregnancy, 373, 376
    for refractory hypertension, 279
  indications for, 385
  interaction with tacrolimus, 340
  as left ventricular hypertrophy
    treatment, 290
  natural, 185, 187
  nondihydropyridine, 448
    drug interactions of, 451
  non-dihydropyridine
    renoprotective effects of, 302,
      303, 304
  renoprotective effects of, 302–303
  side effects of, 448–450, 449, 450,
    451
    gender differences in, 386
    sexual dysfunction, 350, 353
  as stroke prophylaxis, 235
  use in organ transplant recipients,
    339, 340
Caloric intake, for weight loss, 159,
    205
Canadian Consensus Conference on
    Hypertension, 111
Canadian Hypertension Society, 251,
    252–253
Candesartan
  as diastolic dysfunction heart fail-
    ure treatment, 288
  side effects of, 449
Captopril
  antihypertensive efficacy of, in dia-
    betics, 110
  renoprotective effects of, 300, 303

Captopril (*Cont.*)
  as renovascular hypertension treatment, 330
  side effects of, 447
Carbohydrate metabolism, exercise-related improvement in, 215
Cardiac output, in high-normal blood pressure, 121
Cardiac physiology, in obstructive sleep apnea, 91–93
Cardiovascular disease
  in African Americans, 399, 402
  antihypertensive drug therapy prophylaxis for, 105
    optimal blood pressure levels in, 110–113
  economic cost of, 113–114
  isolated systolic hypertension-related, 266–267
  in women, 379–382
Cardiovascular disease risk factors
  novel, **359–368**
    use in risk estimation equations, 365–366
  stratification of, 268–269
  in women, **379–397**
Cardiovascular examination, in blood pressure evaluation, 7
Cardiovascular metabolic abnormalities, high normal blood pressure-related, 121–122, 124
Cardiovascular mortality, 191
  antihypertensive drug therapy prophylaxis for, 113
  high-normal blood pressure-related, 120–121, 122, 123, 124
  perioperative, 421
Cardiovascular physiologic abnormalities, high-normal blood pressure-related, 121–122, 124
L-Carnitine, as peripheral arterial disease treatment, 82
Carotid and Vertebral Artery Transluminal Angioplasty Study (CAVATAS), 75–76

Carotid artery disease (stenosis), 67–76
  assessment of, 74
  asymptomatic, 75
  diagnosis of, 69–70
  medical management of, 70–73
  percutaneous interventions in, 75–76
  revascularization interventions in, 73–75
  risk factor treatment in, 68
  symptomatic, 73–75
  symptoms of, 67–69
Carotid artery syndrome, 69
Carotid duplex imaging, 69, 70
Carteolol, side effects of, 446
Carvedilol
  cardioprotective effects of, 258
  side effects of, 453
  use in organ transplant recipients, 340
Catecholamines, as pheochromocytoma marker, 8, 10
Catheterization, cardiac, racial and sexual bias in recommendations for, 148
Caucasian Americans, hypertension prevalence in, 264
Celecoxib, 429, 430, 431–432
Celecoxib Long-term Arthritis Safety Study (CLASS), 429, 430, 431–432
Celery, antihypertensive effects of, 186, 187, 188
Central a_2-agonists, renoprotective effects of, 303
Central alpha-agonists, side effects of, 450–452
Central nervous system depressants, as orthostatic hypotension cause, 314
Cerebrovascular disease. *See also* Stroke
  in African Americans, 403
CHARM trial, 288

Children
  hypertension in, 411
  microalbuminuria in, 24
Chlorthalidone
  cardioprotective effects of,
    232–233
    in African Americans, 406
  as refractory hypertension treat-
    ment, 281
  side effects of, 350, 352, 450,
    459
Cholesterol. *See also* Dyslipidemia;
    Hypercholesterolemia; Hyper-
    lipidemia
  measurement of, 359
Cholesterol and Recurrent Events
    (CARE) trial, 387
Chronic disease/medical conditions,
    243
  comorbid depression/hyperten-
    sion-related, **191–202**
Chvostek sign, 9
Cilexetil, as diastolic dysfunction
    heart failure treatment, 288
Cilostazol, as intermittent claudica-
    tion treatment, 81–82
Circulation, hyperkinetic, in high-
    normal blood pressure, 121
Citalopram, 196
  side effects of, 198
Claudication
  intermittent, 76–79
    beta-blocker use in, 458
    peripheral arterial disease-
      related, 76–83
    pharmacologic therapy for,
      81–82
    venous, 78
Clinical Hypertension Specialists,
    282
Clomipramine, 197
  side effects of, 198
Clonidine
  as orthostatic hypotension treat-
    ment, 318
  as pregnancy-associated hyperten-
    sion treatment, 373, 376

Clonidine (*Cont.*)
  side effects of, 241, 350, 450–452,
    453
  use in diabetic hypertensive pa-
    tients, 258
Clonidine transdermal patch, as re-
    fractory hypertension treat-
    ment, 279
Clopidogrel, 81
Clopidogrel Vs. Aspirin in Patients at
    Risk of Ischemic Events (CA-
    PRIE) trial, 81
Cocaine abuse
  as antihypertensive drug therapy
    failure cause, 239
  as hypertension cause, 5, 280
Coenzyme Q10 (ubiquinone),
    185–186, 188
Compartment syndrome, differenti-
    ated from intermittent claudi-
    cation, 78
Compliance
  with exercise, 215–218
  with hypertension treatment
    individual barriers to, 129–130,
      134–135
    promotion of, 134–135
    sociocultural barriers to, 129,
      131–133
    socioeconomic barriers to, 129,
      130–131
Computed tomography angiography,
    70
Congestive heart failure
  in African Americans, 402, 406
  angiotensin-converting enzyme
    therapy for, 444
  as cilostazol contraindication, 82
  diabetes mellitus-related, 292
  diastolic, 37, 38, 40–44, 288–289
  hypertension-related, **285–296**
    with left ventricular hypertrophy,
      285–291
  incidence and prevalence of, 285,
    286
  left ventricular hypertrophy-
    related, 37, 38, 285–291

Congestive heart failure (*Cont.*)
  metabolic syndrome-related, 243
  peripheral alpha-antagonists-
    related, 450
  prevention of, 290–292
    in African Americans, 406
    antihypertensive drug therapy
      for, 105, 292, 293
    in elderly patients, 291–292
  systolic, antihypertensive drug
    therapy for, 234, 294
Conn's syndrome, 280
Constipation, Valsalva maneuver in,
  315, 316
Continuous positive airway pressure
  (CPAP) therapy, for sleep apnea, 92–93, 94
Contrast agents, nephrotoxicity of, 59
Controlled breathing techniques, as
  hypertension treatment, 226,
  227
Coronary artery disease, hypertension-related, 285
  depression associated with,
    192–193
Coronary heart disease
  antihypertensive drug therapy pro-
    phylaxis for, 113
  high-normal blood pressure-
    related, 120, 124
  as mortality cause, in African
    Americans, 402
  pulse pressure as risk marker for,
    266–267
C-reactive protein
  as coronary heart disease risk fac-
    tor, 362–363, 364
  as peripheral arterial disease risk
    factor, 67
Creatinine levels, in hypertensive patients, 52
Cubulin, 25
Cultural congruence, in medical
  care, **147–154**
Cushing's disease, 9, 10
Cushing's syndrome, 238
Cyclooxygenase-1, 428, 429

Cyclooxygenase-2, 428, 429
Cyclooxygenase-2 inhibitors (coxibs),
  429, 430–432
  as single-dose antihypertensive
    drug therapy failure cause,
    239
Cyclosporine
  alternatives to, 337–338, 339, 340
  drug interactions of, 339–340
  as hypertension cause, 335
    in organ transplant recipients,
      336–337
Cyclothymia, 194–195
Cytochrome P450 system, antihypertensive drug interactions with,
  443

D
DASH diet. *See* Dietary Approaches
  to Stop Hypertension (DASH)
  diet
Depression
  comorbidity with
    hypertension-related chronic
      diseases, **191–202**
    substance abuse, 133
  diagnosis of, 194–195
    barriers to, 195, 199, 200
  epidemiology of, 191
  treatment of, 195–200
    barriers to, 195, 199, 200
"Derby chairs," 319
Desipramine, 197
  side effects of, 198
Desmopressin, as orthostatic hypotension treatment, 317
Diabetes mellitus
  in adolescents, 418, 432
  in African Americans, 402, 403
  antihypertensive drug therapy in,
    254–259
  blood pressure target goals in,
    111, 249–252, 255–256
  cardioprotective effects of,
    110–111, 250–252, 257–258
  cost-benefits of, 114–115
  indications for, 234

Diabetes mellitus (*Cont.*)
  antihypertensive drug therapy in
    (*Cont.*)
    inefficacy of, 258–259
    renoprotective effects of, 250,
      254–257, 300, 301
  as cardiovascular disease risk fac-
    tor, in women, 389–390, 393
  as end-stage renal disease cause,
    403
  high-normal blood pressure in, 270
  hypertension associated with
    blood pressure target goals in,
      107
    combination antihypertensive
      drug therapy for, 234
    comorbid depression in, 192, 193
    as congestive heart failure cause,
      292
    fundoscopic examination in, 7
    isolated systolic hypertension,
      268
    nonpharmacologic interventions
      for, 254
    in postmenopausal women,
      382
    proteinuria in, 53–54
    as sexual dysfunction cause,
      345–346, 347
    treatment of, **249–262,** 390
  hypertriglyceridemia associated
    with, 390
  inadequacy of treatment for, 244
  as metabolic syndrome compo-
    nent, 243, 244, 245, 246–247
  microalbuminuria associated with,
    24
  obesity-related, in elderly patients,
    270
  peripheral arterial disease-masking
    effect of, 79
  risk factor control goals in, 245
  undiagnosed, in African Ameri-
    cans, 402
Dialysis, 114, 244, 297
Dialysis patients, primary diagnosis
  in, 250

Diastolic dysfunction, 37, 38, 40–44,
    288–289
  asymptomatic, 40–41
  definition of, 41
  evaluation of, 42–43
Diclofenac, 430, 431
Diet
  cardioprotective, in women,
    391–392
  as hypertension cause, 182
  Paleolithic, 182
Dietary Approaches to Stop Hyper-
    tension (DASH) diet,
    155–156, 159, 160, 161, 173,
    176, 183, 207, 231–232, 271
  comparison with low-sodium diet,
    174, 175
  as high-normal blood pressure
    treatment, 125
  use by adolescents, 428
  use by African Americans, 404
Dietary interventions
  for hypertension control, 155–156,
    165–180. *See also* Dietary Ap-
    proaches to Stop Hyperten-
    sion (DASH) diet
    in orthostatic hypotension, 316
    in salt-sensitive hypertension,
      270–271
    socioeconomic barriers to, 131
  for weight loss, 206–207
    for refractory hypertension con-
      trol, 278
Dihydroergotamine, as orthostatic
    hypotension treatment, 318
Diltiazem
  drug interactions of, 339–340,
    444, 450, 451, 458
  as hypertension treatment
    in initial combination treatment,
      240–241
    for refractory hypertension, 279
    for supine hypertension, 321
  renoprotective effects of, 258,
    303
  use in organ transplant recipients,
    339–340

Diuretics. *See also* specific diuretics
  action mechanism of, 457–458
  cardioprotective effects of, 233
  in combination therapy, 457
  as congestive heart failure prophy-
    laxis/ treatment, 291, 292,
    294
  contraindication as high-normal
    blood pressure treatment,
    |126
  cost of, 142
  as diastolic dysfunction heart fail-
    ure treatment, 288
  dosages of, 457
  as hypertension treatment
    in African Americans, 404, 405,
      407
    contraindication in adolescent
      athletes, 414
    in diabetic patients, 255–256
    efficacy of, 233, 457
    in initial combination treatment,
      240
    for isolated systolic hyperten-
      sion, 271–272
    in postmenopausal women, 382,
      384
    in pregnancy, 373
  loop-type
    as hypertensive emergency treat-
      ment, 293
    as Liddle's disease treatment,
      439–440
    side effects of, 459
    as thiazide-type diuretics alter-
      natives, 241
    use in organ transplant recipi-
      ents, 339
    use in renal dysfunction patients,
      302
  as metabolic acidosis cause, 53
  as microalbuminuria treatment, 32
  natural, 187
  pharmacologic features of, 444
  as potassium loss cause, 51, 53
  potassium-sparing, side effects of,
    445

Diuretics (*Cont.*)
  as renovascular hypertension treat-
    ment, 330
  side effects of, 444, 445
    elevated blood glucose, 126
    gender differences in, 386
    impaired lipid metabolism, 126
    sexual dysfunction, 345, 350,
      352, 353, 355
  thiazide-type
    antihypertensive effects of, 232
    cardioprotective effects of,
      232–233
    in combination therapy, 233
    decreased efficacy in renal dys-
      function, 302
    dosages of, 241
    as hypokalemia cause, 439–440
    indications for, 385
    as initial hypertension treatment,
      138, 231, 233, 384
    as Liddle's disease treatment,
      439–440
    as pregnancy-associated hyper-
      tension treatment, 376
    as refractory hypertension treat-
      ment, 279, 281
    as renal disease prophylaxis,
      235
    sexual function effects of, 352,
      355
    as stroke prophylaxis, 73, 235
    use in African Americans, 406
    use in elderly diabetic patients,
      257–258
    use in postmenopausal women,
      384
    vasopressor effect of, 443–445
  use during lactation, 377
Docosahexanoic acid, 184
Doppler spectral analysis, pulsed, 70,
  71
Doxazosin
  in combination therapy, 448
  inefficacy as congestive heart fail-
    ure prophylaxis, 292
  pharmacologic features of, 452

Doxazosin (*Cont.*)
  as refractory hypertension treatment, 279
  side effects of, 450
Doxepin, 197
  side effects of, 198
DRASTIC (Dutch Renal Artery Stenosis Intervention Cooperative) trial, 331
Drug interactions. *See also* names of specific drugs
  of antidepressants, 195
  of antihypertensive drugs, 457
  as single-dose antihypertensive drug therapy failure cause, 239
Drugs. *See also* names of specific drugs
  adverse reactions to, in hypertensive patients, **443–454**
    as single-dose antihypertensive drug therapy failure cause, 239
  as hypertension cause, 5
  as orthostatic hypotension cause, 314, 315
Dysautonomia, as orthostatic hypertension cause, 311–312, 315
Dyslipidemia. *See also* Hyperlipidemia; Hypertriglyceridemia
  isolated systolic hypertension-associated, 269–270
  metabolic syndrome-associated, 246, 247
  in women, 379, 386–389
    pharmacologic treatment of, 386–389
Dysthymia, 194, 195

E
Echocardiographic Heart of England Screening study, 45–46
Echocardiography
  in asymptomatic hypertensive patients, 47
  for blood pressure evaluation, 10

Echocardiography (*Cont.*)
  Doppler, for left ventricular diastolic function assessment, 42–44
  for ejection fraction measurement, 44–45
  for hypertensive patient evaluation, 46
  for left ventricular hypertrophy evaluation, 37, 39–40, 46–47
Edema
  combination hypertension therapy-related, 240–241
  pulmonary
    diastolic heart failure-related, 41
    flash, 280
    hypertensive emergency-related, 293, 294
    renovascular hypertension-related, 59
Eicosapentaenoic acid, 184
Ejection fraction, left ventricular
  depressed, 45–46, 47
  measurement of, 44–45
Elderly patients
  antihypertensive drug therapy in
    as combination therapy, 255–256, 302
    as orthostatic hypotension cause, 281
  diabetic, thiazide diuretic use in, 257–258
  hypertension in
    alcohol use-related, 271
    congestive heart failure prevention in, 291–292
    gender differences in, 379–380
    as isolated systolic hypertension, 106
    lifetime risk of, 265
    as secondary hypertension, 238
Electrocardiography
  for blood pressure evaluation, 10
  for hypertensive heart disease evaluation, 37
  for hypertensive patient evaluation, 46

Electrocardiography (*Cont.*)
for left ventricular hypertrophy
evaluation, 37, 38, 39,
40, 46
Electrolytes, as renal function indicators, 51–53
Enalapril, side effects of, 447
Enalaprilat
as hypertensive emergency treatment, 293
as perioperative hypertension treatment, 445
Endarterectomy
carotid, 73–75
as renal artery stenosis treatment,
63
Endothelial dysfunction
as erectile dysfunction cause, 345,
347–348
as essential hypertension cause,
181, 183
obstructive sleep apnea-related,
93
treatment of, 247–248
Endothelin, sleep apnea-related increase in, 92–93
Ephedra, as refractory hypertension
cause, 280
Ephedrine, as stroke cause, 239
Ephedrine sulfate, as orthostatic hypotension treatment, 317
Eplerenone, 280–281
Eprosartan, side effects of, 449
Erectile dysfunction
endothelial dysfunction-related,
345, 347–348
hypertension-related, 345, 346,
347–355
Erythropoietin, as anemia treatment,
318
Escitalopram, 196
side effects of, 198
Esmolol, pharmacologic features of,
446
Essai Multicentrique Medicaments v.
Angioplastie (EMMA) trial,
331

Estrogen replacement therapy
as endothelial dysfunction treatment, 247–248
as hypertension risk factor, 382
lack of cardioprotective effects of,
392–394
serum lipid effects of, 386
side effects of, 393
Ethacrynic acid, side effects of, 445
Ethnic/minority groups. *See also*
African Americans; Asians;
Hispanics; Mexican Americans
barriers to hypertension control in
sociocultural barriers, 129,
131–133
socioeconomic barriers, 129,
130–131
premature deaths in, 149
European Carotid Surgery Trial
(ECST), 73
Exercise
aerobic
contraindication during pregnancy, 375
as hypertension treatment, 384
barriers to, 219
cardioprotective effects of, 215,
221
in women, 391, 392
definition of, 216
as endothelial dysfunction treatment, 247–248
as high-normal blood pressure
treatment, 126
for hypertension control, 155,
215–222 231, 232, 384
in diabetic patients, 254
in orthostatic hypotension, 316,
319–320
promotion of, 158–159, 160
socioeconomic barriers to, 131
as left ventricular dysfunction treatment, 290
as peripheral arterial disease treatment, 81
quantification of, 215, 218–219

Exercise (*Cont.*)
   terminology of, 216
   transtheoretical ("stages of change")
      model of, 215–218, 221
   for weight management, 126, 159,
      207–208
Exercise testing, prior to exercise pro-
      grams, 161

F

Falls, orthostatic hypotension-related,
      315
Family history, 5
Fat, dietary, 184–185
Felodipine, interaction with grape-
      fruit juice, 449–450, 451
Fenoldopam, as hypertensive emer-
      gency treatment, 293
Fiber, dietary, 182, 185, 188
Fibrates, use in women, 389
Fibrinogen, 362
Fibromuscular dysplasia, as renovas-
      cular hypertension cause, 57,
      58, 59, 60, 62, 325, 327,
      330–332
Fitness, definition of, 216
FITT exercise prescriptions, 158–159,
      218
Flexibility, definition of, 216
9a-Fludrocortisone, as orthostatic hy-
      potension treatment, 317
Fluoxetine, 196
   side effects of, 198
Folate deficiency, 69, 364
Food and Drug Administration, 16
Fosinopril, side effects of, 447
Fosinopril Amlodipine Cardiac
      Events Trial (FACET), 258
Framingham Heart Study, 40, 46,
      204, 265, 267, 292, 360, 361,
      394
Fundoscopic examination, in blood
      pressure evaluation, 6–7
Furosemide
   as refractory hypertension treat-
      ment, 279
   side effects of, 445

G

Gamma linoleic acid, 188, 184–185
Garlic, antihypertensive activity of,
      185, 187, 188
Gender differences. *See also* Women
   in hypertension
      in adolescents, 416–418
      in older adults, 379–380
Glomerular filtration rate
   decreased
      blood pressure target goal in,
         235
      smoking-related, 32
   estimation of, 50–51
Glomerulonephritis, dialysis treat-
      ment for, 250
Glucose intolerance, isolated systolic
      hypertension-associated,
      269–270
Glycosuria, 53
Gout, diuretics-related, 386
Grapefruit, interaction with calcium
      channel blockers, 449–450,
      451
Guanabenz, side effects of, 453
Guanafacine, side effects of, 453
Gynecomastia, antihypertensive drug
      therapy-related, 351

H

Hawthorne berries, antihypertensive
      effects of, 187, 188
Healthy People 2000, 106, 114
Healthy People 2010, 114
Heart and Estrogen/progestin Re-
      placement Study (HERS),
      392–393
Heart failure. *See also* Congestive
      heart failure
   hypertensive emergency-related,
      293
   renovascular hypertension-related,
      59
Heart murmurs, 7
Heart Outcomes Prevention Evalua-
      tion (HOPE), 72–73,
      382–383

Heart Outcomes Prevention Evalua-
    tion (HOPE) trial, 243–244,
    256, 272, 406–407
Heart Outcomes Prevention Evalua-
    tion (MICRO-HOPE) trial,
    256, 301
Heart rate
    during exercise, 126
    in high-normal blood pressure,
        121
    in obstructive sleep apnea, 92
Heat stroke, orthostatic hypotension-
    related, 315
HELLP syndrome, 372
Helsinki Heart Study, 361
Hemoglobin A1c levels, in metabolic
    syndrome, 243–244, 245, 246
Hemorrhage, subarachnoid, calcium
    supplementation-related, 172
Herbal remedies, 132
    as antihypertensive drug therapy
        failure cause, 239
High-density lipoprotein (HDL)
    gender differences in, 386
    optimal level, for stroke prophy-
        laxis, 72
    propranolol-related decrease in,
        246
Hirsutism, minoxidil-related, 386
Homeopathy, as hypertension treat-
    ment, 223
Homocysteine, as coronary heart dis-
    ease risk factor, 363–364, 365
Hormone replacement therapy. See
    Estrogen replacement therapy
Hydralazine, 453
    as pregnancy-associated hyperten-
        sion treatment, 373, 376,
        453
    as refractory hypertension treat-
        ment, 279
    side effects of, 350, 454
    as supine hypertension treatment,
        321
    use during lactation, 377
    use in diabetic hypertensive pa-
        tients, 258

Hydrochlorothiazide
    dose-response effect of, 443–444
    as left ventricular hypertrophy
        treatment, 290
    low dosages of, 443
    side effects of, 445
Hydrodiuril. See Hydrochloroth-
    iazide
Hydroton. See Chlorthalidone
3-Hydroxy-3-methylglutaryl coen-
    zyme A inhibitors
    alternatives to, 402–403
    cardioprotective effects of, in
        women, 386–388
    as carotid disease treatment, 72
    side effects of, 388–389
    as stroke prophylaxis, 72
    use in peripheral arterial disease
        patients, 81
Hyperaldosteronism
    as hypertension cause, 9
    primary
        hypertension-associated,
            403–404
        versus secondary, 53
Hypercholesterolemia, metabolic
    syndrome-associated, 243
Hypercoagulable states
    as ischemic stroke cause, 69
    metabolic syndrome-related, 244
Hyperinsulinemia, microalbumin-
    uria-related, 23, 31–32
Hyperkalemia, angiotensin-convert-
    ing enzyme inhibitors-related,
    257, 301, 447
Hyperlipidemia
    diabetes mellitus-related, 245
    metabolic syndrome-related, 244
    microalbuminuria-related, 23,
        30–31
Hyperparathyroidism, as hyperten-
    sion cause, 9, 10
Hypertension
    age of onset, racial differences in,
        399
    amiloride-sensitive (Liddle's dis-
        ease), **435–441**

Hypertension (*Cont.*)
 arteriolar hyperresponsiveness in,
  123–124
 blood pressure treatment goals in,
  105–118
  historical background of, 138,
   141
  physician factors as obstacles to,
   141–143
  physicians' noncompliance
   with, 141
 borderline, 119
 combination treatment approach
  in, 181, 182
 complicated, treatment of126
 controlled, 137, 138
  patient characteristics in, 139,
   140
  prevalence of, 106
 definition of, 137, 411
 diagnostic blood pressure levels in
  in adolescents, 411, 412
  in adults, 411
 dysmetabolic syndrome of,
  347–348
 economic cost of, 113–115
 essential, in adolescents, 411–412
 gender differences in
  in adolescents, 416–418
  in adults, 379–380
 gestational, 379, 380. *See also*
  Pregnancy, hypertension during
 isolated systolic, **263–276**
  arterial stiffness as cause of,
   265–266
  as cardiovascular disease risk
   factor, 266–267
  as congestive heart failure cause,
   291, 292, 294
  definition of, 263
  in elderly patients, 106, 107,
   263–277, 380
  epidemiology of, 263–265
  primary, 265
  secondary, 265
  treatment of, 267–273

Hypertension (*Cont.*)
 lifespan trends in, 123
 low-renin (Liddle's disease),
  435–441
 metabolic syndrome-associated,
  204, 243, 244, 245
 nocturnal, ambulatory blood pressure measuring in, 4
 oral contraceptives-related,
  416–417
 prevalence of, 399
  in postmenopausal women,
   380–381
  racial differences in, 399–400
 refractory/resistant, **277–284**
  in African Americans, 403–404
  ambulatory blood pressure measuring in, 4
  consultations for, 282
  control or elimination of, 281
  evaluation of, 277–281
  obstructive sleep apnea-related,
   93, 95
  as secondary hypertension,
   279–281
 renovascular, **325–334**
  in adolescents, 417–418
  arteriosclerosis-related, 62–63
  atherosclerosis-related, 325,
   326, 327–328, 330
  clinical features of, 57–59
  diagnosis of, 59, 61–62
  fibromuscular dysplasia-related,
   57, 58, 59, 60, 62, 325, 327,
   330–332
  medical management of,
   330–332
  pharmacological management
   of, 60
  renal artery occlusive disease-related, **57–66**
  surgical management of, 60,
   62–63, 327–328, 331, 332
 salt-sensitive
  dietary interventions for,
   270–271
  hidden, 281

Hypertension (*Cont.*)
  salt-sensitive (*Cont.*)
    licorice-related, 280
    racial differences in, 399
  secondary
    in adolescents, 411–412
    age factors in, 5
    antihypertensive drug therapy
      failure in, 238–239
    racial factors in, 5
    as refractory hypertension,
      279–281
  stage 1, 2
  stage 2, 2
  stage 3, 2
  stepped care approach to, 138,
    240
  supine
    management of, 320–322
    orthostatic hypotension-associ-
      ated, **309–324**
  in surgical patients, **421–426**
    enalaprilat treatment for, 445
  treatment of
    blood pressure target goals in,
      105–118
    historical background of, 138,
      141
    inadequacy of, 244
    with lifestyle modification, 384,
      385
    pharmacologic. *See* Antihyper-
      tensive drug therapy
  uncontrolled, 129, 137, 138
    in organ transplant recipients,
      339, 340
    patient characteristics in, 137,
      139, 140
  undiagnosed, 137, 138
    patient characteristics in, 139,
      140
  untreated, 137, 138
    in the elderly, 380
    patient characteristics in, 139,
      140
  "white coat," 239
    in adolescents, 413

Hypertension (*Cont.*)
  "white coat" (*Cont.*)
    ambulatory blood pressure mea-
      surement in, 4
    antihypertensive drug therapy
      for, 227
    behavioral treatment of, 224,
      227
    blood pressure measurement in,
      278–279
    home blood pressure measure-
      ment in, 3
    as refractory hypertension,
      278–279
  wide pulse pressure, untreated,
    265
Hypertension in African Americans
    Working Group (HAWW),
    405–406
Hypertension Optimal Treatment
    (HOT) study, 108, 110–113,
    251–252, 258, 259, 299
Hypertension specialists
  list of, 241
  referrals to, 241, 282
    of diabetic hypertensive patients,
      258–259
Hypertension treatment. *See also* An-
    tihypertensive drug therapy
  patient barriers to, **129–136**
    individual barriers, 129–130,
      134–135
    overcoming, 134–135
    sociocultural barriers, 129,
      131–133
    socioeconomic barriers, 129,
      130–131
Hypertensive emergencies, 293
  treatment for, 452–453
    adverse outcomes in, 111
Hyperthyroidism, 8, 238
Hypertriglyceridemia
  as coronary heart disease risk fac-
    tor, 361
  gender differences in, 389
  diabetes mellitus-related, in
    women, 390

Hypertriglyceridemia (*Cont.*)
  isolated systolic hypertension-
    associated, 269–270
Hyperuricemia, 52, 53
Hypoaldonsteronism, Liddle's dis-
    ease-related, 435, 438, 439
Hypokalemia
  diuretics-related, 51, 53,
    439–440
    gender differences in, 386
  Liddle's disease-related, 435, 436,
    438, 439, 440
  as orthostatic hypotension cause,
    314
  thiazide diuretics-related, 439–440
Hyponatremia, diuretics-related,
    386
Hypopnea, 89
Hypotension
  antihypertensive drug therapy-
    related, 111
  orthostatic
    a_1-antagonists-related, 241
    antihypertensive drug therapy-
      related, 281, 314
    causes of, 310–311
    definition of, 309, 312
    in elderly patients, 281
    neurogenic, 311–312, 314,
      315
    non-neurogenic, 314
    supine hypertension associated
      with, **309–324**
    transient, 309, 311
    treatment for, 316–320, 321
Hypothyroidism, 8, 238
Hypovolemia, as orthostatic hypoten-
    sion cause, 314
Hypoxia, as orthostatic hypotension
    cause, 314

I

Ibuprofen, 430, 431
Imipramine, 197
  side effects of, 198
Immunosuppressive drugs
  as hypertension cause, 335–339

Immunosuppressive drugs (*Cont.*)
  nonhypertension-inducing, 336,
    337–339, 340
Indapamide, side effects of,
    445
Individual Data Analysis of Antihy-
    pertensive intervention data-
    base, 382, 383
Indomethacin, 431
  as orthostatic hypotension treat-
    ment, 317
Inflammation
  arterial, metabolic syndrome-
    related, 244
  cyclooxygenase-2-related,
    429
Inflammatory markers, for coronary
    heart disease risk, 362–363,
    366–367
INSIGHT trial, 281
Institute of Medicine, 243, 244
Insulin resistance
  in African Americans, 402
  definition of, 402
  metabolic syndrome-related in-
    crease in, 244, 247
  propranolol-related increase in,
    246
Insulin resistance syndrome. *See*
    Metabolic syndrome
Insulin therapy, as weight gain cause,
    246
Internal carotid artery
  atherosclerosis of, 69
    imaging of, 69–70, 71
  emboli to, 68
International Society of Hyperten-
    sion, 251
International Society on Hyperten-
    sion in Blacks (ISHIB),
    405–406
Irbesartan
  renoprotective effects of, 301
    in diabetic patients, 257
  side effects of, 449
Irbesartan Diabetic Nephropathy
    Trial (IDNT), 254, 257

Ischemia, cerebral, 68–69
Isradapine, 451

J
J-curve phenomenon, 111, 272–273
Joint National Committee on Prevention, Detection, Evaluation, and Treatment of High Blood Pressure (JNC), 226–227
  I, 138
  II-IV, 138
  VI, 1, 2, 107, 109, 110, 119, 126, 138, 141, 183, 249–250, 251, 254, 297, 407

K
Kringles, 360–361

L
Labetalol
  as hypertensive emergency treatment, 452–453
  as pregnancy-associated hypertension treatment, 372, 373
  side effects of, 453
  use during lactation, 377
  use in organ transplant recipients, 340
Laboratory evaluation, of hypertensive patients, 7–10
Lactation, hypertension treatment during, 377
Lasix. See Furosemide
Left ventricular failure, hypertensive emergency-related, 293
Left ventricular hypertrophy, 37–41
  in adolescents, 415, 416
  antihypertensive drug therapy for, 47, 105
  concentric, 40, 41
  as congestive heart failure cause, 37, 38, 285–291
  diagnosis of, 415
  eccentric, 40, 41
  echocardiographic evaluation of, 37, 39–40, 46–47

Left ventricular hypertrophy (Cont.)
  electrocardiographic evaluation of, 37, 38, 39, 46
  geometric patterns of, 40, 41
  high-normal blood pressure associated with, 270
  increased aortic pulsatile load-related, 266
  pathophysiology of, 287–289
  as refractory hypertension cause, 278, 279–280, 281
  regression of, 289–290
Leotards, as orthostatic hypotension treatment, 319
Licorice, as hypertension cause, 280
Lifestyle modifications. See also Dietary interventions; Exercise; Smoking cessation; Weight loss
  for diabetic patients, 254
  for high-normal blood pressure control, 125–126
  for hypertension control, 231–232, 384, 385
    in adolescents, 416
    in African Americans, 404, 407
    behavioral strategies for, 157–158
    in isolated systolic hypertension, 270–271
    patient resources for, 162–163
    promotion of, **155–164**
    in women, 384
Lipid-lowering therapy
  in endothelial dysfunction, 247–248
  in high-normal blood pressure, 126
  in metabolic syndrome, 243–244
  in peripheral arterial disease, 81
  as stroke prophylaxis, 72
Lipid metabolism
  antihypertensive drug therapy-related impairment of, 126
  exercise-related improvement in, 215
Lipid Research Clinic Program, 361

Lipoprotein (a), 359, 360–361
Lisinopril
    cardioprotective effects of,
        232–233, 406
    as isolated systolic hypertension
        treatment, 271
    side effects of, 447
Losartan
    cardioprotective effects of, gender
        differences in, 383
    as isolated systolic hypertension
        treatment, 272
    as left ventricular hypertrophy
        treatment, 290–291
    renoprotective effects of, 301
    sexual activity effects of, 351,
        353–354
    as stroke prophylaxis, 72–73
Losartan Intervention For Endpoint
    reduction in hypertension
    (LIFE) trial, 72–73, 257, 272,
    290–291, 383
Lotrel, use in diabetic hypertensive
    patients, 255
Low-density lipoprotein (LDL)
    gender differences in, 386
    optimal level of, 72
    oxidized, 359, 361
Low-density lipoprotein subparticles,
    359, 360–361
Lycopene, antihypertensive effects of,
    185

M
Macroalbuminuria, in diabetic pa-
    tients, screening for, 253
Macronutrients, 181–182
Magnesium
    antihypertensive effects of, 172,
        174, 184
    cardioprotective effects of, 174
Magnetic resonance angiography,
    carotid, 70
Major depression, 192, 194
Mania, 194–195
Massachusetts Male Aging Study,
    347

Medical care
    culturally-congruent, **147–154**
    lack of access to, 130–131
Medical history, in blood pressure
    evaluation, 4–6
Medroxyprogesterone acetate, 392
Megalin, 25
Menopause. See also Women, post-
    menopausal
    dyslipidemia during, 386
Metabolic syndrome, **243–248**
    in adolescents, 415–416
    in African Americans, 25
    as cardiovascular disease risk fac-
        tor, 401
    inadequacy of treatment for, 244
    medical management of, 244–248
    microalbuminuria associated with,
        23, 31–32
    obesity associated with, 243, 244,
        246
        in women, 390, 391
    symptoms of, 204
    in women, 390
Metformin, 246–247
Methyldopa
    as pregnancy-associated hyperten-
        sion treatment, 372, 373, 376
    side effects of, 350, 453
    use during lactation, 377
    use in diabetic hypertensive pa-
        tients, 258
Methylphenidate, as orthostatic hy-
    potension treatment, 317
Metolazone, side effects of, 459
Metoprolol
    renoprotective effects of, 303
    side effects of, 446
Mexican Americans, hypertension
    prevalence in, 264
Microalbuminuria, **23–35**
    assessment of, 10
    as cardiovascular disease risk fac-
        tor, 23, 30, 33, 253
    definition of, 23, 28, 299
    in diabetic patients, screening for,
        253

Microalbuminuria (*Cont.*)
  essential hypertension-associated, 24, 28–30
  in ethnic populations, 24–25
  evaluation of, 23, 26–28
  false-positive test results in, 26, 299
  as hyperinsulinemia risk factor, 23, 31–32
  pathogenesis of, 28–30
  as renal disease risk factor, 23, 24, 28–30, 29, 30, 33, 253, 298
  as serum lipid abnormalities risk factor, 23, 30–31
  treatment of, 32–33
Micronutrients, 181–182
  recommended dietary intake of, 175–176
Midodrine, as orthostatic hypotension treatment, 317, 320
Minority groups. *See* Ethnic/minority groups
Minoxidil
  in combination therapy, 241
  as refractory hypertension treatment, 279
  side effects of, 350, 386, 453–454
Mirtazapine, 196
  side effects of, 198
Modification of Diet in Renal Disease Trial (MDRD), 108–109, 297, 299
Moexipril, side effects of, 447
Multiple Risk Factor Intervention Trial (MRFIT), 120, 122, 250, 251, 360
Muscle deconditioning, as orthostatic hypotension cause, 314
Mycophenolate, 338, 339, 340
Myocardial infarction
  annual economic cost of, 114
  antihypertensive drug therapy following, 234–235
  congestive heart failure-related, 285
  diabetes mellitus-related, 245
  metabolic syndrome-related, 246
  metformin prophylaxis for, 246

Myocardial ischemia, perioperative, 421, 422, 423, 424, 425

N
Nadolol, 446
Naproxen, cardioprotective effects of, 430, 431
National Board of Medical Examiners, 282
National Cholesterol Education Program (NCEP), 81
National Health and Nutrition Examination Surveys (NHANES), 24, 106, 137, 138, 168, 263, 264, 272, 279, 399
National Heart, Lung, and Blood Institute, 168
National High Blood Pressure Education Program, 175–176
National Kidney Foundation, 111, 251, 252–254, 255
National Stroke Association, stroke prevention guidelines of, 70
Natural compounds, with antihypertensive activity, 181–190
Nephrectomy
  laparoscopic, 337
  as renal artery stenosis treatment, 63
Nephrologists, referrals to, 303, 304–306
Nephropathy
  diabetic, 234
  ischemic, 325
Nephrosclerosis, hypertensive, in African Americans, 301
Nephrotic syndrome, 305–306
Nerve root pain, differentiated from intermittent claudication, 78
Neurologic examination
  in blood pressure evaluation, 6
  in orthostatic hypotension evaluation, 313
Neuropathic pain, differentiated from intermittent claudication, 78
Niacin, as statin alternative, 388–389
Nicardipine, 451

Nifedipine
    as congestive heart failure prophy-
        laxis, 291
    as pregnancy-associated hyperten-
        sion treatment, 373
    as supine hypertension treatment,
        321
Nimodipine, 451
Nisoldipine, 451
Nitrates, contraindication in orthosta-
    tic hypotension, 315
Nitric oxide
    impaired synthesis/activity defects
        in
        as metabolic syndrome risk fac-
            tor, 245
        in obstructive sleep apnea, 93
        in renal dysfunction, 24, 29
    as penile erection mediator, 348,
        349
Nitric oxide donors, as erectile dys-
    function treatment, 345
Nitroprusside, as hypertensive emer-
    gency treatment, 293
Noncompliance
    with hypertension treatment,
        129–130, 238–239
    with latest hypertension control
        criteria, 141
Nonsteroidal anti-inflammatory drugs
    cardioprotective effects of,
        427
    as hypertension cause, in organ
        transplant recipients, 336
    prostaglandin-inhibiting activity of,
        428–429
    as refractory hypertension cause,
        280
    use in hypertensive patients,
        427–433, 441–456
Norepinephrine, in borderline blood
    pressure, 121
North American Symptomatic
        Carotid Endarterectomy Trials
        (NASCET), 73
Nortriptyline, 197
    side effects of, 198

Nurses' Health Study, 172, 203–204,
        389, 391
Nutraceuticals, 181, 183–188. *See
        also* Dietary interventions
Nutrient-gene interactions, 181
Nutritional counseling, 157, 161
Nutritional programs, for weight re-
        duction, 391–392

O
Obesity
    antihypertensive drug dosages in,
        279
    bariatric surgical treatment for,
        205, 210, 211, 279
    body mass index in, 203–204
    as borderline blood pressure
        cause, 122
    as cardiovascular/coronary disease
        risk factor, 401–402
        in women, 379, 391–392
    in elderly patients, 270
    as hypertension cause, 203–204
        in adolescents, 411, 415–416
        in African Americans, 401–402
        definition of, 203
        of isolated systolic hypertension,
            269–270, 271
        management of, **203–214**
        measurement of, 203–204
        in postmenopausal women, 381
        of refractory hypertension, 278,
            279
        weight loss management of, 204–
            211, 254, 270, 271, 278, 392
    metabolic syndrome-related, 243,
        244, 246
    microalbuminuria associated with,
        31
    obstructive sleep apnea associated
        with, 93
Octreotide, as orthostatic hypoten-
        sion treatment, 318
Older adults. *See also* Elderly patients
    hypertension prevalence in, 263,
        264, 265
    isolated hypertension in, 263–275

Olive oil, cardioprotective effects of, 184–185
Olmesartan, side effects of, 449
Olmsted County (Minnesota) study, 43–44, 46
Omega-3 fatty acids, 184–185, 187
Omega-9 fatty acids, 184–185, 187
Ophthalmic artery, emboli to, 68
Oral contraceptives, 280, 390, 416–417
Orange juice, interaction with felodipine, 450
Organ transplantation, hypertension associated with, **335–343**
  assessment and management of, 339–341
  causes and mechanisms of, 335–337
Orlistat (Xenical), 209, 278
Osteoporosis, hormone therapy prophylaxis for, 394
Over-the-counter drugs
  as orthostatic hypotension cause, 315
  as refractory hypertension cause, 280
  as single-dose antihypertensive drug therapy failure cause, 239
Overweight. See also Obesity
  body mass index in, 204

P
Parathyroid hormone, 10
Paroxetine, 196
  side effects of, 198
Penbutolol, pharmacologic effects of, 446
Pentoxyifylline, as peripheral arterial disease treatment, 82
Percutaneous interventions. See also Angioplasty, percutaneous
  as carotid artery disease treatment, 75–76
  as renovascular hypertension treatment, 326–327, 328–330
Perindopril, as stroke prophylaxis, 72

Perindopril, side effects of, 447
Perindopril Protection Against Recurrent Stroke Study (PROGRESS), 72
Peripheral arterial disease, 75–83
  diagnosis of, 77–79
  management of, 80–84
  risk factors for, 67, 68
  symptoms of, 76–77
Peripheral vascular resistance, aging-related increase in, 265
Personal digital assistants, body mass index calculators for, 203
Phenylephrine, as orthostatic hypotension treatment, 318
Pheochromocytoma, as hypertension cause, 8, 238
Phosphodiesterase inhibitors, as erectile dysfunction treatment, 345
Physical activity. See Exercise
Physical examination, in blood pressure evaluation, 6–7
Physician-based Assessment and Counseling for Exercise (PACE) study, 158–159
Pindolol
  as orthostatic hypotension treatment, 318
  pharmacologic features of, 446
PIUMA study, 44
Placebo effect, in hypertension control, 224–225
Potassium
  antihypertensive effects of, 155, 184, 188
    clinical trials of, 169, 170
    in diabetic patients, 254
  cardioprotective effects of, 184
  diuretic-related decrease in, 51, 53
  in hypertension, 51, 52, 53
  recommended daily intake of, 176
  as stroke prophylaxis, 169–170
Practical Guide: Identification, Evaluation, and Treatment of Overweight and Obesity in Adults, 207

Pravastatin, cardioprotective effects of, in women, 387

Prazosin, pharmacologic features of, 452

Preeclampsia, 370, 371–372
chronic hypertension-associated, 370, 373
distinguished from preexisting hypertension, 369, 371
risk factors for, 369, 370
superimposed on chronic hypertension, 370, 373, 376
as sustained hypertension risk factor, 60

Pregnancy
angiotensin-converting enzyme inhibitor contraindication in, 386
angiotensin-receptor blocker contraindication in, 386
hypertension during, 5, **369–378.** *See also* Preeclampsia
classification of, 369, 370
hydralazine treatment for, 453
pre-pregnancy evaluation of, 374–375
recurrent, 369, 371
treatment for, 373, 375–376
in renal disease patients, 370, 376
smoking cessation during, 391

Pre-hypertension, in African Americans, 404

Priapism, antihypertensive drug therapy-related, 351

Propranolol
pharmacologic features of, 446
as orthostatic hypotension treatment, 318
side effects of, 246, 350
use during lactation, 377

Prostaglandins
as peripheral arterial disease treatment, 82
physiologic effects of, 427–429, 441–443

Protein, dietary
nephrotoxicity of, 108–109
non-animal, 184, 187

Protein-to-creatinine ratio, 52, 53–54

Proteinuria
blood pressure target goals in, 107
definition of, 299
estimation of, 53–54
preeclampsia-related, 371
reduction of, 32–33
with angiotensin-converting enzyme inhibitors, 300–301, 304
with angiotensin-receptor blockers, 51, 52, 53, 301–302, 304
with beta-blockers, 303, 304
with calcium channel blockers, 302–303, 304
with diuretics, 302, 304
effect on progression to end-stage renal disease, 253–254
as renal disease marker, 298
smoking-related, 32

Pseudoaldosteronism, 438

Pseudoclaudication, 78

Pulmonary vein flow, in diastolic function, 42, 43

Pulse, assessment of, 7

Pulse pressure
aging-related increase in, 263
as cardiovascular risk marker, 266–267

Q

Quality of life, effect of sexual dysfunction on, 353, 354

Quinapril, side effects of, 447

R

Racial factors. *See also* African Americans; Asians; Hispanics; Mexican Americans
in medical care, 147–149

Rales, pulmonary, 7

Ramipril
cardioprotective effects of
in African Americans, 406
in postmenopausal women, 382–383

Ramipril (*Cont.*)
  renoprotective effects of, 298,
    300–301, 302–303
    in diabetic patients, 256
  side effects of, 447
Ramipril Efficacy in Nephropathy
  (REIN) trial, 298, 300–301,
  302–303
Raynaud's phenomenon, beta-
  blocker use in, 458
Recommendations for a National
  Blood Pressure Program Data
  Base for Effective Antihypertensive Therapy, 138
Reduced Sodium Dietary Approaches
  to Stop Hypertension trial,
  167–168
Reduction of Endpoints in NIDDM
  with the All Antagonist Losartan (RENAAL) trial, 243–244,
  254, 257
Referrals
  to hypertension specialists, 241,
    258–259, 282
  to nephrologists, 303, 304–306
Relaxation techniques, as hypertension treatment, 223, 224–227
Remnant particles, 359
Renal artery stenosis
  as angiotensin-converting enzyme
    inhibitor contraindication,
    446–447
  as angiotensin-receptor blocker
    contraindication, 448
  arteriosclerosis-related, 57, 58,
    60
    surgical treatment for, 62–63
  critical, 57
  diagnosis of, 238
  differentiated from renovascular
    hypertension, 325–326
  evaluation of, 7
  fibromuscular dysplasia-related,
    57, 59, 60, 62, 63, 325, 327,
    330–332
  as refractory hypertension cause,
    280

Renal artery stenosis (*Cont.*)
  as renovascular hypertension
    cause, 8, **57–66**
  surgical treatment for, 326–327
  of transplanted kidneys, as hyper-
    tension cause, 336, 337, 340
  treatment for
    with percutaneous transluminal
      angioplasty, 62–63
    with revascularization, 63, 326,
      327–328, 331, 332
    with stenting, 62–63, 327–330,
      332
Renal disease, hypertension-related,
  6
  in adolescents, 417–418
  blood pressure goals in, 108–110
  diabetes mellitus-related, 252–253
  end-stage
    in African Americans, 402, 407,
      417
    depression associated with, 192,
      193
    inadequacy of risk reduction in,
      244
    prevalence of, 297
  hypertension management in, 235,
    297–308
  during pregnancy, 370, 376
  racial differences in, 399
  as refractory hypertension cause,
    279
  smoking-related, 32
  stages of, 51
Renal function assessment, in hypertension, **49–56**
Renal impairment, blood pressure
  target goals in, 107
Renal insufficiency
  angiotensin-converting enzyme in-
    hibitors-related, 459, 460–461
  Liddle's disease-related, 435, 436,
    440
  during pregnancy, 376
Renal parenchymal disease, 9
Renal transplantation, annual economic cost of, 114

Renal transplant patients
hypertension in, 335–341
assessment and management of, 339–341
causes and mechanisms of, 335–337
pregnancy in, 376
Renin
in high-normal blood pressure, 121
as hypertension cause, in organ transplant recipients, 336
in primary *vs.* secondary aldosterone excess, 53
renal artery stenosis-related release of, 57
as renovascular hypertension indicator, 61–62
Renin-angiotensin-aldosterone system
diuretics-related stimulation of, 457
in left ventricular hypertrophy, 286, 287
Renin-angiotensin-aldosterone system blocking agents. *See also* Angiotensin-converting enzyme inhibitors; Angiotensin-receptor blockers
as complicated hypertension treatment, 406–407
as microsalbuminuria treatment, 32, 33
as renovascular hypertension treatment, 326
use in diabetic patients, 255
Renin assay, of peripheral and renal venous blood, 61–62
Renography, isotopic, 61
Reserpine, 241
Resistance training
definition of, 216
for weight management, 207–208
RespeRate, 227
Respiratory disturbance index (RDI), 89

Retinopathy, diabetic, in African Americans, 402
Revascularization
as carotid stenosis treatment, 73–75, 83–84
as peripheral arterial disease treatment, 83–84
as renovascular disease treatment, 63, 326, 327–328, 331, 332
Rofecoxib (Vioxx), 429, 430, 431

S
Salt. *See* Sodium
San Diego Claudication Questionnaire, 77
SAPPHIRE study, 76
Sarcoplasmic reticulum calcium ATPase enzyme (SERCA), 41
Scandinavian Simvastatin Survival Study, 400–401
Scottish and Newcastle trials, 331
Seaweed, antihypertensive effects of, 185, 187
Second Australian National Blood Pressure (ANBP2) trial, 233
Sedentary lifestyle, as hypertension cause
in adolescents, 415–416
in women, 381, 391, 392
Selective serotonin reuptake inhibitors, 195, 196
side effects of, 198
Sertraline, 196
side effects of, 198
Seven Countries Study, 360
Sexual dysfunction, in hypertensive patients, **345–358**
Sibutramine, 210
Simpson's rule, 44–45
Simvastatin, cardioprotective effects of, 386–388
Sirolimus, 339, 340
Sleep apnea, **89–98**
in African Americans, 403
central, 89

Sleep apnea (*Cont.*)
obstructive, 89–95
hypertension associated with,
89, 90–95
as refractory hypertension cause,
278
Sleep Heart Health Study, 90
SMART acronym, for lifestyle modification goals, 157–158
Smoking
as cardiovascular disease risk factor, 379, 390–391
contraindication during pregnancy,
375
as hypertension risk factor, 5, 139
as renal disease risk factor, 32
Smoking cessation
by adolescents, 416
as endothelial dysfunction treatment, 247–248
by peripheral arterial disease patients, 81
by women, 390–391
Social isolation, as barrier to hypertension control, 130, 131, 133
Sociocultural factors, in hypertension
treatment compliance, 129,
131–133
Socioeconomic factors, in hypertension treatment compliance,
129, 130–131
Sodium
as orthostatic hypotension treatment, 316, 317
recommended daily intake of, 168,
175
as single-dose antihypertensive
drug therapy failure cause,
239
Sodium channels, epithelial
mutations in, 438
amiloride-sensitive hypertension-related, 435, 436–437,
439
in salt-sensitive hypertension, 281
Sodium handling, racial differences
in, 399

Sodium nitroprusside, as hypertension treatment
in hypertensive emergencies, 293
in pregnancy, 373
Sodium restriction
antihypertensive effects of, 155,
165–168, 173, 183, 231, 232
clinical trials of, 166–168
comparison with the DASH diet,
174, 175
in diabetic patients, 254
promotion of, 160–161
cardioprotective effects of, 165,
168
as left ventricular dysfunction treatment, 290
as Liddle's disease treatment, 435,
439
as microalbuminuria treatment, 33
during pregnancy, 375
as stroke prophylaxis, 168
Sodium-retaining genes, in African
Americans, 399
Soluble intracelluar adhesion molecules, 363, 364
Sphygmomanometers, electronic, 15
Spironolactone
as congestive heart failure treatment, 294
as hypertension treatment
in aldosteronism-related hypertension, 280
in initial combination treatment,
240
side effects of, 350, 445
Statins. *See* 3-Hydroxy-3-methylglu-
taryl coenzyme A inhibitors
Stenting
of carotid artery, 75–76
of renal artery, 62–63, 327–330,
332
Steroids, as hypertension cause, in
organ transplant recipients,
335, 336
Stress reduction techniques, for hypertension control,
223–229

Stroke
  in African Americans, 403
  as antihypertensive drug therapy
      indication, 234
  calcium as risk factor for, 172
  carotid artery narrowing-related,
      67, 68
  ephedrine-containing neutraceuti-
      cals-related, 239
  estrogen replacement therapy-
      related, 393
  high-normal blood pressure-
      related, 120
  hypertension-related
    annual economic cost of,
        114
    depression associated with, 192,
        193
    racial differences in, 399
  ischemic, 68–69
    in African Americans, 403
  lacunar, 69
  metabolic syndrome-related,
      243
  prevention of, 70, 72
    with antihypertensive drug ther-
        apy, 72–73, 105, 113, 234,
        235
    with diuretics, 53
    with high-potassium diet,
        169–170
    with low-sodium diet, 168
  systolic blood pressure as risk fac-
      tor for, 108, 109
Strong Heart Study, 43
Studies of Left Ventricular Dysfunc-
    tion (SOLVD), 46
Study of Hypertension and the Effi-
    cacy of Lotrel in Diabetes
    (SHIELD), 255
Substance abuse, comorbidity with
    depression, 133
Suicide, depression-related,
    191
Support stockings, as orthostatic hy-
    potension treatment,
    319

Surgical patients, hypertension in,
    421–426
  perioperative management of,
      423–425
  postoperative, 422–423
Swedish Trial in Old People with Hy-
    pertension (STOP), 291, 292
Sympathetic nervous system, diuret-
    ics-related stimulation of, 443
Syndrome of insulin resistance. See
    Metabolic syndrome
Systolic dysfunction, 44–46,
    288–289
Systolic Hypertension in Europe Trial
    (Syst-Eur), 252, 258, 267–268,
    272
Systolic Hypertension in the Elderly
    Program (SHEP), 108, 109,
    252, 269, 273, 291, 292
Systolic Hypertension in the Elderly
    (SHEP), 267–268

T
Tacrolimus
  drug interactions of, 340
  as hypertension cause, in organ
      transplant recipients, 336–337
Takayasu's arteritis, differentiated
    from intermittent claudication,
    78
Target organ damage, in hyperten-
    sion, 181, 182
Taurine, antihypertensive effects of,
    186, 187
Terazosin
  in combination therapy, 448
  pharmacologic features of, 452
Third Report of the Expert Panel on
    Detection, Evaluation, and
    Treatment of High Blood Cho-
    lesterol in Adults (ATP III),
    388, 389
Thromboangiitis obliterans, differen-
    tiated from intermittent claudi-
    cation, 78
Thromboembolism, estrogen replace-
    ment therapy-related, 393

Thrombosis, deep venous, differentiated from intermittent claudication, 78

Thromboxane A_2, physiologic effects of, 427–429

Thyroid disorders, as hypertension cause, 8, 10

Timolol, as open-angle glaucoma treatment, 60

Torsemide, side effects of, 459

Trandolapril, side effects of, 447

Transforming growth factor-b1, 29

Transient ischemic attacks, 67, 68, 69

Transtheoretical ("stages of change") model, of exercise, 215–218, 221

Trazodone, 197
  side effects of, 198

Treatment of Hypertension According to Home or Office Blood Pressure (THOP) trial, 17

Treatment of Mild Hypertension Study (TOMHS), 398

Trial of Nonpharmacologic Interventions in the Elderly (TONE), 166–167, 168

Triamterene
  as Liddle's disease treatment, 435, 436, 437, 439, 440
  side effects of, 459

Triazolopyridines, side effects of, 198

Tricyclic antidepressants, 195, 197
  side effects of, 198

Trousseau's sign, 9

U

Ubiquinone (coenzyme Q10), 185–186

Ultrasonography
  deep abdominal renal artery, 61
  duplex
    of carotid stenosis, 69–70, 71, 74
    of renal artery stenosis, 10
  high-frequency B-mode, 69–70, 71

Underweight, body mass index in, 204

United Kingdom, blood pressure target goals in, 110

United Kingdom Prospective Study (UKPDS), 110, 114, 250–251, 292, 299, 303

Uric acid levels, in hypertensive patients, 52, 53

Urinalysis, in hypertensive patients, 52, 53–54

Urography, for renovascular hypertension diagnosis, 61

Uropathy, obstructive, 238, 241

V

Valsalva maneuver
  avoidance of, 208
  defecation/urination-related, 315

Valsartan, side effects of, 350–351, 449

Valsartan Heart Failure Trial, 294

Vascular disease, as sexual dysfunction cause, 345

Vascular insufficiency, as sexual dysfunction cause, 345–346

"Vasculopath," 280

Vasodilators, direct
  natural, 187
  side effects of, 453–454

Venlafaxine, 196
  side effects of, 198

Ventricular remodeling, 288–289

Verapamil
  drug interactions of, 339–340, 444, 450, 451
  as refractory hypertension treatment, 279
  renoprotective effects of, 303
    in diabetic patients, 258
  as supine hypertension treatment, 321
  use in organ transplant recipients, 339–340

Very low-density lipoprotein, 360

Veterans Administration Cooperative study, 73, 105
VIOXX Gastrointestinal Outcomes Research (VIGOR) trial, 429, 430, 431
Vitamin B$_6$ deficiency, 364
Vitamin B$_{12}$ deficiency, 69, 364
Vitamin B6 (pyridoxine), antihypertensive effects of, 185, 187, 188
Vitamin C, antihypertensive effects of, 185, 187
Vitamin E
  antihypertensive effects of, 187
  as coronary heart disease prophylaxis, 361

W

Waist circumference, as obesity indicator, 204
Water ingestion, as postprandial hypotension treatment, 316
Weight loss
  exercise-related, 126, 159, 207–208
  for high-normal blood pressure control, 125, 126
  for hypertension control, 155, 157, 204–211, 231, 232, 270, 271, 384
    in diabetic patients, 254
    promotion of, 158, 159–160
    in refractory hypertension, 278
  as left ventricular dysfunction treatment, 290
  as sleep apnea treatment, 93
  in women, 392
Weight loss (bariatric) surgery, 205, 210, 211

Weight loss medications, 209–210, 278
Weight maintenance, 159
Weight-training regimens, as hypertension cause, 427
Wisconsin Sleep Cohort Study, 90
Women
  cardiovascular disease risk factor reduction/prevention in, **379–397**
  hypertension in
    antihypertensive drug therapy for, 382–386
    obesity-related, 203–204
    as renovascular hypertension, 58
    as sexual dysfunction cause, 345, 346, 347
  minority-group, noncompliance with hypertension control, 133–134
  postmenopausal
    cardiovascular event rates in, 392
    estrogen replacement therapy in, 392–394
Women's Health Initiative (WHI), 380–381, 391, 392
Women's Health Study, 172
World Health Organization, 251

Y

Yohimbine, as orthostatic hypotension treatment, 317

Z

Zinc, antihypertensive effects of, 187